Topical Reviews in
Accident Surgery

Topical Reviews in

Accident Surgery

Volume 1

EDITED BY

N. Tubbs FRCS

Department of Surgery
The General Hospital, Steelhouse Lane, Birmingham

AND

P. S. London MBE, FRCS

Birmingham Accident Hospital
Bath Row, Birmingham

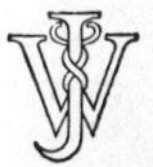

Bristol
John Wright & Sons Ltd
1980

Published by John Wright & Sons Ltd., 42–44 Triangle West, Bristol BS8 1EX.

British Library Cataloguing in Publication Data

Topical reviews in accident surgery.
   Vol. 1
   1. Wounds – Treatment
   2. Surgery
   I. Tubbs, N II. London, Peter Stanford
   617′.1   RD93

ISBN 0 7236 0534 3

Printed in Great Britain by John Wright & Sons Ltd.,
at The Stonebridge Press, Bristol BS4 5NU

Contributors

S. P. Allison MD, FRCP
Consultant Physician, General Hospital, Nottingham NG1 6HA

J. P. Bull CBE, MD, FRCP
Director, M.R.C. Unit, Birmingham Accident Hospital, Bath Row, Birmingham B15 1NA

D. J. Dandy FRCS
Kennels Farmhouse, Great Wilbraham, Cambridge CB1 5JW

E. M. Eagling FRCS
Consultant Ophthalmic Surgeon, Birmingham and Midland Eye Hospital, Church Street, Birmingham B3 2NS

T. R. Fisher FRCS
Consultant Orthopaedic Surgeon, Hartshill Orthopaedic Hospital, Hartshill Road, Stoke-on-Trent ST4 7NZ

E. T. Mays MD
Professor, Department of Clinical Surgery, University of Kentucky, Lexington, Kentucky 40506, USA

W. M. Steel FRCS
Consultant Orthopaedic Surgeon, Hartshill Orthopaedic Hospital, Hartshill Road, Stoke-on-Trent ST4 7NZ

G. Teasdale MRCP, FRCS
Institute of Neurological Science, Southern General Hospital, Glasgow GS1 4TF

C. H. Thomas FFARCS
Consultant Anaesthetist, Birmingham Accident Hospital, Bath Row, Birmingham B15 1NA

Preface

Accidents and injury continue to take their toll in mortality and morbidity. In the Western World a variety of different methods of dealing with this problem have evolved; in the medical sphere this has varied from providing general care physicians (casualty consultants), through various specialities such as accident surgery, to committee management with a specialist such as an orthopaedic surgeon in charge. However, the injuries remain the same and pose the two problems of overall care and of special regional care. The specialist must be aware of the advances in overall care while the general physician or surgeon must be aware of the advances in what may be called specialist disorders.

Examples of advances in both these fields are to be found in this volume of Topical Reviews and are intended to be of interest and value to everyone concerned with care of the injured.

Nigel Tubbs
P. S. London

Contents

Foreword

Accident surgery covers many specialities and therefore requires diversified knowledge in a wide range of subjects.

This book, *Topical Reviews in Accident Surgery,* presents relevant advances in many specialities and I recommend it to the physician who is looking for advice on the treatment of the injured patient.

The title *Topical Reviews* indicates that the authors must be selective, rather than comprehensive, and suggests that the process of selection and presentation will be repeated, as it needs to be from time to time.

With two English Editors it is not surprising that the emphasis is on British experience in this field. However, American readers will find numerous references to American publications.

The authors are well known in England as well as in the United States and are respected for their contributions to the treatment of trauma and to the literature on trauma.

Mr P. S. London has been recognized by the American Association for the Surgery of Trauma, having been elected to Honorary Fellowship in that organization.

I believe that *Topical Reviews* is a very worth while contribution and should be read by all surgeons interested in the surgery of trauma. It is a pleasure to wish this new publication well.

Frank E. Stinchfield MD
Professor, Orthopaedic Surgery Columbia Presbyterian Medical Center
New York, New York, USA

J. P. Bull

1 Epidemiology of Accidents and Injuries

INTRODUCTION

If we are to reduce the toll of injuries we need to aim for improvements in both prevention and clinical care. For prevention to be effective it needs to be informed by knowledge of circumstances and causes. Clinical information is essential if we are to see these causes in perspective and in return the clinician can be helped in understanding individual patients as well as in planning accident services.

Death due to different kinds of accidents can usefully be compared with deaths from all causes at different ages per million at risk (*Fig. 1.1*). The particular significance of road accidents in adolescents and young adult males is then evident together with a similar but less prominent peak in females. Domestic accidents make an appreciable contribution to mortality in childhood and in old age. Occupational accidents are not very prominent as causes of death; in males of working age they are on average easily exceeded by road accidents. The mortality rate is about equal to that for domestic accidents, which itself is low at these ages.

The outstanding importance of accidents and in particular road traffic accidents in deaths among young persons (15–29 years) can be seen by comparing them with other classified causes of death (*Fig. 1.2*). For both males and females accidents are the leading cause of death in this age period, and in young men road accidents alone cause more deaths than any other class of disease. Taking all age groups together, in the UK and in most industrialized countries, road accidents cause nearly half of the total of accidental deaths. Most of the remainder are due to domestic accidents and the majority of these affect elderly persons and are caused by falls. These deaths are commonly not due to the injury itself but occur secondarily from complications such as chest infection and pulmonary embolism. Fatal industrial injuries account for about 5 per cent of the total accidental deaths.

Non-fatal Injuries

It is less easy to compare different causes of non-fatal injuries because of lack of uniformity in criteria for notification. In the UK, for instance, industrial accidents become notifiable when they cause absenteeism. Injuries from road accidents are all nominally notified if they involve motor vehicles but the definition of severity is based on admission to hospital. No standard notification procedure applies to domestic accidents.

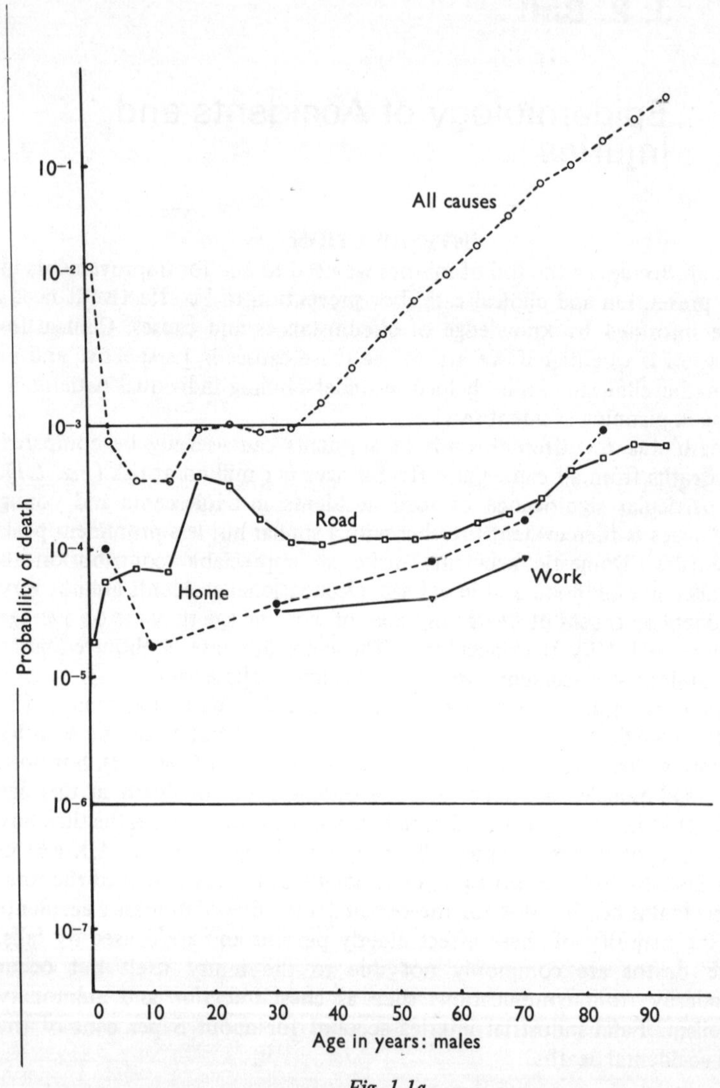

Fig. 1.1a

Direct comparisons of national figures for these main sources of injury is
therefore not possible. National hospital discharge samples based on the
Hospital In-patient Enquiry for 1973 (DHSS, 1977) suggest that about
equal numbers of road and domestic injuries cause admission as in-patients.
Males exceed females by about 2 : 1 in road accidents and females exceed
males by about 3 : 2 in domestic accidents. For all injury admissions males

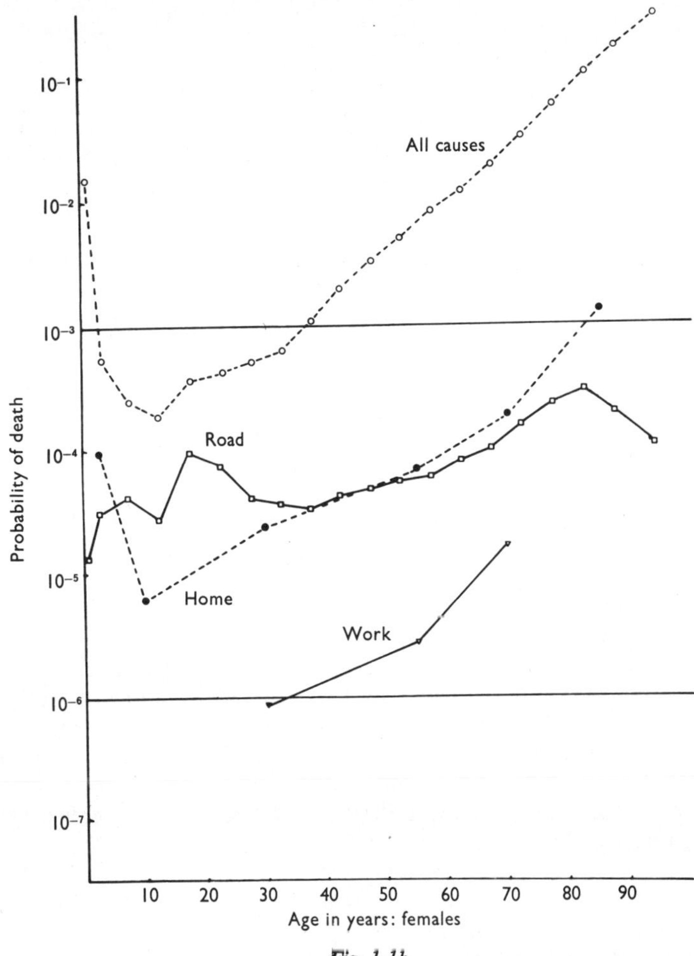

Fig. 1.1b

Fig. 1.1 Deaths from accidents at different ages compared with deaths from all causes. (Rates per head of population at risk. England and Wales 1975.) (Data from O.P.C.S. DH2 No. 2 and DH4 No. 2, 1977.)

exceed females by about 5 : 4. The in-patient survey estimates that there are about half a million patients admitted annually from accidents and poisonings with an average stay of 11 days. These injuries vary greatly in severity; for instance fractures, dislocations and sprains with a peak incidence in young adults have a mean stay of 22 days. Poisonings with a peak incidence in young children have an average stay of less than 3 days. Surveys made at the Birmingham Accident Hospital confirm these figures and show that the proportions of different circumstances of accidents vary

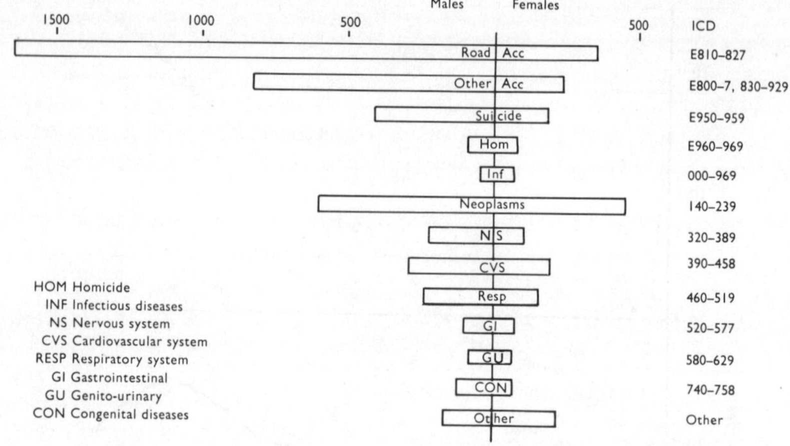

Fig. 1.2. Classified causes of death in persons aged 15–19 years (England and Wales 1975). A key is given of some of the more uncommon abbreviations from ICD (International Classification of Diseases). (Data from O.P.C.S. DH2 No. 2, 1977.)

greatly as one considers different levels of severity. Of in-patient admissions 21 per cent were from road vehicle accidents and a further 6 per cent from other accidents occurring in the street, making a total of 27 per cent related to the use of roads. In the same series domestic accidents accounted for 30 per cent of admissions and industrial accidents 13 per cent. Sport, recreation and school accidents together produced 8 per cent of the cases. Of these cases the more severe are treated in the Major Injuries Unit and of 220 cases admitted there in one year 153 (70 per cent) were from road accidents and 23 (11 per cent) were industrial. About 50 per cent of the road traffic accident cases had severe multiple injuries, a further 25 per cent were primarily head injuries and a further 20 per cent were primarily lower limb injuries. By comparison few of the industrial injuries were multiple, so that the severe injuries which demand most intensive medical and surgical care even in an industrial urban area are primarily from road accidents. A similar conclusion comes from consideration of the causes of the most severely disabling injuries, for instance amongst those patients with severe brain damage road accidents are the most common cause of the injury.

No systematic national figures are available for slight injuries. The sample of Birmingham Accident Hospital cases showed that non-admitted injury cases were nine times as frequent as in-patient admissions and the leading circumstances of these accidents were industrial (26 per cent), domestic (23 per cent), road vehicle accidents (6 per cent) with a further 9 per cent from accidents in the street not involving vehicles. Apart from these hospital cases other minor injuries are treated by general practitioners and, in the case of industrial injuries, by factory medical departments and first-aid posts. A study in the Wessex Region showed that for each hospital case three others were treated by general practitioners at health centres.

To summarize what is known from national and local hospital studies, it seems that road traffic and domestic accidents contribute about equally to fatal injuries and greatly exceed industrial accidents. Among the most severe injuries treated in hospital road traffic accidents predominate and among in-patient admission cases road and domestic accidents are about equal and each accounts for about one-third of admissions, industrial cases about one-eighth and recreation and school accidents about one-twelfth. Among slight injuries (not admitted) industrial and domestic each accounted for about one-quarter, with relatively few road traffic cases.

In most industrial countries before 1973, the trend was for the numbers of occupational and domestic accidents to remain constant or to fall while, with increasing traffic, road accidents tended to increase. The crisis in oil supplies of 1973 caused big changes in the use of road vehicles, the rise in fuel price stimulated economies, road traffic decreased and speed limits were introduced. These changes were followed by a drop in road accident deaths of about 15 per cent. In countries which benefited from the rise in oil prices road accidents have increased greatly along with the new prosperity, the increase in the number of cars and new drivers. In western countries road deaths are again beginning to rise; a feature of this is that a greater use of motor cycles was stimulated by the fuel crisis and to this has been added a further fashion for the 'leisure' use of these machines by young people. An increase in deaths and injuries among motor cyclists is now causing world-wide concern.

MECHANISMS OF INJURY AND THE INJURED PERSON

Accidents cause energy to be wrongly applied and human tissues have limited tolerance to mechanical, thermal or chemical trauma. The ordinary activities of life use energy in quantities only just sufficient to cause appreciable injury but a slightly excessive exposure can easily cause more problems. Falls on the level usually cause little or no injury in young people. In elderly people the threshold is more easily exceeded as in the common wrist and femoral neck fractures. Even in the young these moderate quantities of energy will injure if their application is concentrated on sharp objects such as knives or broken glass. These familiar examples illustrate variations in the two important factors: the injured person and the injuring object.

Most of the personal variables are related to age though not necessarily directly. There are characteristic ages at which new and potentially dangerous techniques are learned. The child learns to walk, to climb stairs, to use sharp objects, at each stage he encounters new possibilities of injury. Soon he starts to use the road as a pedestrian. A recent series of studies by Howarth et al. (1974) has thrown light on the relation of age, experience, exposures and risk for child pedestrians. When the child first starts to use the road there is the highest risk per crossing. This risk diminishes with experience but the frequency of exposures rises faster so that peak accidents occur at about seven years of age. Exposure continues to rise after this but is combined with a lower unit risk. The peak incidence of accidents is thus neither when children first use the road nor when they most often use the road, it occurs instead when (exposure × risk) is at a maximum. The same principles have been shown for motor cyclists and doubtless underlie the early age-related peaks which are found in each category of road user during the development of competence (*see Fig. 1.3*). The age-specific risk per exposure may, of course, have other elements than learned proficiency. There can be a further deliberate risk-taking, particularly among young male drivers, which may entail high accident rates when the driving techniques have already been thoroughly mastered. At the other end of the age span the age-specific risk rises again corresponding to diminished sensory and motor abilities. Frequency of exposure usually falls but not as much as to prevent a rise in accident rate. The added factors of reduced thresholds for injury and increased liability to death for a given injury contribute further to the rise in mortality from accidents in the elderly (Bull, 1978).

Alcohol in Relation to Road Accidents

Alcohol can greatly increase the risk of accident in all types of exposure and the relation to road accidents has been particularly thoroughly investigated. The classic study by Borkenstein et al. (1964) estimated that liability to cause an accident is ten times greater at a blood alcohol of 100 mg per cent (0·1 g per cent). The introduction of an 80 mg per cent limit in the UK in 1967 was followed by a sharp reduction in accidents, particularly at night when a combination of drinking and driving is most common. This improvement has since greatly diminished; it seems that enforcement is now inadequate since high alcohol levels are again commonly found in drivers in crashes, for instance about 40 per cent of fatally injured drivers aged 20–29 years have blood alcohol levels above the legal limit (Sabey, 1978). Recent studies have also shown the importance of alcohol in pedestrian accidents with, as might be expected, rather lower risks for given blood alcohol levels (Clayton et al., 1977). Information from industrial and domestic accidents is incomplete but almost certainly high alcohol levels produce high accident risks.

Disabilities

Chronic medical conditions are not prominent as factors in road accidents. In most countries certain severe diseases are a bar to obtaining a licence but it seems that people with moderate medical disabilities usually take the precaution of not driving beyond their competence, for instance they avoid heavy traffic and night driving. A few accidents are directly related to acute attacks of illness but it is doubtful if many of these could usefully be detected by previous medical examination (Ysander, 1970). The chronic illnesses and disabilities of old age do, however, contribute to pedestrian accidents and to many of the resulting deaths (*Fig. 1.3*) and even more so to domestic accidents (*Fig. 1.1*).

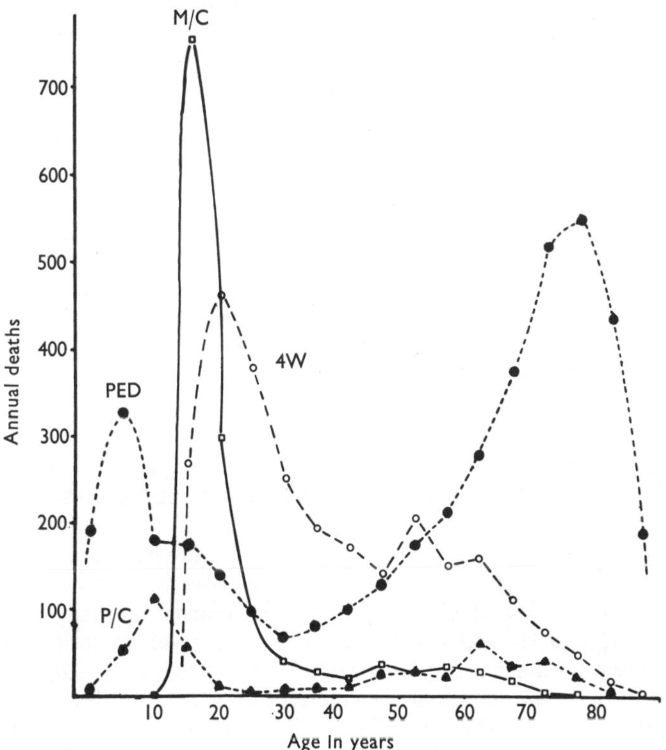

Fig. 1.3. Deaths of different categories of road user in relation to age (1975–6 England and Wales). Ped – pedestrians, P/C – pedal cyclists, M/C – motorcyclists, 4W – drivers of 4-wheeled vehicles. (Data from O.P.C.S. DH2 Nos. 2 and 3, 1977.)

Falls, whether due to neurological or other disabilities, become common in many elderly people and some of these falls cause injury. In younger adults as well, epilepsy and other types of unconsciousness are fairly common causes of burns and scalds. The Biblical patient who 'oft times falleth into the fire and oft times into the water' is still with us. About 13 per cent of in-patient burns and scalds in adults occur in epileptic attacks and a further 10 per cent are associated with other types of unconsciousness (Bull et al., 1964).

Psychology of 'Personal Error'

It is widely agreed that 'personal error' is a very common cause of accidents but the underlying psychology has been interpreted in many different ways. Early work during and after World War I led to the concept of 'accident proneness'. In highly repetitive work certain operators were shown to have more than their expected share of accidents even after all known personal and exposure variables had been excluded. This concept is often incorrectly used in popular parlance when variations in exposure or other factors are more important and might indeed be more readily corrected. In studies of bus and tram drivers in Helsinki, Haakinen (1958) was able to confirm that accident proneness existed and could be correlated with the results of certain psychological tests. Others claim that such proneness may be transient. If so, job selection based on such tests may be unfair and in any case many eligible applicants would be excluded since the correlation is not exact. An appropriate field for such tests is the selection of persons to train as air-line pilots.

It may be more useful to classify persons by their behaviour on the hazardous task. This was done by Quenault (1967) for car drivers. He found for instance that a proportion of drivers, his 'dissociated active' group, rarely used the rear view mirror and drove as though other road users could be ignored; not surprisingly they had more accidents. A related but more fundamental approach which is now being developed again is to investigate the psychology of 'risk taking'. This distinguishes between the perceived and actual risk and investigates what determines changes in the thresholds of risk acceptance. This may suggest better ways for presenting dangerous occurrences and perhaps for training in safer behaviour.

Those convicted of serious driving offences have been shown to have committed more than their share of the other crimes and many of them when interviewed showed selfish and even ruthless self interest (Willett, 1965). These findings are in line with the earlier work of Tillman and Hobbs (1949) who found that accident-repeaters had histories of various forms of antisocial behaviour, far more often than did accident-free controls. They coined the phrase that 'a man drives as he lives'. Though this may well be true it is less easy to suggest practical action. Even withdrawal of a driving licence does not keep some antisocial drivers off the road.

PREVENTION

Methods of prevention can usefully be seen as attacking different parts of the energy—exposure—injury sequence. For different types of accidents different links in this chain can be most readily broken. Haddon (1973) has given an analysis of the different preventive strategies. He distinguishes several levels of action by which either the energy may be prevented from release, the subject may avoid exposure, or the effect of exposure may be mitigated. For instance, in road accidents the limitation of speed will reduce the available energy, a pedestrian precinct will prevent exposure, a seat belt will mitigate injury, and finally a good accident service will minimize disability should injury happen.

These approaches emphasize ways in which accidents and injuries can be prevented without necessarily requiring voluntary change of behaviour from the person involved. This is in contrast to much 'safety' propaganda which exhorts people to be 'more careful'. On the surface it also seeks to contradict the studies which show that personal error is more important in accidents than are mechanical or environmental factors. Personal error, however, causes injury because the mechanical and environmental factors permit it and many studies have shown that the effects of propaganda in altering behaviour on the roads have been disappointing. Engineering changes, which incidentally often also entail changes in behaviour, are by contrast often successful (e.g. separation of opposing traffic by divided highways) as also are appropriate legal changes provided that enforcement is ensured (e.g. alcohol limits).

A recent study of the possible prevention of road accidents by the application of present knowledge estimates that one-fifth of injury accidents could be saved by changes in road environment, for instance, by improvements in junction design and traffic management, a further quarter by changes in the vehicle, including antilock brakes, safer tyres and obligatory wearing of seat belts, and a further third by changes in driver behaviour including enforcement of alcohol limits and safer speeds (Transport and Road Research Laboratory, 1978). Prevention of domestic and industrial accidents can be tackled in the same way, taking into account the epidemiological background, the modes of energy release and the most feasible strategies for action.

REFERENCES

Borkenstein R. F., Crowther R. R., Shunate R. P., Zeil W. B. et al. (1964) The role of the drinking driver in traffic accidents. Indiana University.

Bull J. P. (1978) Measures of severity of injury. *Injury* **9**, 184–7.

Bull J. P., Jackson D. M. and Walton C. (1964) Causes and prevention of domestic burning accidents. *Br. Med. J.* **2**, 1421–27.

Clayton A. B., Booth A. C. and McCarthy P. E. (1977) *A Controlled Study of the Role of Alcohol in Fatal Adult Pedestrian Accidents.* TRRL Supplementary report 332. Bracknell, Transport and Road Research Laboratory.

Department of Health and Social Security (1977) *Report on Hospital In-patient Enquiry for 1973.* London, HMSO.

Haakinen S. (1958) *Traffic Accidents and Driver Characteristics.* Finnish Institute of Technology Scientific Research 13.

Haddon W. (1973) Energy damage and the ten countermeasure strategies. *J. Trauma* **13**, 321–31.

Howarth C. I., Routledge D. A. and Repetto-Wright R. (1974) An analysis of road accidents involving children. *Ergonomics* **17**, 319.

Office of Population Censuses and Surveys (1977) *Mortality Statistics 1975 DH2 No. 2 and DH4 No. 2.* London, HMSO.

Quenault S. W. (1967) *Driver Behaviour: Safe and Unsafe Drivers. Road Research Laboratory LR 70.* Bracknell, Transport and Road Research Laboratory.

Sabey B. E. (1978) A review of drinking and drug taking in road accidents in Great Britain. *Proc. 22nd AAAM and 7th IATM Conference.* Morton Grove, Illinois, American Association for Automotive Medicine, pp. 188–98.

Tillman W. A. and Hobbs G. E. (1949) Accident-prone automobile drivers: Study of psychiatric and social background. *Am. J. Psychiatry* **106,** 321–31.

Transport and Road Research Laboratory (1978) *Potential for Accident and Injury Reduction in Road Accidents.* TRRL LF684. Bracknell, Transport and Road Research Laboratory.

Wessex Regional Hospital Board (1973) *Report on the Accident and Emergency Services.* Winchester.

Willett T. C. (1965) *The Criminal on the Road. A study of serious motoring offences and those who commit them.* London, Tavistock.

Ysander L. (1970) Sick and handicapped drivers. *Acta Chir. Scand.* Suppl. 409.

S. P. Allison

2 Metabolic Aspects of Injury

INTRODUCTION

With the improvement in management during the shock phase of injury, most patients now survive this part of their illness. They therefore present a major challenge to the clinician who has to carry out supportive management until the underlying illness is resolved by surgery and natural healing. In recent years it has been realized that proper nutrition and detailed attention to water, electrolyte and metabolic balance are as important for success as adequate cardiorespiratory support. This chapter will be devoted first to nutrition of injured patients and secondly to some aspects of fluid balance as they affect patients after the shock phase of injury. Practical aspects of treatment follow logically from a consideration of the pathophysiological changes.

Before considering the problems of feeding patients, it is relevant to discuss the evidence that starvation and weight loss are detrimental. In normal subjects rapid loss by dehydration of more than 10 per cent of the normal body weight impairs work capacity. In experimental animals loss of one-third of the lean body mass is fatal and early studies by Studley (1936) showed that weight loss was an important risk factor in patients undergoing gastric surgery. Studies of survival under starvation conditions show a rising mortality with weight loss in excess of 40 per cent, and if such weight loss is rapid and associated with acute illness or injury, the risk of even 25 or 30 per cent weight loss may be substantial (Keys et al., 1950; Lawson, 1965; Kinney et al., 1970). Protein malnutrition also impairs immune response (Cannon et al., 1943; Law et al., 1973). Unfortunately there is very little reliable information in terms of controlled studies of starvation and the effect on the clinical outcome of injured patients. There is much convincing anecdotal evidence however, in a number of clinical circumstances, particularly in the management of inflammatory bowel disease. Current knowledge indicates that small degrees of weight loss do not significantly affect the clinical outcome, but where weight loss is rapid and in excess of ten per cent, active nutritional treatment is required. The injured patient is exposed to the twin problems of starvation and the catabolic response to injury. An understanding of the physiological responses to starvation and injury may therefore be helpful in guiding management.

PHYSIOLOGY OF STARVATION AND INJURY

Energy Requirements

Energy expenditure is measured in terms of oxygen consumption. It may also be expressed in terms of kilocalories or kilojoules and related to the requirements for carbohydrate (4 kcal/g), fat (9 kcal/g) and protein (4·5 kcal/g). Its magnitude depends upon age, sex, weight, height, physical activity and associated illness (Kinney, 1975; Wilmore, 1978). The resting metabolic expenditure of an average adult lying in bed is approximately 25 kcal/kg and is increased by 20 per cent when the patient is ambulatory (Kinney, 1975). Early studies of Coleman and Dubois (1915) on febrile patients showed an increase of 14 per cent in energy expenditure for every 1 °C rise in temperature. In his classic studies of long bone fractures, Cuthbertson (1930) described an increase in oxygen consumption proportional to the degree of injury. The changes in energy expenditure associated with increasing severity of injury are shown in Table 2.1. To

Table 2.1 Changes in Energy Requirements of a 70 kg Man with Injury

	Percentage increase in metabolic rate	*Energy expenditure (kcal)*	*Required energy intake (kcal)*
Normal at rest		1 800	2 200
Postoperative	0–10	1 800–2 000	2 700
Multiple injuries	+ 20	2 200	3 200
Major sepsis	+ 40	2 500	3 500–3 800
Major burn	+ 80–100	3 200–3 500	4 500–5 000

Adapted from Kinney (1975)

account for such factors as specific dynamic action and the cost of healing and resynthesis of tissue, the energy value of food supplied should be between 20 and 50 per cent higher than the estimated energy expenditure. Theoretical considerations suggest that it is cheaper in energy terms to preserve tissue than to resynthesize it once it has been broken down. This accords with clinical experience that it is easier, during acute illness, to preserve body weight than to restore it once it has been lost. Wilmore (1978) has published excellent Tables from which it is possible to calculate more precisely the energy requirements of any individual patient.

Metabolic Changes in Starvation

The theoretical fuel reserves of a man weighing seventy kg are shown in Table 2.2 (Cahill and Owen, 1968). Were he to be completely starved under basal conditions (1 800 kcal per day) he would have consumed all his body tissues in ninety-two days. Such an occurrence would be impossible in view of the limitations imposed on survival by weight loss which have been discussed above, and as the capacity to survive starvation is enhanced by adaptive changes which take place. The work of authors such as Lehman, Dubois, Benedict, Keys and Cahill reviewed by Levenson et al., (1975) have led to our present knowledge of this adaptation which takes place in starved man to conserve essential tissues. Fat reserves provide more than 90 per cent of the energy requirements, the remainder being derived from protein. The stores of glycogen (approximately 400 g) are too small to make more than a transient contribution. The triglyceride of adipose tissue is broken down by lipolysis and the resulting fatty acids and

Table 2.2. Theoretical Fuel Reserves of a Man Weighing 70 kg

	kg	*kcal*
Fat (adipose triglyceride)	15	141 000
Protein (mainly muscle)	6	24 000
Glycogen−muscle	0·12	480
Glycogen−liver	0·07	280
Glucose−extracellular fluid	0·02	80
Total		165 840

Adapted from Cahill and Owen (1968)

glycerol are released into the circulation and taken up by cells for use as fuel. A continuing supply of carbohydrate is essential for the energy metabolism of the nervous system and blood cells and for the supply of important metabolic intermediates. Although the glycerol derived from adipose tissue can be reconverted to glucose, much of the new glucose synthesized by the liver is derived from muscle amino acids which are deaminated, the amino groups being converted to urea, while the carbon fragments enter the gluconeogenic pathway. The branched-chain amino acids leucine and isoleucine are oxidized within muscle after transfer of their amino groups to pyruvate, forming alanine, a major gluconeogenic precursor. Muscle amino acids also provide a continuing source for hepatic protein synthesis, e.g. for albumin production.

During starvation adaptations take place to minimize loss of protein. There is an overall decrease in metabolic rate which is greater than would be expected on the grounds of weight loss alone. After three to five days of starvation, lipolysis and the consequent high concentrations of acetyl CoA lead to the formation of ketone bodies from which the brain can derive a substantial proportion of its energy. Muscle can also oxidize ketones instead of the branched-chain amino acids, which again spares protein. There is therefore, less demand for glucose and the rate of gluconeogenesis from protein decreases by 50 per cent.

Kinney et al. (1970) compared the rates of weight loss following injury with those found by Benedict (1915) during starvation. He showed that major injury, associated with approximately 50 per cent of the required calorie intake, gives the same rate of weight loss as Benedict found during total starvation without injury. This emphasizes yet again the rapidity with which severely ill patients can reach lethal degrees of malnutrition.

Kinney also studied the changes in body composition after injury and starvation. He showed that in both conditions, the contribution of protein to weight loss was only 12 per cent during a period of twenty-one days. The contribution of adipose tissue was very much dependent upon the calorie intake but was up to 25 per cent. The greatest contribution came from loss of body water which was between 63 and 74 per cent of the weight lost. In this respect it is important to remember that total starvation is associated with an early diuresis whereas following injury there is a tendency to retain salt and water if this is given in excess (*vide infra*). Also, adipose tissue is virtually anhydrous whereas muscle tissue consists of 75 per cent water. Thus, one kilogram of muscle contributes only 250 g of protein giving 1 000 kcal whereas one kilogram of adipose tissue yields virtually pure fat and 9 000 kcal.

Response to Injury
Ebb Phase
Cuthbertson described the metabolic response to injury in two phases. During the ebb or shock phase there is a fall in metabolic activity. In clinical conditions this period is dominated by the problems of cardio-respiratory resuscitation. Experimental work on animals has confirmed that during this period there is a fall in oxygen consumption, hyper-glycaemia and diminished glucose oxidation. After a variable time, usually hours, the ebb phase gives way to the flow phase of injury.

Flow Phase
The changes in this phase contrast strikingly with those seen after starvation. The metabolic rate rises in proportion to the degree of injury and its complications, and net catabolism of protein is accelerated causing increased losses of nitrogen in the urine. Kinney et al. (1970) showed that in the absence of food 80–90 per cent of the energy requirements are met from fat reserves. They also found that the amino acids released from muscle are largely taken up by the liver for new glucose production rather than being used indiscriminately as fuel to meet energy demands. During starvation, glucose infusion inhibits hepatic gluconeogenesis immediately, but after injury the point at which a rise in blood sugar switches off gluconeogenesis is set at a higher level. The teleological question as to why injured patients need such a high rate of endogenous glucose production may have been answered by the studies of Wilmore (1977) who showed that the injured tissues of a burned leg have a far higher glucose uptake than those of the opposite normal limb suggesting that injured tissues have a high obligatory requirement for glucose.

Mediation of the Response to Injury
The response to injury is mediated by the central nervous and endocrine systems (Wilmore et al., 1976a). The response to minor injury can be blocked by interruption of the nerve supply of the injured area. With major soft tissue injury such as burns, division of the cervical spine fails to block the response, although drugs such as morphine, which depress the hypothalamus, cause inhibition: this suggests that there are factors released into the circulation from major injuries which act directly at hypothalamic level. The hypothalamus controls the release of catecholamines which have a dominant role in mediating the response to injury. Following moderate injury the surge of catecholamine release may be relatively brief, but in conditions such as major burns, markedly elevated catecholamine secretion may be detected for several weeks until healing takes place (Birke et al., 1957). The hypothalamus, by its releasing factors which are transmitted to the pituitary through a portal system, also controls the release of pituitary hormones. In his Harveian oration Albright (1943) likened the response to injury to the changes seen in Cushing's syndrome and when Cope et al. (1943) demonstrated elevated levels of corticosteroids after injury, it was suggested that these hormones might be the dominant mediators. Subsequent work (Mason, 1955) revealed that patients who had undergone adrenalectomy or hypophysectomy and were receiving basal substitution therapy showed a normal response to injury, although in experimental animals removal of the adrenal cortex abolished the response. This suggested that corticosteroids play a permissive rather than a primary role. Growth hormone secretion is also increased after injury (Ross et al., 1966). Thyroid hormone levels are decreased with a rise in the relatively inactive reverse T3 (Burr et al., 1975; Becker et al., 1976).

Endocrine pancreatic secretion is strikingly altered. In the acute phase of injury there is a catecholamine mediated suppression of insulin release, but after the shock phase there are elevated levels of plasma insulin in the presence of persisting glucose intolerance which suggests a resistance to insulin action (Allison et al., 1967, 1968). During the course of his illness a severely burned patient may show episodes of septicaemia and hypovolaemia, each of which is associated with a reversal to the shock phase pattern with a fall in insulin secretion. Glucagon secretion is increased (Wilmore et al., 1974a). It should be noted that the alpha-adrenergic receptors which mediate a suppression of insulin release also mediate an increase in glucagon secretion. There is thus a reciprocal relationship between the secretion of these two hormones which is reflected in their metabolic effects.

Relationship between Endocrine and Metabolic Response
The relationship between endocrine and metabolic response is illustrated in *Fig. 2.1*. Throughout intermediary metabolism insulin has an anabolic or storage effect in the sense that it causes large molecules to be

synthesized from small molecules. Following injury, since insulin secretion and then activity are diminished and the secretion of other hormones, which have catabolic effects are increased, it has been suggested that this altered endocrine pattern is responsible for the metabolic changes observed. The changes in carbohydrate metabolism include hyperglycaemia, glucose intolerance, glycogenolysis and accelerated gluconeogenesis, all of which

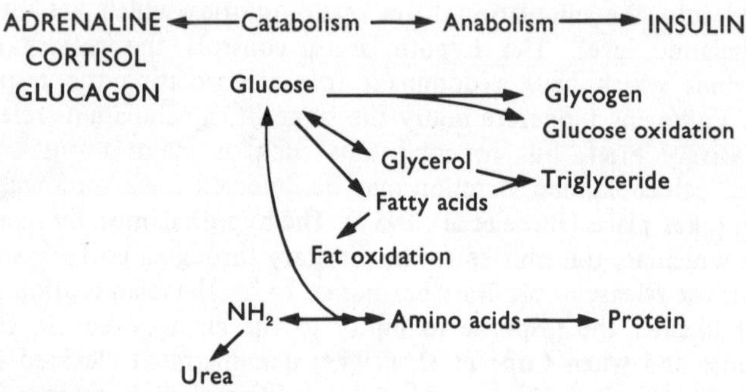

Fig. 2.1. Diagrammatic representation of the interrelationships between some important intermediary metabolites and of the influence of hormones on anabolic and catabolic processes. (Reproduced from Allison, 1974, by kind permission of Academic Press.)

are compatible with this hormonal pattern. It should be noted that although in the ebb phase the oxidation of glucose is diminished, in the flow phase, it is increased. These changes are understandable if one considers that the purpose of the response to injury is to mobilize metabolic reserves for use at the site of injury. High levels of catabolic hormones and of insulin, with a high set point for hepatic gluconeogenesis, ensure a plentiful supply of gluconeogenic precursors, a continuation of gluconeogenesis, and preferential utilization of glucose at peripheral sites. Wilmore (1978) suggested that this apparently rather costly process in energy terms may be partly responsible for the increased oxygen consumption and heat production of injured patients. In fat metabolism, insulin enhances the synthesis and storage of triglyceride whereas lipolysis is excited by catecholamines, glucagon, ACTH and growth hormone. The endocrine response thus ensures the mobilization of endogenous fat reserve. In protein metabolism, insulin has been shown to enhance the muscle uptake of amino acids and also their incorporation into protein. Cortisol enhances the reverse process and also induces gluconeogenic enzymes in the liver. Glucagon also has potent gluconeogenic effects.

PRINCIPLES OF TREATMENT

In order to have evolved, the biochemical changes which characterize the response to injury must have proved advantageous. The paradox is, however, that the changes which might ensure the survival of a moderately injured man or animal deprived of food, also carry the seeds of destruction after severe injury. It may therefore be less useful to try and block a response which is obligatory for survival than to minimize it by removing additional stimuli such as hypovolaemia, infection, pain, fear and cold. This approach has been extremely fruitful and will be examined in more detail later. The second approach has been to combine an adequate nutritional programme with hormonal treatment which alters the endocrine and substrate pattern of the patient. This allows the patient's metabolic demands to be met whilst preserving his own tissues intact.

Minimizing the Response

There has been considerable interest in the role of environmental temperature as a factor in the metabolic response to injury. Experimental work has shown that injured patients nursed in the thermoneutral zone (approximately 30 °C) have a lower oxygen consumption and nitrogen loss than those nursed at normal room temperature (20–22 °C). This is particularly striking in the case of severe burns. Davies and Liljedahl (1970) reported metabolic changes in four cases of severe burns. They showed a significant reduction in catecholamine secretion and in nitrogen and potassium losses when the patients were nursed at 32 °C as compared with normal room temperature. Wilmore (1977) found that the central temperature set point of patients with major burns is approximately 2 °C higher than normal even in the absence of invasive infection. Thus, the metabolic work required to maintain this temperature in the face of a low environmental temperature is considerable, particularly when the increase in heat loss due to conduction, convection and evaporative water loss from the burned surface is taken into consideration. Wilmore further showed that when burned patients were invited to alter their own environmental temperature by operating the heat controls they tended to select a temperature in excess of 30 °C. This evidence provides a firm basis for recommending that all injured patients should be nursed in a comfortably warm environment and that all burns units should have the capacity to control the environmental temperature around the individual patient's bed.

Aggressive treatment of invasive infection, circulatory inadequacy, anoxia, pain and anxiety also limits the extent of the metabolic response to injury.

Nutrition

A two or three day fast following minor injury may be of little clinical consequence, but in major injuries and extensive burns the catabolic rate may be so high that it is important to start an adequate feeding regimen as soon as possible after the initial stage of resuscitation. It was suggested in the past that feeding alone could not alter the negative nitrogen balance of injury, but recent experience suggests that this view is incorrect and that the maintenance of zero or even positive nitrogen balance after injury is quite possible providing the feed is both qualitatively and quantitatively adequate. The oral route which is to be preferred at all times may be unsuccessful because of failure to consider palatability and the individual patient's preferences and also because of anorexia. Sip feeding where the patient is encouraged to take small amounts of liquid supplement every 15–30 minutes requires continual encouragement of the patient but may obviate the use of more invasive methods of feeding. Severely catabolic patients should not be allowed to have any drink which does not contain nutritional value in terms of energy or nitrogen. If the patient is unable or unwilling to swallow, but the gastrointestinal tract is functioning normally, nasogastric tube feeding may be employed. Only in the presence of gastrointestinal failure is it necessary to use intravenous feeding. The principles of nutrition are the same whichever route is used.

Energy Requirements (*see* Table 2.1)
As described above, the basal energy expenditure is 25 kcal/kg. Appropriate adjustments should be made for the degree of injury, e.g. multiple injuries with sepsis cause a 50 per cent increase in metabolic rate and an energy expenditure of 37·5 kcal/kg. The appropriate energy intake is 45 kcal/kg. A major burn with a 100 per cent increase in metabolic rate expends 50 kcal/kg and requires an intake of 65 kcal/kg. It is preferable, in clinical nutrition to calculate the energy intake in terms of non-protein calories since the purpose of feeding is to cause protein to be used anabolically instead of being wasted as mere fuel. Although, during starvation, fat and carbohydrate are equally protein sparing (Jeejeebhoy et al., 1976) in the catabolic patient glucose is far more sparing than fat by virtue of its capacity to excite an insulin response (Long et al., 1977; Woolfson et al., 1979).

Nitrogen Requirements (*Protein in grams = 6·25 × nitrogen in grams*)
Injured patients have different nitrogen requirements from starved individuals. Experiments on fasting normal adults have shown that if 100 per cent of energy expenditure is met, zero nitrogen balance can be achieved with an intake of only 7 g of nitrogen and a calorie to nitrogen ratio of 300 : 1. In similar experiments upon adult burned patients, in whom 100 per cent of the energy expenditure was met, Wilmore and MacDougal (1977) found that the nitrogen requirement for zero balance is 25 g per day, giving a calorie to nitrogen ratio of 150 : 1. Most patients need something between these two extremes, and a diet containing a calorie to nitrogen ratio of 200 : 1 is suitable for most patients.

Hormonal Treatment
Various attempts have been made using hormonal treatment to inhibit protein catabolism after injury. Growth hormone has been found to have

protein sparing effects by Liljedahl et al. (1961) and Wilmore et al. (1974b). However, growth hormone is scarce and expensive. Anabolic steroids have proved only moderately effective (Johnston, 1978). Wilmore et al. (1976a) have shown that in some severely burned patients catecholamine exhaustion may occur and that this is swiftly followed by collapse and death. It seems unwise, therefore, to think in terms of adrenergic blockade.

Pursuing the hypothesis outlined above, in which it is proposed that many of the metabolic changes are determined by an alteration in balance between insulin and the catabolic hormones, Hinton et al. (1971) used insulin in the treatment of burned patients and showed that insulin and glucose produced striking falls in nitrogen excretion. However, these studies fail to distinguish between the effect of insulin *per se* and that of additional carbohydrate calories. Further studies by Woolfson et al. (1979) have shown that insulin has a potent protein-sparing effect which is additional to carbohydrate calorie supply. These authors speculated that insulin acts to inhibit net muscle protein catabolism rather than acting directly on gluconeogenesis and ureagenesis in the liver. The metabolic demand for glucose is at the same time met by glucose infusion. It is also vital to give an ample supply of amino acids for protein synthesis otherwise insulin would starve the liver of its endogenous amino acid supply, thus ensuring a 'kwashiorkor-like' state with an accelerated fall in serum albumin levels.

It is our practice to give glucose as 50 ml of 50 per cent glucose per hour by constant infusion pump. The insulin is administered intravenously by syringe pump at a rate of 4–20 units per hour according to the degree of insulin resistance prevailing. The blood sugar may be checked using finger-prick blood and glucose oxidase sticks in combination with either an Ames Eyetone Meter or a Boehringer Reflomat. The rate of insulin infusion is then altered by the nursing staff while the glucose infusion rate remains constant. Potassium and phosphate supplements must also be given with this regimen. One litre of 50 per cent glucose is given with 30–40 mmol of potassium dihydrogen phosphate daily with 100–200 mmol of potassium chloride, according to the plasma potassium levels and the potassium balance. In cases of acute oliguric renal failure it may be necessary to give little or no additional potassium.

Exercise
Paralysed or inactive muscles waste. However well managed their nutritional treatment, patients with motor dysfunction following head injury undergo muscle wasting. On the other hand, early mobilization and exercise have anabolic effects on muscle and should be encouraged.

PRACTICAL ASPECTS OF NUTRITION
Nasogastric Tube Feeding
In acutely ill patients it is important to establish that the stomach is emptying properly before full nasogastric feeding is established. Therefore

a Ryle's tube is used initially, giving 60 ml of water per hour down the tube and aspirating four-hourly. If, after twenty-four hours, it is clear that most of the water is passing on and not remaining in the stomach, a half-strength feed is given for the next twenty-four hours followed by full strength thereafter. During this time the stomach may be aspirated intermittently to ensure that gastric emptying is continuing satisfactorily. The Ryle's tube may then be removed and a fine bore nasogastric tube introduced. We have used a 1 mm internal diameter radio-opaque plastic tube with a wire introducer (Roussel Ltd). Although aspiration is not possible with this tube, it has several advantages over the Ryle's tube. It is passed much more readily and with less discomfort to the patient. When it is in place the patient is hardly aware of it and can swallow and cough quite easily. Although it may occasionally become obstructed it is easily cleared using a 2 ml syringe of water. A continuous drip system is used in which the feed is placed in one litre glass or plastic bottles and infused via a specially designed giving set. This method has the advantage over the old bolus injection method by saving an enormous amount of nursing time and by causing less diarrhoea.

Materials

Proprietary feeds of known content have the advantage over liquidized ward diets in that they are less viscous and therefore can be used in a drip system. The fact that their composition is known accurately may be important in terms not only of nitrogen, but also of electrolyte and mineral balance.

The importance of a high carbohydrate intake has already been emphasized. Recovery of small bowel function after surgery or injury is more rapid than is sometimes realized and water and salt absorption can be enhanced by the presence of glucose. Glucose however, as a monosaccharide, can be given only in a very dilute form without making the feed extremely hypertonic and likely to cause diarrhoea. Caloreen, a glucose polymer of average chain length five molecules has proved ideal in this respect being only one-fifth the osmolality of glucose in solution, weight for weight. It is also far less sweet than glucose and can be tolerated in high concentration in supplementary oral feeds.

Many proprietary feeds already contain fat. There is no advantage of medium chain triglycerides over other fat sources and indeed they may be more liable to cause diarrhoea.

The use of so-called 'elemental diets', i.e. those containing amino acids rather than whole protein has been built upon mythical foundations. Since half the route of nitrogen absorption is in the form of di- and tripeptides, giving amino acids cuts out one route of absorption of nitrogen. Weight for weight, amino acids exert a higher osmotic pressure than whole protein in solution. There is also no foundation for the suggestion that amino acid preparations have lower residue than whole protein.

Since amino acids are far more expensive than whole protein there seems to be no case for the use of elemental diets in the management of injured patients. We have used either Complan or Clinifeed as our nitrogen source.

Table 2.3. Basic Tube Feed Composition

Nutrient	Non-nitrogen energy (kcal)	Nitrogen (grams)	Na mmol	K mmol
Complan 300 g Caloreen 250 g NaCl 2·5 g	2 071	9·6	4·6	53
5 cans Clinifeed 400 Caloreen 250 g	2 700	12	57	62·7

The feeds are usually made up to 3 litres with water. More electrolytes are added to meet clinical requirements, although KCl has to be administered separately as it tends to curdle whole protein feeds.

The latter is already in liquid form and is not only convenient but passes readily down the fine bore tube. Our basic formulae are shown in Table 2.3.

Complications

The complications of nasogastric feeding, mainly diarrhoea, have prevented this technique being used as much as it deserves. Feeding by continuous drip rather than by bolus administration lessens the problem. Broad spectrum antibiotics are an important factor. Feeds of high tonicity cause intestinal hurry and in this respect Caloreen and whole protein have an advantage over glucose and amino acids. In some patients it is necessary to add codeine phosphate syrup to control diarrhoea. Regurgitation of liquid and aspiration into the lungs can be avoided by ensuring that the stomach is emptying properly before the full feed is administered. However, paralysed patients on ventilators and in the horizontal position may have trouble with this symptom, in which case it may be necessary to pass a feeding tube into the small bowel or to have recourse to intravenous feeding. It is hoped to avoid the problems of oesophagitis using the fine bore tube and both this and stress ulceration of the stomach may be helped by the use of cimetidine either by tube or intravenously.

A high plasma osmolality induced by intravenous feeding is an indication of mismanagement, and may be produced by administration of large amounts of carbohydrate to injured patients who, owing to their response to injury, are glucose intolerant. Testing the urine for glucose and frequent blood sugar estimation allow this complication to be observed early and appropriate treatment started with a sliding scale of soluble insulin injections. High protein intake unaccompanied by sufficient calories induces a high urea production rate. If this is also combined with inadequate water intake to excrete the excess urea produced, this may also lead to a hyperosmolar state. A too rapid introduction of feeds at full volume and strength may result in nausea during the early stages and necessitate a reduction in the rate of administration.

Many patients, particularly those with burns, suffer from anorexia, and although able to swallow they will not willingly eat enough to cover their nutritional needs. In these circumstances feeding with a fine bore tube overnight may be sufficient to bring their food intake to the required amount. A fine bore tube can be left in place during the day since it does not prevent the patient from swallowing comfortably.

INTRAVENOUS FEEDING

Technique

Intravenous feeding should be reserved for those patients in whom gastro-intestinal dysfunction precludes any other method. It is possible to use peripheral veins with isotonic preparations of amino acids, fat and carbo-hydrate, but this method necessitates frequent changing of the drip site and it is now customary to use central venous catheters for this technique. A long catheter may be introduced via an arm vein, although in skilled hands the subclavian approach may be preferred. The details of the technique have been elaborated elsewhere but it must be emphasized that meticulous attention to detail is necessary if serious complications of intravenous feeding are to be avoided.

The cannula should, if possible, be inserted in an operating theatre, but in any case the most scrupulous aseptic technique must be employed. If the subclavian route is used, a subcutaneous tunnel will help to prevent infection entering the circulation around the cannula. An antibiotic and antifungal cream should be applied to the site of entry into the skin and the whole covered with a sterile dressing. The drip set should be changed daily and the cannula and its connections handled using aseptic technique. The proper position of the cannula in the superior vena cava or right atrium should be ascertained radiographically and any malpositioning corrected. It has been suggested that the cannula should be changed every seven days or whenever fever suggests invasive infection. With improved techniques it has been possible to leave the cannula in position for long periods, sometimes for many months. It cannot be stressed too strongly that the incidence of septicaemia and thrombophlebitis is inversely proportional to the care and skill employed in some specialized units has beeen reduced to negligible proportions.

Principles

The principles of design of an intravenous feed are no different from those outlined above. The non-catabolic patient should receive two-thirds of his energy requirements as glucose and one-third as fat whereas the hyper-catabolic patient, e.g. after major burns, should receive at least sixty per cent if not all his caloric requirement as glucose with additional insulin. The nitrogen source should consist of amino acids since whole protein is not used efficiently for anabolic purposes and should be reserved for plasma volume expansion. There are a number of suitable preparations on the market which have proved very satisfactory in practice. Our own experience has been with Vamin and Table 2.4 shows examples of two of our typical programmes; one for a non-catabolic patient and one for a catabolic patient.

Table 2.4. Basic Intravenous Feeding Regimens for Adult Patients

Non-Catabolic Adult	*Volume (ml)*	*Non-N energy (kcal)*	*Nitrogen (grams)*	*Na (mmol)*	*K (mmol)*
Nutrient					
Glucose 20 per cent	1 500	1 200	–	–	–
Intralipid 20 per cent	500	1 000	–	–	–
Vamin glucose	1 000	400	9·4	50	20
Totals	3 000	2 600	9·4	50	20
Additives	KH$_2$ PO$_4$ 20 mmol Soluvit, Lipovit KCl 60 mmol Folate (15 mg i.m. weekly) NaCl if necessary				
Catabolic Adult	*Volume (ml)*	*Non-N energy (kcal)*	*Nitrogen (grams)*	*Na (mmol)*	*K (mmol)*
Nutrient					
Glucose 50 per cent Insulin 4–20 units/hr	} 1 000	2 000	–	–	–
Intralipid 20 per cent	500	1 000	–	–	–
Vamin glucose	2 000	800	18·4	100	40
Totals	3 500	3 800	18·4	100	40
Additives	KH$_2$ PO$_4$ 30–40 mmol, Soluvit, Lipovit KCl as required. Folate (15 mg i.m. weekly).				

Blackburn et al. (1973) suggested the use of isotonic amino acid infusions in the feeding of surgical patients. They argued that glucose infusion excites insulin release, diminished lipolysis and prevents ketosis with resulting adaptation to starvation (*vide supra*). If isotonic amino acids were substituted for dextrose, ketosis would develop and the amino acids would be used anabolically, the patient using his own fat stores as the energy source. Although they showed that amino acids alone produced a less negative nitrogen balance than dextrose alone, their conclusion that amino acids with glucose gave a worse nitrogen balance than amino acids alone seems unwarranted from their own data and has been refuted by others (Greenberg et al., 1976).

Minerals

The importance of mineral supplements has been emphasized in recent years. The phosphorylation of large quantities of glucose may cause dangerous hypophosphataemia unless inorganic phosphate supplements are supplied. Some of the old casein hydrolysate amino acid mixtures contain phosphate, as does Intralipid, in the form of phospholipid, but some of the modern synthetic amino acid solutions contain little or no phosphate. It has been our practice therefore, to add between 5 and 10 mmol of potassium dihydrogen phosphate with each 100 g of glucose. supplied. Further requirements are then decided upon by measurement of plasma and urinary phosphate levels. Magnesium is supplied in the form of 12 mmol of the sulphate per day. This must be given in a solution separate from phosphate in order to prevent precipitation. Zinc is particularly essential to healing tissues and recent work has suggested that injured patients, particularly with major burns, may become seriously deficient in the element. Adamel, a proprietary mineral mixture, meets many of the basic requirements although additional amounts of the above mentioned minerals and of iron may be required.

Vitamins

Comparatively little is known about vitamin requirements of ill people. We use the proprietary preparations Soluvit (water soluble vitamins) and Lipovit (fat soluble vitamins for adding to Intralipid). We also give additional folate 15 mg weekly by intramuscular injection since ill people quickly run short of this vitamin and may manifest pancytopenia as a consequence (Wardrop et al., 1975).

WATER AND ELECTROLYTES

Normal Physiology

Before considering the abnormalities which occur in disease it may be useful to review the normal distribution of body fluids. The total body water of an average man is 60 per cent of the body weight. This proportion is lower in obese subjects and higher in infants. The body water is divided between the intracellular and extracellular spaces, which are in osmotic equilibrium across the cell membranes. The sodium pump ensures that the chief osmotic cation in the extracellular space is sodium. In order to maintain electrical neutrality in the presence of negatively charged proteins, which are unable to pass the cell membrane barrier, potassium is retained in the intracellular space. The extracellular space is further divided into the intravascular fluid (plasma) and the interstitial fluid. The capillary membrane prevents the plasma proteins, particularly albumin, from passing freely from the intravascular to the interstitial space and thus ensures the integrity of the plasma volume.

Table 2.5 shows normal values for a man weighing 70 kg.

The values for exchangeable electrolytes represent the amounts with which infused electrolytes readily equilibrate in a short time. The exchangeable potassium lies chiefly in muscle and may thus be used as an index of lean body mass.

From these considerations the effects of infused liquids can readily be calculated. One litre of 5 per cent dextrose solution will, after metabolism of the glucose, be distributed throughout the whole body water, expanding it to 43 l until the kidneys can excrete the overload. The ECF and plasma

Table 2.5. Normal Values for a Man Weighing 70 kg

	Percentage body weight	Volume (litres)	mmol	mmol/kg
Total body water	60	4·2	–	–
Intracellular fluid	43	30	–	–
Extracellular fluid	17	12	–	–
Interstitial fluid	13	9	–	–
Plasma volume	4·3	3	–	–
Exchangeable sodium	–	–	2 940	42
ECF sodium	–	–	1 750	–
Exchangeable potassium	–	–	3 300	–

volume will be expanded by 285 ml and 70 ml respectively. One litre of 0·9 per cent saline will be confined to the ECF which will thus be expanded to 13 l, the plasma volume receiving an addition of 250 ml. Plasma or its substitutes will be retained within the intravascular space, provided that capillary permeability is normal. Haemacel or dextran 70, the most frequently used substitutes, have half lives in the circulation of 6 hours or less and are thus of use only in acute resuscitation. For the hypoalbuminaemic hypovolaemia seen during prolonged severe illness, the use of plasma or plasma proteins is mandatory to achieve more prolonged volume expansion.

These facts may appear obvious, but it is surprising how often they are forgotten in a welter of loose thinking and inappropriate treatment. Terms such as 'dehydration', 'fluid' or 'hypovolaemia' have precise meanings but they are often used imprecisely. If diagnosis is couched in precise terms such as 'plasma deficit', 'water lack', 'sodium and water lack', 'sodium and water excess' etc. then logical treatment will follow. One often sees saline being administered to an oliguric oedematous patient when the condition is one of lack of intravascular fluid combined with interstitial salt and water overload. The presence of oedema, which cannot be ascribed to inflammation or venous or lymphatic obstruction, must signify salt and water excess. Conversely the signs of diminished skin turgor, dry mouth and sunken eyes *may* be due to lack of salt and water but are more often due to weight loss and mouth breathing.

In health, the kidneys have an enormous capacity to vary the amount and composition of urine formed, in order to preserve the body fluids in a constant state. Volume and osmoreceptors govern the secretion of anti-diuretic hormone and aldosterone which control water and salt excretion. Changes in blood flow distribution within the kidney and possibly a third factor also govern sodium excretion. Oligaemia is the most potent stimulus to liberation of both ADH and aldosterone, overriding osmotic stimuli if both are present. After injury, these normal responses are modified in a way which prevents the patient being able to compensate for any medical carelessness in fluid administration.

Response to Injury
Since the observations of Pringle et al. (1905), it has been known that anaesthesia and operation produce oliguria. With the introduction of regular intravenous infusion in the 1930s, it was found that postoperative patients were unable to excrete the large amounts of salt and water administered and became oedematous (Coller et al., 1944). Further observations by Wilkinson et al. (1949), LeQuesne and Lewis (1953), and Moore (1959) confirmed that postoperative or injured patients tend to retain salt and water which are then excreted during recovery. Moore coined the terms 'sodium retention phase' and 'sodium diuresis phase' to describe these two periods of illness. When the illness is prolonged and beset by complications, the sodium and water retention phase persists and may be exacerbated by hypoalbuminaemia and associated fall in plasma volume (Hinton et al., 1972, 1973). The view that salt and water should be restricted in such patients received a setback from the observation of Shires et al. (1961), using $^{35}SO_4$ as a marker, that there is a 25 per cent fall in 'functional' extracellular fluid volume after trauma. Partly as a consequence of this and other work, sodium crystalloid solutions came to be used extensively in resuscitation from shock in burns and other injuries. Thousands of casualities in Vietnam were treated in this way with success, but many died and at autopsy were found to have pulmonary oedema. The response to haemorrhage includes mobilization of fluid and protein reserves to expand the plasma volume with resultant fall in haematocrit. There is therefore, some logic in providing the liquid component for this response in the form of crystalloid. It has also been argued, that in view of the generalized increase in capillary permeability seen in major burns, colloid has no advantage over crystalloid solution in these patients.

I have strong reservations about the use of crystalloid solutions after injury for the following reasons. Firstly, Roth et al. (1969) showed that Shires' observations were an artefact of the method he used. Using other, more valid techniques, they also showed that no ECF deficit exists after injury. Secondly, in the discussion of normal physiology (*vide supra*), it has been shown that to get a 1 litre expansion of plasma volume using saline, 4 l must be infused, causing interstitial oedema of 3 l. On the other hand, one litre of colloid solution would produce the same result without unnecessary expansion of interstitial volume. The increase in capillary permeability after burns does not, in my view, invalidate the argument. Early recovery is associated with a returning capacity to excrete any interstitial overload. However, if there are complications, the patient, rescuscitated with crystalloid solutions, is left with oedematous tissues, including the lungs. Thirdly, crystalloid infusions dilute the plasma albumin and therefore lower the level of left arterial pressure at which pulmonary oedema forms.

In his pioneer work Blalock (1930) demonstrated the loss of plasma and blood into injured tissue and emphasized the role of colloid in re-suscitation. His conclusion, that it is appropriate to replace that type of fluid which has been lost, seems singularly simple and valid, in spite of all attempts to find alternatives. Even after the shock phase, it may be necessary to sustain intravascular volume by repeated blood or plasma transfusions, since many burned and other severely ill patients seem unable to sustain plasma volume, and easily become underperfused (Hinton et al., 1972). Blood and plasma volume measurements are a poor guide to transfusion requirements as, particularly in the presence of sepsis, it is often necessary to transfuse to a greater than normal blood volume in order to produce functional improvement. The appearance of the peripheral tissues, central venous pressure and the volume and sodium content of the urine are better indices of circulatory adequacy (Hinton et al., 1972, 1973).

Water and electrolyte administration should match losses, remembering the inability of injured patients to excrete any excess water or sodium.

Potassium
Potassium is excreted in increased amounts after injury (Wilkinson et al., 1950) partly as a result of mineralocorticoid action but chiefly because of protein catabolism. As the negatively charged protein is broken down, so the positively charged potassium ions are released from the cells and excreted in the urine. Conversely, with feeding and, one may hope, protein anabolism, it is necessary to provide potassium supplements to avoid an acute deficit which may not be apparent until tissues are being re-synthesized.

Mediation of Electrolyte Changes
Both ADH and aldosterone secretion are elevated after injury but local haemodynamic factors within the kidney may be as important. A re-distribution of blood flow from cortex to medulla under the influence of catecholamines would increase sodium reabsorption. Any factors which diminish renal perfusion will exacerbate these changes and conversely, adequate and *continuing* treatment of any hypovolaemia or cardiac insufficiency will limit them.

Hyponatraemia and 'Sick Cells'
A limited capacity to dilute the urine may persist until the convalescent phase is reached. Excessive infusion of hypotonic solutions will therefore

result in hyponatraemia, and is the most common cause of this phenomenon. Severely ill patients also develop defective cell membranes so that sodium accumulates within the cells. These changes have been called the 'sick cell syndrome', a subject which has been discussed in detail by Flear and Singh (1973). In some burned patients with this syndrome Hinton et al. (1973) found that both blood volume expansion and insulin and glucose infusion resulted in sodium diuresis and rise of the plasma sodium to normal levels.

Renal Failure

The kidneys of injured patients not only lose their capacity to dilute the urine but in many cases there is marked loss of concentration ability amounting to polyuric renal failure. Such patients may be able to increase their urine volume while retaining a fixed urine to plasma ratio of less than 10 : 1. Our management of such patients includes the use of insulin and glucose to maintain a low urea production rate and a high salt and water input with frusemide intravenously to maintain a forced diuresis. At the same time we ensure that the plasma volume is fully expanded in order to remove any pre-renal factors. This is vital because in the presence of an inadequate circulating volume, the high crystalloid load will be retained and the patient will not respond to frusemide. The blind use of diuretics without some estimate of circulatory function and water balance is to be deplored. With improved treatment of shock, acute reversible oliguric renal failure is fortunately rare but is characterized by a urine output of less than 400 ml per day and a urine—to—plasma urea ratio of less than 14 : 1 (Luke and Kennedy, 1967). In such patients dialysis is usually mandatory.

MONITORING METABOLIC CHANGES

Weight

Many modern intensive care units throughout the world now have bed scales which greatly ease the management of critically ill patients. In view of calibration problems it is better to have weight sensing devices permanently attached to each bed with perhaps a single central monitor for economy. Short-term changes in weight represent gain and loss of water in a way which cannot be monitored satisfactorily by any other means. Water balances are notoriously inaccurate although input and output charts are still useful for indicating fluid administration and urinary output. Long-term weight gain in the absence of oedema may be interpreted as real body tissue gain.

Examination of the Patient

It is a common experience to find crystalloid solutions being administered in large amounts to patients who are oedematous. This is usually on the nebulous grounds of 'dehydration' diagnosed because of a dry mouth, diminished skin turgor and sunken eyes. The first of these is usually caused by mouth breathing and the second two signs can be caused by age, weight loss and cold as well as lack of salt and water. A good idea of central venous pressure may be obtained by estimating the height of jugular venous distension above the clavicle when the patient is at an angle of 45°. With intravascular volume deficiency the neck veins may not be apparent whereas they will of course be elevated if the patient has been over-transfused or is in heart failure. The signs, therefore, of fluid overload are more reliable than those of fluid lack.

If the thickness of a fold of skin over the triceps is measured and subtracted from the circumference of the arm at this level it allows one to recognize changes in the proportions of fat and muscle.

Urine Volume and Composition

Urine volume may be a helpful guide to fluid administration in the shock phase of injury and thereafter may continue to be a manifestation of intravascular volume deficit. If the patient becomes oliguric (less than 400 ml/24 hr with a urine—to—plasma urea ratio of less than 14 : 1), this is a sign of intrinsic rather than pre-renal failure. Estimation of the 24 hour excretion of urea and electrolytes allows calculation of the urea production rate reflecting the degree of protein catabolism and also allows a crude nitrogen balance to be estimated using the following formula.

Urine urea (g/24 hr) $\times$ 28/60 $\times$ 5/4 = nitrogen output (g)
A correction is made for changes in plasma urea as follows.
Change in plasma urea (g/litre) $\times$ whole body water (60 per cent body weight) $\times$ 28/60
(60 = MW of urea; 28 = wt of two atoms of nitrogen, 5/4 is a correction factor to allow for the fact that urea = 4/5 of the nitrogen excreted).

Estimation of sodium and potassium in the urine allows balances of these electrolytes to be kept. Measurement of urinary sodium excretion gives a useful reflection of the patient's progress. If the urinary sodium excretion falls in spite of continuing sodium administration this usually implies some change in the patient which requires therapy, i.e. onset of infection, hypovolaemia or other complications. Restoration of the capacity to excrete sodium implies satisfactory clinical progress. Since the blood level of phosphate and of magnesium is under renal control, deficiency of these minerals leads to their disappearance from the urine. Conversely, adequate replacement therapy is reflected by overspill of considerable amounts into the urine.

Blood Estimations

The frequency of blood estimations will depend upon the clinical situation. Frequent haemoglobin, white count and platelet counts may be necessary although one- or twice-weekly estimations may in some cases be sufficient. The frequency of estimation of plasma, urea and electrolytes will also depend upon the clinical conditions.

Twice-weekly measurements of serum albumin are usually sufficient. Decreasing values may imply inadequate protein intake although it takes up to three weeks to increase low albumin, even with intensive feeding. Other proteins such as transferrin have been suggested as better indices of nutrition. Plasma levels of calcium, phosphate and magnesium may be measured once weekly but sometimes need to be estimated more frequently. Patients receiving large amounts of carbohydrate should have their urine frequently tested for glucose, using Clinitest. The results should be recorded on a standard diabetic urine chart.

Blood glucose can be conveniently measured on the ward using glucose oxidase sticks and a Boehringer Reflomat or Ames Eyetone Meter, with occasional laboratory estimations as confirmation.

Acid base disturbances are outside the scope of this chapter, but the necessity for measurement of more than venous plasma bicarbonate will depend on other factors in the clinical situation.

Future Developments

Owing to improvement in resuscitation methods most patients now survive the shock phase of injury. Improved supportive measures after shock now ensure a good survival rate of injured patients in most centres. There remains however, a hard core of patients who become severely ill in spite of all efforts. The problems presented by this group of patients have recently been reviewed by Border et al. (1976) who have described them as suffering from multiple systems organ failure. The reader is referred to their recent discussion on the subject. Perhaps when this condition becomes better understood treatment will prove more effective. Since Border has postulated that this syndrome may be associated with failure of energy production at cellular level, the introduction by Baue (1977) of ATP infusions may be a hopeful development. In the meantime an infinite capacity for taking pains is not only the mark of good practice in the operating theatre, but also in the postoperative and post-injury period.

REFERENCES

Albright F. (1943) Cushing's syndrome: Its pathology, physiology, its relationship to adrenogenital syndrome and its connection with problems of reaction to body injurious agents (alarm reaction by Selye). Harvey Lecture **38**, pp. 123–186.

Allison S. P. (1974) In: Lee H. A. (ed.), *Parenteral Nutrition in Acute Metabolic Illness.* London. Academic, p. 167.

Allison S. P., Hinton P. and Chamberlain M. J. (1968) Intravenous glucose tolerance; Insulin and free fatty acid levels in burned patients. *Lancet* **2**, 1113.

Allison S. P., Prowse K. and Chamberlain M. J. (1967) Failure of insulin response to glucose load during operation and after myocardial infarction. *Lancet* **1**, 478.

Baue, A. E. (1976) Metabolic abnormalities in shock. *Surg. Clin. North Am.* **56**, 1059.

Becker R., Johnson D. W., Woeber K. A. et al. (1976) Decreased serum T3 following thermal injury. *Fed. Proc.* **35**, 216.

Benedict F. G. (1915) A study of prolonged fasting. Carnegie Institute of Washington, Publ. No. 203.

Birke G., Duner H., Liljedahl S. O., et al. (1957) Histamine, catecholamines and adrenocortical steroids in burns. *Acta Clin. Scand.* **114**, 87.

Blackburn G. L., Flatt J. P. and Clowes G. H. A. jun. (1973) Protein sparing therapy during periods of starvation and sepsis or trauma. *Ann. Surg.* **177**, 588.

Blalock A. (1930) Experimental shock: the cause of the low blood pressure produced by muscle injury. *Arch. Surg.* **20**, 959.

Border J. B., Chenier R., McMenamy R. H. et al. (1976) Multiple systems organ failure. Muscle fuel deficit with visceral protein malnutrition. *Surg. Clin. North Am.* **56**, 1147.

Burr W. A., Griffiths R. S., Black E. G. et al. (1975) Serum T3 and reverse T3 concentrations after surgical operations. *Lancet* **2**, 1277.

Cahill G. F. and Owen O. E. (1968) In: Dickens F., Randle P. J. and Whelan W. J. (ed.), *Carbohydrate Metabolism and its Disorders*. London, Academic, p. 497.

Coleman W. and DuBois E. F. (1915) Calorimetric observation on the metabolism of typhoid patients with and without food. *Arch. Intern. Med.* **15**, 887.

Coller F. A., Campbell K. N., Vaughan A. H. et al. (1944) Postoperative salt intolerance. *Ann. Surg.* **119**, 533.

Cope O., Nathanson I. T., Rourke G. M. et al. (1943) Metabolic observations on shock. *Ann. Surg.* **117**, 937.

Cuthbertson D. P. (1930) Effect of Injury on metabolism. *Biochem. J.* **24**, 1244.

Davies J. W. L. and Liljedahl S. O. (1970) Protein catabolism and energy utilization in burned patients treated at different environmental temperatures. In: Porter R. and Knight J. (ed.), *Energy Metabolism in Trauma* (Ciba, Foundation Symposium). London, Churchill, p. 59.

Flear C. T. G. and Singh C. M. (1973) Hyponatraemia and sick cells. *Br. J. Anaesth.* **45**, 976.

Greenberg G. R., Manliss E. B., Anderson H. G. et al. (1976) Protein sparing therapy in postoperative patients. *N. Engl. J. Med.* **294**, 1411.

Hinton P., Allison S. P., Farrow S. et al. (1972) Blood volume changes and transfusion requirements of burned patients after the shock phase of injury. *Lancet* **1**, 913.

Hinton P., Allison S. P., Littlejohn S. et al. (1971) Insulin and glucose to reduce catabolic response to injury in burned patients. *Lancet* **1**, 767.

Hinton P., Allison S. P., Littlejohn S. and Lloyd J. (1973) Electrolyte changes after burn injury and the effect of treatment. *Lancet* **1**, 218.

Jeejeebhoy K. N., Anderson G. H., Nakhooda A. G. et al. (1976) Metabolic studies in total parenteral nutrition. *J. Clin. Invest.* **57**, 125.

Keys A., Brozek J., Henshel A. et al. (1950) *The Biology of Human Starvation*, Vol. 1, Minneapolis, Minnesota Press, p. 329.

Kinney J. M. (1975) Energy requirements of the surgical patient. In: Ballinger W. F., Collins J. A., Drucker W. R. et al. (ed.), *Manual of Surgical Nutrition*. Philadelphia, Saunders, p. 223.

Kinney J. M., Duke J. H., Long C. L. et al. (1970) Tissue fuel and weight loss after injury. *J. Clin. Pathol.* **23**, suppl. 4, 65.

Lawson L. J. (1965) Parenteral nutrition in surgery. *Br. J. Surg.* **52**, 795.

LeQuesne L. P. and Lewis A. A. G. (1953) Postoperative water and sodium retention. *Lancet* **1**, 153.

Levenson S. M., Crowley L. V. and Seifter E. (1957) In: Ballinger W. F., Collins J. A., Drucker W. R., Dudrick S. J. and Zeppa R. (ed.), *Manual of Surgical Nutrition*. Philadelphia, Saunders, p. 236.

Liljedahl S. O., Gemzell C. A., Plantin L. O. et al. (1961) Effect of human growth hormone in patients with severe burns. *Acta Chir. Scand.* **122**, 1.

Long J. M., Wilmore D. W., Mason A. D. jun. et al. (1977) Effect of carbohydrate and fat intake on nitrogen excretion during *Ann. Surg.* **185**, 417.

Luke R. G. and Kennedy A. C. (1967) Prevention and early management of acute renal failure. *Postgrad. Med. J.* **43**, 280.

Mason A. S. (1955) Metabolic response to total adrenalectomy and hypophysectomy. *Lancet* **2**, 632.

Moore F. D. (1959) *Metabolic Care of the Surgical Patient.* Philadelphia, Saunders.

Pringle H., Maunsell R. C. B. and Pringle S. (1905) Effects of ether anaesthesia on renal activity. *Br. Med. J.* **2**, 942.

Ross H., Johnstone I. D. A., Welborn T. A. et al. (1966) Effect of abdominal operation on glucose tolerance and serum levels of insulin, growth hormone and hydrocortisone. *Lancet* **2**, 563.

Roth E., Lax L. C. and Maloney J. V. (1969) Ringers lactate solution and extracellular fluid volume in the surgical patient: a critical analysis. *Ann. Surg.* **169**, 149.

Shires T., Brown F. T., Canizaro P. C. et al. (1961) Distributional changes in extracellular fluid during acute haemorrhagic shock. *Surg. Forum* **11**, 115.

Studley H. O. (1936) Percentage of weight loss. A basic indicator of surgical risk in patients with chronic peptic ulcer. *J.A.M.A.* **106**, 458.

Wardrop C. A. J., Heatley R. V., Tennant G. B. et al. (1975) Acute folate deficiences in surgical patients on amino acid − ethanol intravenous nutrition. *Lancet* **2**, 640.

Wilkinson A. W., Billing B. H., Nagy C. et al. (1949) Excretion of chloride and sodium after surgical operations. *Lancet* **1**, 640.

Wilkinson A. W., Billing B. H., Nagy C. et al. (1950) Excretion of potassium after partial gastrectomy. *Lancet* **2**, 135.

Wilmore D. W. (1978) *Metabolic Management of the Critically Ill.* New York, Plenum.

Wilmore D. W. and MacDougal W. S. (1977) In: Richards J. R. and Kinney J. M. (ed.), *Nutritional Aspects in the Care of the Critically Ill.* London, Churchill Livingstone, p. 583.

Wilmore D. W., Long J. M., Mason A. D. jun. et al. (1976a) Catecholamines as mediators of the metabolic response to thermal injury. In: Wilkinson A. W. and Cuthbertson D. (ed.), *Metabolism and the Response to Injury,* London, Pitman Medical, p. 287.

Wilmore D. W., Moylan J. A., Pruitt B. A. et al. (1974a) Hyperglucagonaemia after burns. *Lancet* **1**, 73.

Wilmore D. W., Moylan J. A. jun. Bristow B. F. et al. (1974b) Anabolic effects of human growth hormone and high caloric feeding following thermal injury. *Surg. Gynecol. Obstet.* **138**, 875.

Wilmore D. W., Taylor J. W., Hander E. W. et al. (1976b) Central nervous system function following thermal injury. In: Wilkinson A. W. and Cuthbertson D. (ed.), *Metabolism and the Response to Injury,* London, Pitman Medical, p. 274.

Woolfson A. M. J., Heatley R. V. and Allison S. P. (1979) Insulin to inhibit protein catabolism after injury. *New Engl. J. Med.* **300**, 14.

C. H. Thomas

3 Treatment and Aggravation of the Pulmonary Complications of Injury

INTRODUCTION

Severe injury commonly causes abnormalities of the respiratory system, even if the thorax has not been involved in the original insult. Direct injury of the chest may cause respiratory disturbances because of damage, e.g. pulmonary contusion, inhalation of smoke or because of disruption of the normal mechanism of alveolar ventilation. The lungs may be damaged by complications to the original injury, for example fat embolism, aspiration of vomit, pulmonary oedema after head injury, or by complications of treatment such as fluid overload, infection and oxygen toxicity. The extent of direct or indirect respiratory injury may vary from sub-clinical hypoxaemia (detectable only by blood gas analysis) to frank, life-threatening respiratory failure present at the time of admission to hospital. At the two extremes the choice of appropriate treatment is not difficult. In the intermediate stages, where the patient is on the verge of respiratory failure, the decisions are more complex and problems may arise from unnecessarily delayed or overzealous treatment.

Pulmonary injuries, whether direct or indirect, have certain common features. There are abnormalities of alveolar ventilation and pulmonary capillary perfusion and intrapulmonary shunts are often increased. Pulmonary compliance is reduced and the work of breathing is increased, often at a time when the patient is least able to respond to the increased demand. There is an increased susceptibility to pulmonary oedema and alveoli may be collapsed due to bronchial blockage with blood, mucus, or foreign material. More alveoli may be occluded by intra-alveolar haemorrhage and exudates.

Treatment of the different forms of pulmonary injury has several common objectives: maintenance of an adequate supply of oxygen to the tissues by attending to all aspects of oxygen transport, avoidance of aggravation of the pulmonary lesion and control of complications which may develop. Recovery is usually spontaneous but may be delayed or prevented by fluid overload, infection, etc. Sufficient time for recovery must be provided by controlling respiratory failure.

Consideration of the management of the crushed chest provides a good example of how treatment can help or hinder a respiratory injury. Crushed chest injuries, particularly with a flail segment, are often considered to be an indication for mechanical ventilation which would normally last for fourteen days, after which the rib fractures are said to be stabilized. This philosophy causes too many patients to be ventilated artificially and any paradoxical respiratory movements present when ventilation starts will still be present when it is discontinued two or even four weeks later. A ventilator has been described as providing internal pneumatic stabilization of rib fractures (Avery et al., 1956). Like other forms of splinting, its use should be limited to patients who need it while definitive therapy to control the underlying problem is established; it should then be discontinued as soon as possible.

Mechanical ventilation can undoubtedly save the life of a patient in respiratory failure who fails to respond to more conservative methods. Unfortunately it is also potentially dangerous, partly because the medical profession has failed to establish, and then maintain, adequate safety standards. Ventilators are still manufactured without an effective method for locking the tubing securely in place. Newspaper reports from coroner's courts periodically show that disconnection of tubing and other forms of mechanical failure can be fatal. Ventilator alarms are helpful but not foolproof. Infection and damage caused by an artificial airway increase the risks of intermittent positive-pressure ventilation (IPPV) accordingly there must be hope of substantial benefit before the risks of treatment are justified.

The principles of the treatment of crushed chest injuries were clearly stated by Lloyd et al., 1965; Reid and Baird, 1965; Campbell, 1966. There have been variations of the original protocols in later years, with some authors recommending increased use of IPPV (Gibbons et al., 1973; James et al., 1974) and others advocating minimal use (Trinkle et al., 1975; Shackford et al., 1976). There is general agreement that the magnitude of the anatomical deformity (especially the number of fractured ribs) is a poor indicator of the severity of the injury. The main indicator is how well the patient breathes and coughs on his own, when given good analgesia, adequate transfusion, etc. The first requirement is proper resuscitation particularly to restore the blood volume to normal, control pain and treat any pulmonary compression due to pneumothorax or haemothorax. Obvious respiratory failure must be controlled by tracheal intubation and artificial ventilation. After resuscitation the patients may be classified into three groups according to the observed functional disability.

(1) In the first group pain is the main problem but with adequate analgesia the patients are able to breathe and cough effectively. Continuous thoracic epidural analgesia and intercostal nerve blocks have been enthusiastically recommended by many of the authors already referred to. Oxygen is given to maintain a satisfactory arterial oxygen tension (PaO_2).

(2) The second group consists of patients who are able to breath spontaneously but cannot cough adequately. They require tracheobronchial suction to keep their lower airway cleared of mucus. An artificial airway is commonly required, in which case the inspired gases must be humidified. Additional oxygen and analgesia are also required, as in the first group.

(3) The most severe injuries constitute the third group. They are characterized by respiratory failure despite conservative support, and this makes artificial ventilation necessary. The main features are clinical signs of respiratory distress and fatigue with deteriorating blood gas tensions.

The main objective of treatment is to diminish the effect of the underlying pulmonary disorder and prevent the onset of respiratory failure. Paradoxical respiratory movements should not be regarded as an indication for mechanical ventilation. When paradox was rejected as an indication the frequency of use of IPPV on patients with a flail segment fell from 88 per cent to 46 per cent (Shackford et al., 1976). Associated injuries, particularly of the head or upper abdomen, may increase the need for ventilator therapy. Pre-existing disease such as obesity, chronic lung disease and advanced age may also precipitate respiratory failure. The original classification can only be provisional because patients may deteriorate or improve and thus move from one category to another. Surgical fixation of broken ribs is usually impracticable or unnecessary. In a discussion of the indications for surgical intervention after chest injury, Brown (1972) recommended surgical fixation of double uncomminuted fractures on one side if accessible through a single incision, particularly after a thoracotomy.

When assessing the success of this treatment two main facts emerge. First, the mortality is almost nil in the first and second groups and always higher in the third; this is to be expected as group 3 consists of the more seriously injured patients. The expectation of survival is dependent on the patient's health before the injury and other injuries sustained in the accident, e.g. severe head injury and damage to major blood vessels.

The second major conclusion is that the use of mechanical ventilators is associated with an increased complication rate (Trinkle et al., 1975; Shackford et al., 1976), particularly damage to the upper airway and infection. Complications of tracheostomy were reported as a cause of death although others have not shared this experience (James et al., 1974). The patients who require ventilator therapy after pulmonary injury are more susceptible to infection because of the lung damage and there can be little doubt that the risk is increased by the use of an artificial airway and mechanical ventilation.

Thus one form of therapy may save the life of one patient but would prejudice the life of another for whom the risks are unwarranted. Although the example used has concentrated mainly on the hazards of mechanical ventilation similar dilemmas are to be found in other aspects of management of respiratory injuries.

PROBLEMS OF ARTIFICIAL AIRWAYS

There are many reasons why an endotracheal tube or a tracheostomy tube may be required after injury. The airway may be severely damaged or reflex protection of it may be impaired in unconscious patients. Artificial

airways are essential for IPPV when the airway must be sealed off from the
pharynx to keep the inspired air in and the pharyngeal contents out.

Tracheostomy is usually considered if the endotracheal tube is required
for more than 3–7 days (Bain, 1972); possible damage to the larynx is the
usual indication for the change. Patient comfort is greater with a tracheostomy and, in rare cases, anatomical disruption of the upper airway can
make tracheostomy unavoidable (*Fig. 3.1*). When an endotracheal tube is

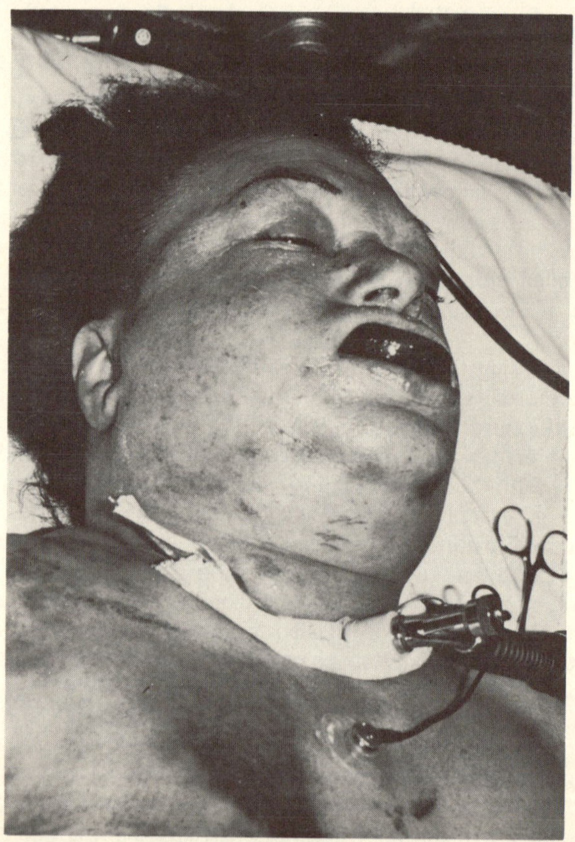

Fig. 3.1. Tracheostomy after a massive haematoma of the tongue caused total airway
obstruction.

removed following a prolonged period of intubation the patient suffers a
temporary inability to cough effectively, and ability to co-operate with a
physiotherapist is therefore essential. If co-operation is not possible
because of persisting coma, tetraplegia or general muscular weakness,
tracheostomy is indicated. When there is no special indication for

tracheostomy, endotracheal intubation is sufficient for most cases which require an artificial airway after injury.

Endotracheal tubes may cause ulcers between, and over, the arytenoid cartilages, ulcers and granulomas on the vocal cords and ulcers of the cricoid cartilage. Sore throat and difficulty with coughing are common but normally resolve within a few days after extubation. Laryngeal and tracheal stenosis are infrequent complications. Obstruction by post-intubation granulomas is very rare and can be very difficult to treat, however, rapid regression of granulation tissue has been reported after oral zinc sulphate (Pullen, 1970; Marshak and Marshak, 1973).

By contrast, tracheostomy is often disfiguring and causes some degree of stenosis in almost all cases (Friman et al., 1976), although it is often insignificant. Stenosis usually occurs at the site of the stoma (Pearson and Fairley, 1970; Friman et al., 1976) but, in common with endotracheal tubes, it may also occur at the level of the cuff or tip of the tube. Tracheostomy wounds are commonly infected and the infection has direct access to the trachea and the damaged lung. Laryngeal damage is also possible as a result of tracheostomy and tracheo-oesophageal fistulae are associated with a high mortality.

Problems caused by artificial airways made of irritant materials have been reduced by the development of non-irritant, polyvinyl chloride tubes which are quality controlled by implantation into rabbits and tissue cultures. The non-irritant properties are lost with the normal methods of sterilization used in hospital, therefore the tubes should be used once only and then discarded.

Developments in cuff designs have resulted in large volume, 'floppy' cuffs on endotracheal and tracheostomy tubes, which reduce tracheal damage by the cuff (Cooper and Grillo, 1969; Mathias and Wedley, 1974). The larger cuffs exert a much lower pressure on the tracheal mucosa but overinflation will cause high intracuff pressures and tracheal damage (Ching and Nealon, 1974; Mackenzie et al., 1976). Fryer and Marshall (1976) recommended that the minimum volume of air required to inflate the cuff should be recorded and that the same volume should be used whenever the cuff is reinflated. High pressures can be more reliably avoided by measuring the pressure as the cuff is inflated, using manometers produced for the purpose. Magovern et al. (1972) have described an integral safety device designed to prevent overinflation. The safe pressure is approximately 3·5 kPa (25 mmHg) which is above the 2 kPa (15 mmHg) that is necessary to prevent aspiration of pharyngeal contents (Carrol, 1973) but low enough to allow capillary perfusion of the tracheal wall. When the patient breathes spontaneously the cuff pressure may have to be higher to prevent aspiration (near 7 kPa, 50 mmHg) (Pavlin et al., 1975). This may also apply when a patient is fighting the ventilator, although fighting has been shown to increase intracuff pressures above the desired level.

Improved materials and high compliance cuffs will not protect the larynx and trachea from any damage caused by intubation (Bowes et al., 1973) therefore considerable care must be used during intubation. In the author's experience, many cases of difficulty arise from failure to observe the basic rules of intubation, particularly failure to raise the head onto a pillow, an item often absent from an intensive care unit bed. Tracheal stenosis following the use of a low pressure cuff has been described (Bradbeer et al., 1976); the patient had been intubated three times before and a tight fit with an 8 mm tube was recorded.

Endobronchial intubation with an unnecessarily long tube is a well recognized hazard. A long tube may also cause damage to the carina with subsequent granulomas; this is a rare complication but has been described as a cause of tracheal obstruction in a child (Abeyewickreme and Simpson, 1977).

MECHANICAL VENTILATION

Mechanical ventilation should be used after injury if there is uncontrolled respiratory failure, to help control intracranial hypertension, occasionally in the early postoperative period, and as one part of the treatment of septicaemia (Milligan et al., 1974; Halmagyi and Kinney, 1975). When it is indicated care must be taken to obtain the maximum benefit with the minimum of complications. The tragedy of morbidity, or even mortality, caused by ventilator therapy can be avoided only by constant attention to detail. Probably the greatest single safeguard for the patient is the presence of a nurse at the bedside; the patient must never be out of sight. Young et al. (1974) have shown that mortality is reduced by treating all patients with severe respiratory problems in a specialized unit. Mechanical problems with the ventilator or the patient's circuit can be reliably detected with pressure sensitive alarms if they are properly connected to the circuit and switched on. All tube connections, to the patient and the machine should be firmly secured to prevent inadvertent disconnection; simple push-on connections are not suitable.

Even if the patient's lungs are normal, abnormalities will develop when mechanical ventilation is used. The functional residual capacity is reduced, thus increasing airway closure particularly in the elderly and obese (Weenig et al., 1974; Hedenstierna et al., 1976); the same is probably true for a damaged lung, which often has an increased tendency to airway closure. Anatomical dead space is decreased by an artificial airway but is increased again by IPPV (Hedenstierna and Lundberg, 1975). Forrest (1972) has demonstrated rapid deterioration of lung compliance in guinea-pigs that were hyperinflated and showed that there was an associated decrease in alveolar surface activity.

Variations of the ventilator flow waveform do not have a marked effect on pulmonary gas exchange (Adams et al., 1970; Baker et al., 1977). Changes of tidal volume, rate of ventilation and inspiration to expiration time ratio (I : E ratio) are important. Large tidal volumes with high airway pressures and an increased I : E ratio reduce venous return and cardiac output (Morgan et al., 1966). These adverse effects can be mitigated by careful blood volume expansion and by avoiding hyperventilation (Morgan et al., 1969). When transfusion is used to maintain the cardiac output the patient's blood volume may be increased to above normal; this may cause overloading of a failing heart when ventilation is discontinued. Visick et al. (1973) showed that large tidal volumes are preferable to small tidal volumes for efficient gas exchange with IPPV. Large tidal volumes with slow respiratory rates were also shown to reduce changes in physiological dead space, compliance and intrapulmonary shunt (Hedenstierna and McCarthy, 1975; Baker et al., 1977). Molnar and Refsum (1974) raised the PaO_2 by increasing the tidal volume with a simultaneous increase of the ventilator dead space to maintain a normal $PaCO_2$. Unlike most studies of the effects of ventilation, Molnar and Refsum's study included patients on ventilators due to post-traumatic respiratory failure.

Controlled ventilation and assisted ventilation have recently been joined by intermittent mandatory ventilation (IMV) to assist patients with respiratory failure. The technique allows patients to breathe spontaneously from a circuit in which humidified air and oxygen are flowing. A ventilator is also incorporated in the circuit and is set to inflate the patient at regular, but increasing intervals until full independence is achieved. The method was first used for neonates and later it was used on adults with respiratory failure to aid weaning from a ventilator (Downs et al., 1973, 1974b). This method was recommended for treating flail chests and Cullen et al. (1975) claimed a reduction in the duration of mechanical ventilation. The technique allows sedation to be substantially reduced and encourages spontaneous respiratory efforts while preventing alveolar hypoventilation. If a raised expiratory pressure is used with IMV the gases must be delivered at pressures higher than the expiratory pressure; this maintains an adequate gas flow without extra work for the patient (Brach et al., 1976).

Occasionally the pulmonary lesion which has caused the respiratory failure is wholly unilateral and the inspired gas is distributed to the normal (more compliant) lung only. The damaged lung tends to collapse while the normal lung becomes hyperinflated. The dilemma may be overcome by using a double lumen tube; this allows proper ventilation of the normal lung while the collapsed lung is reinflated using higher airway pressures (Glass et al., 1976; Powner et al., 1977). Currently available double lumen tubes are all potentially irritant to the tracheal mucosa which limits the duration of the treatment. Bronchial obstruction must be excluded before differential ventilation of the lungs is attempted.

When a patient is intubated, particularly when he is on a ventilator, it is necessary to replace the normal cough mechanism to prevent accumulation of tracheal secretions. Efficient sputum control is essential therapy for any bronchial infection; failure to aspirate non-infected mucus predisposes to

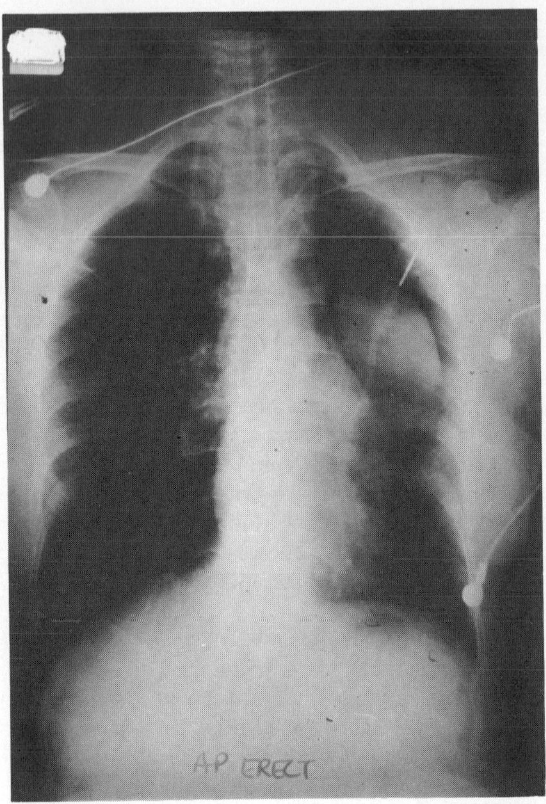

Fig. 3.2. Collapse of the left upper lobe with a pneumothorax after inhalation of smoke.

atelectasis and secondary infection. The usual routines include postural changes, manual hyperinflation of the lungs, vibration of the chest wall and then aspiration of the tracheal contents. Postural changes may be inhibited by skeletal traction after trauma but in most cases full use of posture is possible. Extreme position changes using special beds has been described (Piehl and Brown, 1976; Schimmel, 1977). The possible advantages are improved bronchial drainage, better matching of ventilation and capillary perfusion, and possibly reduced hydrostatic pressures across abnormally permeable pulmonary capillaries. Conversely, changes of position may cause increased perfusion of atelectatic regions which can cause a marked deterioration of the patient's condition (Katz and Barash, 1977).

Severe hypoxia is possible after physiotherapy and tracheal suction, especially in patients with poor cardiovascular reserves or obstructive lung disease (Taylor and Waters, 1971; Gormezano and Branthwaite, 1972).

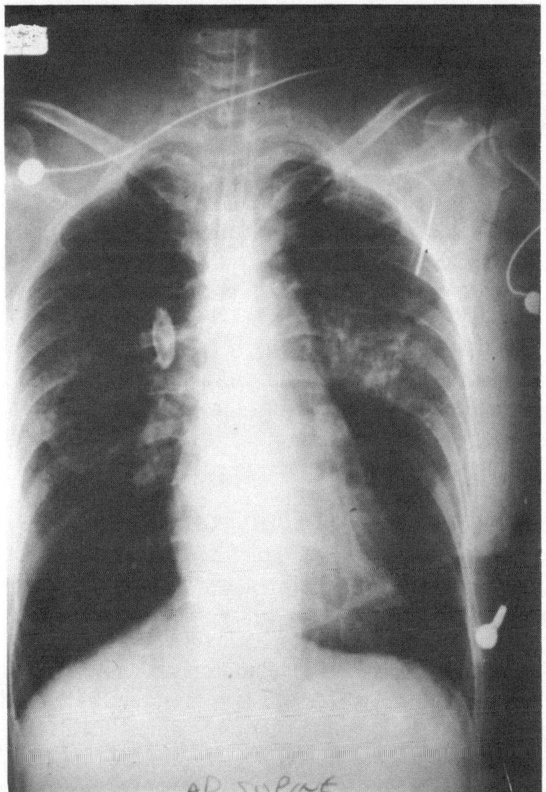

Fig. 3.3. Lung re-expanded after large quantities of carbon-stained mucus and a bronchial cast were removed using a flexible fibreoptic bronchoscope through the endotracheal tube.

Careless use of suction through an endotracheal tube is particularly hazardous; the tracheal pressure will fall significantly if the suction catheter is too large (Rosen and Hillard, 1970). Henville (1977) recommends the following formula.

Diameter of tracheal tube (mm) $\times$ 1·5 = Catheter size (FG).

FLEXIBLE FIBREOPTIC BRONCHOSCOPY

Despite vigorous attempts to clear the tracheobronchial tree a few patients do develop clinical and radiological signs of obstruction. Restricted movement and use of 'portable' X-rays can make diagnosis of atelectasis difficult, particularly in the presence of surgical emphysema and pulmonary contusion. Because of these problems of diagnosis and management the introduction of flexible fibreoptic bronchoscopes into clinical practice has been a welcome development. Their use in the intensive care unit has been reported (Lindholm et al., 1976; Milledge, 1976) and when compared with rigid bronchoscopes they have several advantages which are particularly obvious when there is already an artificial airway in the trachea.

To use a rigid bronchoscope safely it is necessary to starve the patient for several hours; additional injury to an already oedematous airway may be caused by extubation, bronchoscopy and reintubation. During the bronchoscopy the pulmonary damage can make adequate oxygenation difficult to achieve. The flexible bronchoscope is passed into the trachea through the tracheal tube, making starvation and extubation unnecessary, and ventilation can continue without interruption. Although the suction channel is narrow it is possible to remove blood clots and viscous sputum; with care whole lobes or lungs can be re-expanded without seriously disturbing the patient (*Figs. 3.2 and 3.3*). Millen et al. (1978) have re-inflated collapsed lobes by sealing the bronchus with a detachable tracheostomy tube cuff applied around the bronchoscope, the lung was inflated with air blown down the suction channel.

POSITIVE END EXPIRATORY PRESSURE

Over the last decade positive end expiratory pressure (PEEP) has emerged as a useful additional treatment for many forms of pulmonary damage, including some which result from injury. The technique involves raising the airway pressure to above atmospheric level at the end of expiration; it can be applied to patients on a ventilator, on IMV or breathing spontaneouly. Raised expiratory pressure is a more accurate description but there already exists an abundance of terms of which PEEP is most generally accepted. Others include continuous positive pressure breathing/ventilation, positive expiratory pressure plateau and continuous positive/raised airway pressure.

The end expiratory pressure can be achieved by resisting flow from the lungs, thus causing more air than usual to be retained at the end of expiration. Alternatively a pressure sensitive valve can be placed in the expiratory limb of the ventilator circuit; this remains open until the preset pressure is reached and then it closes. Mechanical PEEP valves can stick (and some regularly do) causing dangerously high inspiratory pressures. Such obstruction can be avoided, often with great financial economy, by venting exhaled gases to atmosphere through a column of water. Free movement of air then occurs until the prescribed pressure is reached and the pressure is maintained even if the pattern of ventilation is altered. By avoiding an expiratory resistance in favour of an underwater seal a lower mean intrathoracic pressure is obtained and this reduces the hazards of PEEP (Colgan et al., 1971).

The functional residual capacity (FRC) of the lungs is increased by raising the expiratory pressure; the magnitude of the increase varies with the total compliance and the pressure applied. An increased FRC reduces the tendency for airways to collapse and recruits more alveoli for gaseous exchange (Craig and McCarthy, 1972; West, 1976). Improved matching of ventilation with perfusion causes a rise in PaO_2 for a given inspired oxygen concentration. Inspired oxygen can therefore be reduced in order to diminish the risks of oxygen therapy. PEEP is of greatest value when the FRC is reduced, with a low compliance and a large intrapulmonary shunt, or when there are a substantial number of alveoli with low ventilation: perfusion ratios. It has no benefit if the FRC is normal or above normal as occurs with asthma and emphysema (Ashbaugh and Petty, 1973; Esteban et al., 1974).

PEEP may be used in respiratory distress arising from many conditions such as pulmonary contusion, fat embolism, aspiration of vomit, and sepsis (Ashbaugh et al., 1969; Kumar et al., 1970; Ashbaugh and Petty, 1973; King et al., 1973; Sladen et al., 1973). PEEP has also been found to be potentially useful after near-drowning in salt and fresh water (Ruiz et al., 1973; Modell et al., 1974). Improved alignment of fractured ribs has been described by Sladen et al. (1973) but this should only be accepted as a by-product of treatment; PEEP should only be used to improve pulmonary function. As with mechanical ventilation, PEEP is not a panacea and there are distinct hazards associated with its use. Reduction of the cardiac output and abnormalities of regional blood flow are the main complications and must be balanced against the potential benefits. Fortunately the patient acts as his own control if the effects of PEEP are assessed after each increment of pressure.

The best level of expiratory pressure varies greatly between patients, and at different times in the same patient. If treatment is effective a high level PEEP which was initially indicated, will become too high when the lungs improve. Ideally oxygen transport should be measured with each increment of pressure but this is not always possible. Fortunately Suter et al. (1975) have demonstrated that oxygen transport improves as the total compliance improves but is reduced if PEEP is increased further. Compliance can be assessed at the bedside by maintaining a constant tidal volume and measuring the pressure change in inspiration as PEEP is increased. If a catheter is present in the pulmonary artery assessment of variations of cardiac output or arteriovenous oxygen tension difference help to determine the best level of PEEP. However, pulmonary capillary wedge pressures must be interpreted with caution if the expiratory pressure is raised; if the catheter tip is above the atria the measured pressure will be greatly affected by the airway pressure (Roy et al., 1977).

When PEEP was applied to dogs with normal lungs, the lungs were found to contain more water than usual (Thornton et al., 1975). Even when it was used on dogs with pulmonary oedema it did not reduce the lung water although it did improve function; high pressures did prevent intra-alveolar oedema (Caldini et al., 1975; Hopewell and Murray, 1976).

Intrathoracic pressure rises with the expiratory pressure and in normal lungs there is a consequent reduction of venous return and cardiac output.

As lung compliance deteriorates less of the pressure is transmitted to the great veins, therefore higher pressures can be applied without reducing the cardiac output (Dueck et al., 1972; Philbin et al., 1972). Depression of the cardiac output can be reversed by increasing the blood volume (Qvist et al., 1975). In a manner similar to that already described for IPPV the hypervolaemia used to counteract the undesirable effects of PEEP can overload a weak heart if the pressure is suddenly reduced. If there is any doubt about reserves of the heart then dopamine should be considered to maintain the cardiac output but this may cause the PaO_2 to fall and so reduce the benefit of PEEP (Berk et al., 1977). Although it is possible to plan a gradual reduction of the expiratory pressure, sudden pressure falls during physiotherapy and tracheal suction are unavoidable.

Investigations of renal function have shown that PEEP will cause marked changes in renal blood flow when used in animals with normal lungs. Gammanpila et al. (1977) found a diminished renal blood flow and glomerular filtration rate. Hall et al. (1974) measured reductions in creatinine clearance, salt excretion and urine production; blood flow was not reduced but its distribution was diverted from the cortex to the juxtamedullary zone, which may explain the reduced sodium excretion. Sodium retention is not peculiar to patients on a ventilator or PEEP although it is a feature of both forms of treatment. It is also found after trauma when there is hypovolaemia, heart failure, severe sepsis and unsuitably large infusions of sodium. All of these causes must be excluded before ventilation or PEEP is held to be responsible for increasing oedema. Pilon and Bittar (1973) detected a fall in thoracic duct lymph flow and suggested that it might contribute to the formation of peripheral oedema during the application of PEEP.

Jaundice is not uncommon after major injury. Johnson and Hedley-Whyte (1972) noted a decrease in portal blood flow when PEEP was used on dogs with pulmonary oedema. Increasing jaundice should be regarded as an indication to withdraw PEEP.

Pulmonary injuries are frequently associated with head injuries, therefore it is necessary to consider the effect of raised expiratory pressures on intracranial pressure. Using cats Aidinis et al. (1976) found that PEEP could cause adverse changes in the pupils and the electroencephalogram if it was used in the presence of intracranial hypertension. Pulmonary oedema did protect the brain from the deleterious effects unless the pressures were inappropriately high. If in doubt raised expiratory pressure should be avoided; probably the only safe way to use it in patients with brain injuries is by simultaneously measuring the intracranial pressure.

The usual levels of PEEP found to be useful are between 5 and 15 cmH_2O (King et al., 1973). Occasionally in very severe cases of respiratory distress such levels are ineffective but the patients may respond to much higher pressures used with IMV (Kirby et al., 1975a, b). If very high expiratory pressures are considered then full monitoring facilities must be available to ensure that tissue oxygenation is maintained. High PEEP has been recommended as superior to an extra-corporeal membrane oxygenator (Kirby, 1978) which requires greater technical support and is not free of complications. Very few health services have, or ever will have, sufficient staff or funds to make membrane oxygenators freely available; the rapid expansion of the scope of cardiac surgery is reducing their availability for non-cardiac work.

OXYGEN THERAPY

In 1775 Priestley suggested that oxygen might be useful in medicine but warned that overuse may lead to toxic effects (Leigh, 1973a). Like any other drug, sufficient, and no more, should be used to obtain the desired effect. Leigh (1973a) has clearly described how oxygen has been consistently abused for two centuries, despite the sensible introduction that it received.

After injury some patients are in obvious need of oxygen, being cyanosed or in respiratory failure. However, many more with non-thoracic injuries such as fractures of the lower limb and pelvis, suffer a moderate degree of hypoxia which is detectable only by blood gas estimation (Collins et al., 1968; Simmons et al., 1969; Tachakra and Sevitt, 1975). Oxygen can be given quickly and easily to alleviate either form of hypoxia and, because hypoxic respiratory drive is not a problem after injury, it is without risk. Many of the injuries which cause hypoxia are also associated with severe, systemic fat embolism. It is claimed that fat embolism is more harmful if there is pre-existing hypoxia and if hypoxia is reversed the damage can be minimized (Szabö, 1970). If oxygen is given routinely for the first 48–72 hours to patients at risk from fat embolism the incidence of systemic complications of the syndrome may be reduced.

Although oxygen undoubtedly increases the arterial oxygen pressure it can also cause early or late pulmonary changes which reduce the efficiency of oxygen transfer to the pulmonary capillary blood. As soon as therapy commences there is an increase in the intrapulmonary shunt (Kerr, 1975) possibly due to elevated mixed venous oxygen tensions enlarging shunt blood flow (Smith et al., 1973). West (1976) has also demonstrated that extra inspired oxygen will cause poorly ventilated alveoli to collapse; as the concentration rises so does the minimum ventilation : perfusion ratio (V/Q) that is necessary to preserve alveolar expansion. The effect is more pronounced in patients with a substantial number of alveoli with very low V/Q ratios.

High concentrations of oxygen inhaled over a long period will cause structural damage to the lungs (Kafer, 1971; Winter and Smith, 1972). Assessing the damage caused by oxygen is difficult as many of the changes seen in the lungs after prolonged illness are probably caused as much by the unnatural progression of the underlying illness as the administered oxygen. Modern life-support procedures allow many patients to linger for days or weeks beyond the normal time of death before they eventually die. There is not a well established toxic level but certain guidelines are commonly accepted. Pure oxygen can be tolerated for at least twenty-four hours (Singer et al., 1970); Barber (1970) exposed terminal head injuries to 100 per cent inspired oxygen for an average of forty hours without significant structural change in the lungs. The risk of oxygen toxicity is probably very low if the inspired concentration is below 50 per cent and space travel has shown that oxygen at one-third atmospheric pressure is safe for prolonged periods. Work on the sea bed, at very high pressures for prolonged periods, may provide further information. The original pulmonary injury dictates the minimum inspired oxygen concentration; an acceptable degree of arterial hypoxaemia for an ill patient, with possible central nervous and renal damage, cannot be defined. It is necessary to maintain a PaO_2 that will produce a normal haemoglobin saturation (10 kPa, 75 mmHg). Because the damage caused by hypoxia is rapid in onset, and often permanent, the minimum inspired oxygen concentration should produce a normal PaO_2 under the worst of the prevailing conditions, taking into account changes of position, cardiac output, ventilation, etc.

There are further practical problems associated with oxygen therapy. With conscious, spontaneously breathing patients the method of administration must be accurate and acceptable (Green, 1972; Leigh, 1973a, b). If a mask is uncomfortable it is unlikely to be worn continuously. Nasal prongs have limited accuracy and maximum concentration but they are comfortable and can be worn while eating, talking, expectorating, etc. Many commonly used ventilators do not have automatic oxygen concentration regulators, which means that the concentration will vary with different ventilator settings unless the oxygen flow into the machine is also adjusted.

A useful advance in oxygen therapy, particularly for the critically ill patient, has been the introduction of transcutaneous oxygen electrodes. The sensor is a modified Clarke electrode with a built-in heating element which produces vasodilatation in the skin over which it is applied. It is strapped to the skin under a clavicle or over the sternum and its position must be changed every four hours to allow recalibration and prevent burning. In adults approximately fifteen minutes is necessary for the electrode to equilibrate with the capillary blood. The measured PO_2 is lower than the arterial, but the difference is constant and therefore once measured it can be used to derive the PaO_2 (Rooth et al., 1976; Al-Diaidy et al., 1977).

OXYGEN DELIVERY

The discussion so far has been primarily concerned with the prevention or control of respiratory failure. When securing normal delivery of oxygen to the pulmonary capillaries simultaneous efforts must be made to ensure that the oxygen is transported to the tissues; normal arterial oxygen levels are not confirmation of good oxygen transport. Efficient oxygen flux requires a normal or above normal cardiac output, an adequate haemoglobin concentration, and virtually full saturation of the haemoglobin. Oxyhaemoglobin normally releases oxygen to the tissues when exposed to normal tissue oxygen pressures but hypoxia results if the affinity of haemoglobin for oxygen is increased. Finally, the tissues must be able to use the oxygen presented to them. Assessing early tissue hypoxia is difficult as most of the clinical signs and biochemical lesions occur when hypoxia is established and severe. If consumption increases after each improvement of the transport mechanism then hypoxia must have been present even if delivery was already above normal (Bryan-Brown, 1977).

Changes in cardiac output are common after injury, the most common causes of low output after respiratory damage are probably under-transfusion and inappropriate ventilator therapy (hyperventilation, PEEP etc.). Conditions such as myocardial contusion, tamponade or pre-existing heart disease and acid base abnormalities must be excluded. Inefficiency of the left ventricle will aggravate any tendency to pulmonary oedema; if the cardiac output is clinically inadequate, despite apparently adequate transfusion, the pulmonary capillary wedge pressure should be measured. Central venous pressures may be misleading and pulmonary oedema, due to overtransfusion, can result from reliance on them. Wedge pressures enable a more informed decision to be made regarding further transfusion or the use of inotropic drugs to stimulate an increase in cardiac output.

Haemoglobin is the principal carrier of oxygen, although the normal concentration is approximately 14 g/100 ml it has been shown that haemodilution of 12–14 g/100 ml is associated with increased oxygen delivery (Gruber, 1970). Above 10 g/100 ml the quantity of haemoglobin is less important than the quality, as long as polycythaemia is avoided. Oxyhaemoglobin must dissociate readily in the tissues otherwise hypoxia occurs, or there must be a compensatory rise of the cardiac output. An estimate of the affinity of haemoglobin for oxygen can be made by measuring the oxygen tension when it is 50 per cent saturated (P50). The normal P50 is approximately 3·5 kPa (26·5 mmHg). With a fall of as little as 0·5 kPa tissue hypoxia can be avoided only by a 100 per cent increase of the cardiac output (Ledingham, 1977). Bryan-Brown (1975) described how variations of the affinity of haemoglobin for oxygen can substantially reduce oxygen transport by reducing the quantity of oxygen released in the brain while maintaining a viable tissue PO_2. The volume of oxygen available per unit volume of blood is diminished.

Many factors after injury can adversely affect the affinity of haemoglobin for oxygen. Respiratory alkalosis is common, particularly in artificially ventilated patients, and metabolic alkalosis rapidly develops after a large blood transfusion. Routine use of sodium bicarbonate with transfused blood is unnecessary if resuscitation is prompt and adequate; it should be used only to correct a measured deficit otherwise it will aggravate the usual post-transfusion alkalosis. Transfused blood has a depressed P50 particularly if it is anticoagulated with acid citrate dextrose (ACD) instead of citrate phosphate dextrose (CPD) (Jesch et al., 1975). Severe burns alter the dissociation of oxyhaemoglobin; Greenburg et al. (1976) described the changes as detrimental but Arturson (1975) found the curve shifted to the right. Carbon monoxide poisoning inhibits dissociation as well as reducing the volume of oxygen transported and this should be considered after inhalation of smoke.

Red cell organic phosphate concentrations play a central part in oxyhaemoglobin dissociation, the most important of these being 2,3 diphosphoglycerate (2,3 DPG) (MacDonald, 1977). Blood anticoagulated with CPD retains a higher concentration of 2,3 DPG than blood that has been anticoagulated with ACD, the concentration declines as the storage time increases with either anticoagulant. Unusually high concentrations of 2,3 DPG are possible in specially prepared red cells and these have been shown to be beneficial in post-cardiopulmonary by-pass patients (Dennis et al., 1975). If it is made generally available high 2,3 DPG blood may prove to be very useful to aid oxygen transport in other cases with diminished cardiac reserves.

Intracellular 2,3 DPG concentration is also depressed if the serum inorganic phosphate levels fall. Hypophosphataemia occurs after surgery (Young et al., 1973) and similar falls are also likely after injury. It also occurs when feeding is recommenced after a period of starvation, but is easily controlled by using phosphate supplements (Travis et al., 1971). Several synthetic amino acid solutions used for intravenous feeding are deficient in phosphates and Intralipid does not contain an adequate amount. Even dextrose-saline infusions are capable of causing significant hypophosphataemia during starvation (Guillan et al., 1976). Septicaemia, particularly when caused by Gram-negative bacteria, induces hypophosphataemia and mortality increases as the serum phosphate concentration falls (Riedler and Scheitlin, 1969).

SALT, WATER AND COLLOIDS

After major injury there is commonly a phase of salt and water retention. If the lungs are damaged there is an increased tendency for them to develop interstitial oedema. The oedema forms around the portion that is injured, particularly after pulmonary contusion, but there is also a tendency for more remote parts of the lung to become oedematous. The pulmonary oedema is aggravated by retention of sodium, and pulmonary function often deteriorates before other signs of salt retention appear.

The probability of salt and water retention is greater when the patient is ventilated mechanically; Sladen et al. (1968) noticed that water retention occurred in ventilated patients and that pulmonary oedema resulted. The retention was accompanied with hyponatraemia and weight gain. Although the oedema was generally controlled with diuretics, in one case the necessary diuresis occurred as a result of blood transfusion. A later study (Hinton et al., 1972) has shown the importance of hypovolaemia as a cause of sodium retention in spontaneously breathing, severely burned patients; transfusion produced the desired diuresis. Gett et al. (1971) found that ventilated patients retained sodium and this was associated with a fall in the urine sodium concentration and reversal of the usual sodium : potassium concentration ratio in the urine.

As a part of a series of laboratory studies of pulmonary contusion, Trinkle et al. (1973) found that the associated pulmonary oedema was aggravated by lactated Ringer's solution and low molecular weight dextran but was reduced by diuretic therapy. Water restriction and diuretics were subsequently used to treat pulmonary contusion in humans (Trinkle et al., 1975). Fleming and Bowen (1972) also demonstrated the value of diuretics in the management of pulmonary oedema in injured patients resuscitated with Ringer's lactate solution and blood. If acute renal failure complicates the respiratory injury early dialysis is indicated to prevent water overload as well as for increasing uraemia and hyperkalaemia (Zimmerman, 1971).

Diuretics are usually prescribed to improve alveolar ventilation and lung compliance. Powers et al. (1977) suggested that hypertonic mannitol might improve pulmonary capillary perfusion by reducing endothelial cellular swelling. A bolus of 25 g of mannitol was given to eleven patients with respiratory distress syndrome (eight after major injury). The dead space: tidal volume ratio fell, indicating a possible improvement of perfusion. The effect was not found after frusemide, and was only transient after the mannitol; the effect of further doses of mannitol was not measured, neither was it compared with another form of blood volume expansion.

Although sodium retention is common the usual biochemical anomaly is hyponatraemia, which is not caused by water retention. The hyponatraemia is not accompanied by a fall of plasma osmolality and is probably due to increased permeability of cell membranes to sodium thus allowing it to migrate into the cells (Flear and Singh, 1973). The abnormality usually reverses itself as the patient's condition improves but it can be alleviated by avoidance of tissue hypoxia, control of septicaemia and by adequate nutrition. Hinton et al. (1973) studied the effects of hypertonic glucose, with potassium and insulin, on severely burned patients with the biochemical abnormalities described; there was a rapid increase in sodium excretion and the serum sodium concentration returned to normal as treatment progressed.

There has been a vogue for large volumes of crystalloid solutions to be used for resuscitation of hypovolaemic patients. Plasma colloids play a part in maintaining the normal interstitial water content by encouraging water to return into the blood stream down a colloid osmotic pressure gradient. Large crystalloid infusions dilute the plasma proteins thus reducing the normal pressure gradient. In a study of patients undergoing abdominal aortic surgery there was no demonstrable difference between crystalloids and colloids (Virgillio, 1977). Lowe et al. (1977) could not find any difference between colloidal and non-colloidal solutions for resuscitation of patients after abdominal trauma; however, they excluded all patients with thoracic injuries. Pulmonary oedema did occur in six patients with large infusions of Ringer's lactate which caused the colloid osmotic pressure to fall to within 0·67 kPa (5 mmHg) of the left ventricular filling pressure (Stein et al., 1974). When Ringer lactate solutions were used to treat hypovolaemia in dogs with pulmonary contusion the size of the pulmonary lesion and the surrounding oedema was increased. Plasma did not cause the same deterioration, even if the same volumes were used; plasma was even safer if the volume transfused was equal to the blood lost (Richardson et al., 1974).

In the absence of pulmonary damage and with an efficient left ventricle, it would seem to be relatively safe to substitute crystalloid solutions for colloidal solutions when replacing blood lost. However, the immediate recognition of lung damage may be difficult during the early stages of resuscitation and some pulmonary problems are slow to develop, e.g. inhalation of vomit, pulmonary fat embolism.

Serum albumin concentrations often fall in ill patients and Tonnesen et al. (1977) found that survival was less likely as the albumin titre decreased. However, there was no difference between patients in respiratory failure and those who were not when comparisons were made within the group of survivors and non-survivors. Low serum albumin concentrations could aggravate any tendency to pulmonary oedema and concentrated albumin solutions are commonly used to control oedema. Marty (1974) has reviewed the more recent investigations of Starling's hypothesis and concludes that the usual, simple view of hydrostatic versus colloid osmotic pressure is inadequate. A large part of the albumin stores are extravascular and albumin replacement therapy increases the transfer of albumin from the blood to the interstitial fluid. Pulmonary lymphatic drainage is reduced as the interstitial albumin concentration rises and interstitial oedema may be aggravated by intravenous infusions of albumin, particularly if the capillary permeability is increased.

While low serum albumin concentrations may predispose to pulmonary oedema the converse is also true. Da Luz et al. (1975) discovered diminished plasma colloid osmotic pressures in patients who developed pulmonary oedema after myocardial infarction although there was no difference in the amount of water retention when compared to a similar group without pulmonary oedema. As the pulmonary oedema resolved after treatment with digoxin and diuretics the colloid osmotic pressure returned to normal.

SYNTHETIC GLUCOCORTICOIDS

The place of parenteral glucocorticoids in the management of various forms of pulmonary injury has been debated for many years. Hausmann and Lunt (1955) reported the use of hydrocortisone in two cases of acid pulmonary aspiration syndrome and their impression was that the patients benefited from treatment. Nearly all the evidence supporting the clinical use of steroids is based on similar impressions; unfortunately there has been little hard evidence of their value to humans. Clinical impressions of their beneficial effects have been recorded for adult respiratory distress syndrome of various causes, but the evidence is not convincing (Dines et al., 1961; Vandam, 1965; Ashbaugh and Petty, 1966; Nicholl et al., 1967; Fischer et al., 1971; Petty and Ashbaugh, 1971; Sladen, 1976).

Animal studies of steroid therapy for the pulmonary lesions associated with injury in humans have given conflicting results. Benefit has been reported after pulmonary aspiration of acid (Dudley and Marshall, 1974; Toung et al., 1976) and fat embolism (Wertzberger and Pettier, 1968; Nylén and Sylvén, 1976). In the experiments on fat embolism the steroids were given before the injury; Rokkanen (1974) used methylprednisolone in humans after severe trauma and found an insignificant fall in the incidence of clinical fat embolism; the final outcome was also unaffected. Other trials did not provide laboratory evidence of improvement after acid aspiration (Taylor and Prys-Davies, 1968; Chapman et al., 1974; Downs et al., 1974a) nor after fat embolism (Parker et al., 1974).

Franz et al. (1974) did demonstrate that methylprednisolone could reduce the severity of experimentally induced pulmonary contusion in dogs. The same group successfully used the drug on patients with pulmonary contusion (Trinkle et al., 1975); once again, so many aspects of treatment were included in the study that proper assessment of the contribution of the steroid in humans is impossible. Steroids have been shown to mitigate the effect of inhalation of smoke in animals but superinfection was a problem (Seinfeld et al., 1975; Dressler et al., 1976). Levine et al. (1978) used dexamethasone in a small series of patients with respiratory tract damage after burns and could not demonstrate any advantage.

In the discussion of the difficulties of oxygen transport the importance of the increased affinity of transfused haemoglobin for oxygen was stressed. McConn and Del Guercio (1971) listed steroid therapy as one of the ways of improving the dissociation of transfused oxyhaemoglobin. Palliation of pulmonary contusion and improved oxyhaemoglobin dissociation are two areas where steroid therapy may prove to be useful, but more precise clinical investigation is required. To add to the confusion the recommended dose of drug varies considerably; from a total of 100 mg of hydrocortisone (Hausmann and Lunt, 1955) to 16 000 mg of methylprednisoline (Sladen, 1976).

INFECTION

Infection of lungs that have been damaged is an important life-threatening complication. The risk of infection is greatly increased by retention of tracheo-bronchial secretions and by insertion of an artificial airway. It is one of the main contraindications to tracheostomy and endotracheal intubation. The problem is increased by the fact that the patients at risk are nursed within one unit, often amid other infected patients. The main routes for the transfer of bacteria are through the air, on fomites and on the hands of nurses or other attendants. The hands of the staff are particularly important for the transfer of Gram-negative bacteria, which are so commonly involved in infections that occur in intensive care units (Lowbury et al., 1970; Casewell and Phillips, 1977; Meers et al., 1978).

It is obviously important to take whatever steps are possible to prevent infection spreading among patients at risk in a confined area. Adequate space between beds, use of individual cubicles and efficient ventilation are all desirable, but require considerable capital investment which is often obtained only when the entire hospital is rebuilt. Disciplined observation of precautions to prevent spread of bacteria by hands and fomites, combined with sensible use of antibiotics can reduce cross infection even in old, overcrowded units.

Inanimate objects within the patient's environment can become vectors of bacteria. The risk can be reduced by supplying each patient with a comprehensive range of equipment so that none is used on two different people, unless it has been thoroughly cleaned between use. Infection has also been carried to the patient from areas outside the ward, such as the hospital kitchen (Lowbury et al., 1970), the pharmacy (Baird et al., 1976; Baird and Shooter, 1976) and clinical investigation areas (Epidemiological Research Laboratory, 1977). Mechanical ventilators are an obvious source of infection, although casual sampling may not detect any bacteria, even if complete sterilization has not been achieved (Phillips et al., 1974). Effective protection from ventilator infections is possible by using disposable or autoclavable patient circuits, including the humidifier, and also isolating the patient from the ventilator with bacterial filters (Holdcroft et al., 1974).

The hands of medical staff are a long established mode of transmitting bacteria and brief observation shows that hand washing between patients is often neglected. Though hand washing should be encouraged, further protection is provided by wearing waterproof, disposable gloves and aprons whenever the patient is touched. The use of gloves has two practical advantages; unlike hand washing, failure to comply is obvious and casual visitors are effectively discouraged from handling those who are at risk. Gloves and aprons must be changed between each patient and this depends on good discipline in all members of staff.

Most pulmonary damage caused by injury is not initially infected and therefore antibiotics do not offer any immediate benefit, but they may provide an environment that selectively encourages growth of resistant bacteria. Frequent bacteriological investigation of sputum, urine, wounds and all catheters or tubes removed from the patient will usually permit logical use of antibiotics for known bacteria instead of blind prophylaxis with broad spectrum antibiotics. Regular scrutiny of all bacteriological reports will help to identify the most commonly occurring bacteria in a unit and their probable antibiotic sensitivities. Resistance to even the most powerful antibiotics will occur if they are used frequently within a unit or hospital (Nakahora et al., 1977).

By adopting all the precautions that have been discussed the present author has witnessed almost complete eradication of *Pseudomonas aeruginosa* from an intensive care unit for over two years. Less common bacterial such as *Serratia marcescens* have also been absent but Klebsiella species have not been so well controlled. Pseudomonas has been brought into the unit on several burned patients in respiratory failure, but it has not spread to other patients.

The management of pulmonary injuries and the complications, has developed so that patients with injuries that were once fatal now have an increased chance of survival. Certain aspects of treatment have a well established place in any treatment regimen. Mechanical ventilation can save the life of a patient with progressive ventilatory failure. Sensible use of oxygen is always beneficial and PEEP can cause dramatic improvement of arterial oxygenation, especially when combined with intermittent mandatory ventilation. Pulmonary oedema can be avoided by careful fluid restriction and can be treated with modern diuretics. Other treatments still require further investigation to establish their value, particularly for humans, e.g. albumin replacement therapy and steroids.

Even with the well established methods of treatment abuse may be counter-productive; unnecessary artificial ventilation may result in avoidable secondary infection of damaged lung; PEEP may raise the PaO_2 but reduce oxygen transport. The best results will be obtained only by measuring the effect of each phase of treatment, in every patient, and by continuing to reassess the value of each procedure as the illness progresses. Treatment is not complete until all aspects of oxygen transport have been examined and improved where necessary.

REFERENCES

Abeyewickreme N. and Simpson P. M. (1977) Carinal granuloma after endotracheal granulation. *Br. med. J.* **2**, 868.

Adams A. P., Economides A. P., Finlay W. E. et al. (1970) The effects of variations of inspiratory flow waveform on cardio-respiratory function during controlled ventilation in normo, hypo- and hypervolaemic dogs. *Br. J. Anaesth.* **42**, 818.

Aidinis S. J., Lafferty J. and Shapiro H. M. (1976) Intracranial responses to PEEP. *Anesthesiology* **45**, 275.

Al-Diaidy W., Skeates S. J., Hill D. W. et al. (1977) The use of transcutaneous oxygen electrodes in intensive therapy. *Intens. Care Med.* **3**, 35.

Arturson G. (1975) Oxygen affinity of whole blood in vitro and under standard conditions in patients with severe burns. *Burns.* **1**, 249.

Ashbaugh D. G. and Petty T. L. (1966) The use of corticosteroids in the treatment of respiratory failure associated with massive fat embolism. *Surg. Gynecol. Obstet.* **122**, 493.

Ashbaugh D. G. and Petty T. L. (1973) Positive end-expiratory pressure. Physiology indications and contra indications. *J. thorac. cardiovasc. Surg.* **65**, 165.

Ashbaugh D. G., Petty T. L., Bigelow D. B. et al. (1969) Continuous positive pressure in adult respiratory distress syndrome. *J. thorac. cardiovasc. Surg.* **57**, 31.

Avery E. E., March E. T. and Benson D. W. (1956) Critically crushed chests: A new method of treatment with continuous mechanical hyperventilation to produce alkalotic apnoea and internal pneumatic stabilisation. *J. thorac. cardiovasc. Surg.* **32**, 291.

Bain J. A. (1972) Late complications of tracheostomy and prolonged endotracheal intubation. *Int. Anesthiol. Clin.* **10**, 225.

Baird R. M., Brown W. R. C. and Shooter R. A. (1976) Pseudomonas aeruginosa in hospital pharmacies. *Br. med. J.* **1**, 511.

Baird R. M. and Shooter R. A. (1976) Pseudomonas aeruginosa infections associated with use of contaminated medicaments. *Br. med. J.* **2**, 349.

Baker A. B., Collis J. E. and Cowie R. W. (1977) Effects of varying inspiratory flow waveform and time in intermittent positive pressure ventilation: II, various physiological variables. *Br. J. Anaesth.* **49**, 1221.

Barber R. E., Lee J. and Hamilton W. K. (1970) Oxygen toxicity in man: A prospective study in patients with irreversible brain damage. *N. Engl. J. Med.* **283**, 1478.

Berk J. L., Hagen J. F., Tong R. K. et al. (1977) The use of dopamine to correct the reduced cardiac output resulting from positive end expiratory pressure. A two edged sword. *Crit. Care Med.* **5**, 269.

Bowes J. B., Kelly D. F. and Peacock J. H. (1973) Intubation trauma: Effects of short term endotracheal intubation on the tracheal mucous membrane of the pig. *Anaesthesia* **28**, 603.

Brach B. B., Yin F., Timms R. et al. (1976) Reduced inspiratory effort during intermittent mandatory ventilation with PEEP. *Crit. Care Med.* **4**, 142.

Bradbeer T. L., James M. L., Sear J. W. et al. (1976) Tracheal stenosis associated with a low pressure cuffed, endotracheal tube. *Anaesthesia* **31**, 504.

Brown M. M. (1972) Diagnosis and management of major thoracic injury. *Ann. R. Coll. Surg. Engl.* **50**, 182.

Bryan-Brown C. W. (1975) Consumable oxygen: availability of oxygen in relation to oxyhaemoglobin dissociation. *Crit. Care Med.* **3**, 103.

Bryan-Brown C. W. (1977) Wrecking the machinery? *Crit. Care Med.* **5**, 163.

Caldini P., Leith J. D. and Brennan M. J. (1975) Effect of continuous positive pressure ventilation (CPPV) on oedema formation in the dog lung. *J. appl. Physiol.* **39**, 672.

Campbell D. (1966) The management of chest injuries. *Br. J. Anaesth.* **38**, 298.

Carroll R. G. (1973) Evaluation of tracheal tube cuff designs. *Crit. Care Med.* **1**, 45.

Casewell M and Phillips I. (1977) Hands as route of transmission for Klebsiella species. *Br. med. J.* **2**, 1315.

Chapman R. L. Jr., Modell J. H., Ruiz B. C. et al. (1974) Effects of continuous positive pressure ventilation and steroids on aspiration of hydrochloric acid (pH 1·8) in dogs. *Anesth. Analg. (Cleve.)* **53**, 556.

Ching N. P. H. and Nealon T. F. (1974) Clinical experience with new low pressure high volume tracheostomy cuffs. Importance of limiting intracuff pressure. *N. Y. State J. Med.* **74**, 2379.

Colgan F. J., Barrow R. E. and Fanning G. L. (1971) Constant positive pressure breathing and cardiorespiratory function. *Anesthesiology* **34**, 145.

Collins J. A., Gordon W. C. Jr., Hudson T. L. et al. (1968) In apparent hypoxaemia in casualties with wounded limbs. *Ann. Surg.* **167**, 511.

Cooper J. and Grillo H. C. (1969) Experimental production and prevention of injury due to cuffed tracheal tubes. *Surg. Gynecol. Obstet.* **129**, 1235.

Craig D. B. and McCarthy D. S. (1972) Airway closure and lung volumes during breathing with maintained airway positive pressure. *Anesthesiology* **36**, 540.

Cullen P., Modell J. H., Kirby R. R. et al. (1975) Treatment of flail chest: Use of intermittent mandatory ventilators and positive end expiratory pressure. *Arch. Surg.* **110**, 1099.

da Luz P. L., Shubin H., Weil M. H. et al (1975) Pulmonary oedema related to changes in colloidosmotic and pulmonary artery wedge pressure in patients after acute myocardial infarction. *Circulation* **51**, 350.

Dennis R. C., Vito L., Weisel R. D. et al. (1975) Improved myocardial performance following high 2,3 diphosphoglycerate red cell transfusions. *Surgery* **77**, 741.

Dines D. E., Baher W. G. and Scantland W. A. (1961) Aspiration pneumonitis. Mendelson's syndrome. *J. Am. med. Ass.* **176**, 229.

Downs J. B., Chapmen R. L. Jr., Modell J. H. et al. (1974) An evaluation of steroid therapy in aspiration pneumonitis. *Anesthesiology* **40**, 129.

Downs J. B., Klein E. F., Desantels D. et al. (1973) Intermittent mandatory ventilation: A new approach to weaning patients from mechanical ventilators. *Chest* **64**, 331.

Downs J. B., Perkins H. M. and Sutton W. W. (1974b) Successful weaning after five years of mechanical ventilation. *Anesthesiology* **40**, 602.

Dressler D. P., Shornik W. A. and Kupersmith S. (1976) Corticosteroid treatment of experimental smoke inhalation. *Ann. Surg.* **183**, 46.

Dudley W. R. and Marshall B. E. (1974) Steroid treatment for acid aspiration pneumonitis. *Anesthesiology* **40**, 136.

Dueck R., Wagner R. D. and West J. B. (1977) Effects of positive end expiratory pressure on gas exchange in dogs with normal and oedematous lungs. *Anesthesiology*, **47**, 359.

Epidemiological Research Laboratory (1977) Unusual infection in intensive care unit. *Br. med. J.* **1**, 111.

Esteban A., de Elio J., Cerda E. et al. (1974) Blood gas changes with different end expiratory pressures in patients with chronic bronchitis. *Br. J. Anaesth.* **46**, 159.

Fischer J. E., Turner R. H., Herndon J. H. et al. (1971) Massive steroid therapy in severe fat embolism. *Surg. Gynecol. Obstet.* **132**, 667.

Flear C. T. G. and Singh C. M. (1973) Hyponatraemia and sick cells. *Br. J. Anaesth.* **45**, 976.

Fleming W. H. and Bowen J. C. (1972) The use of diuretics in the treatment of an early wet lung syndrome. *Ann. Surg.* **175**, 505.

Forrest J. B. (1972) The effect of hyperventilation on pulmonary surface activity. *Br. J. Anaesth.* **44**, 313.

Franz J. L., Richardson J. D., Grover F. L. et al. (1974) Effect of methylprednisolone sodium succinate on experimental pulmonary contusion. *J. thorac. cardiovasc. Surg.* **68**, 842.

Friman L., Hedenstierna G. and Schildt B. (1976) Stenosis following tacheostomy. A quantitative study of long term results. *Anaesthesia* **31**, 479.

Fryer M. E. and Marshall R. D. (1976) Tracheal dilatation. *Anaesthesia* **31**, 470.

Gammanpila S., Bevan D. R. and Bhudu R. (1977) Effect of positive and negative expiratory pressure on renal function. *B. J. Anaesth.* **49**, 199.

Gett P. M., Sherwood-Jones E. and Shepherd G. F. (1971) Pulmonary oedema associated with sodium retention during ventilator treatment. *Br. J. Anaesth.* **43**, 460.

Gibbons J., James O. and Quail A. (1973) Management of 130 cases of chest injury with respiratory failure. *Br. J. Anaesth.* **45**, 1130.

Glass D. D., Tonnessen A. S., Gabel J. C. et al. (1976) Therapy of unilateral pulmonary insufficiency with a double lumen endotracheal tube. *Crit. Care Med.* **4**, 323.

Gormezana J. and Branthwaite M. A. (1972) Effects of physiotherapy during intermittent positive pressure ventilation: changes in arterial blood glass tension. *Anaesthesia* **27**, 258.

Green I. D. (1972) Methods of administration of oxygen. *Br. J. hosp. Med.* Equipment Suppl. p. 33.

Greenburg A. G., Frank H. and Peskin G. W. (1976) The left shifted oxyhaemoglobin curve in the burn patient. *J. Trauma* **16**, 573.

Gruber U. F. (1970) Recent developments in the investigation and treatment of hypovolaemic shock. *Br. J. hosp. Med.* **3**, 631.

Guillan P. J., Hill G. L. and Morgan D. B. (1976) Hypophosphataemia: A complication of 'innocuous dextrose-saline'. *Lancet* **2**, 710.

Hall S. V., Johnson E. E. and Hedley-Whyte J. (1974) Renal hemodynamics and function with continuous positive pressure ventilation in dogs. *Anesthesiology* **41**, 452.

Halmagyi D. F. and Kinney J. (1975) Metabolic rate in acute respiratory failure complicating sepsis. *Surgery* **77**, 492.

Hausmann W. and Lunt R. L. (1955) The problem of the treatment of peptic aspiration pneumonia following obstetric anaesthesia (Mendelson's Syndrome). *J. obstet. Gynaecol. Br. Emp.* **62**, 509.

Hedenstierna G. and Lundberg S. (1975) Airway compliance during artificial ventilation. *Br. J. Anaesth.* **47**, 1277.

Hedenstierna G. and McCarthy G. (1975) Mechanics of breathing, gas distribution and functional residual capacity at different frequencies of respiration during spontaneous and artificial ventilation. *Br. J. Anaesth.* **47**, 706.

Hedenstierna G., McCarthy G. and Bergstrom M. (1976) Airway closure during mechanical ventilation. *Anesthesiology* **44**, 114.

Henville J. D. H. (1977) Sunction catheters. *Br. J. hosp. Equip.* **5**, 248.

Hinton P., Allison S. P., Farrow S. et al. (1972) Blood volume changes and transfusion requirements of burned patients after the shock phase of injury. *Lancet* **1**, 913.

Hinton P., Allison S. P., Farrow S. et al. (1973) Electrolyte changes after burn injury and effect of treatment. *Lancet* **2**, 218.

Holdcroft A., Lumley J., Goya H. et al. (1974) Respiratory filters in clinical practice. *Lancet* **2**, 25.

Hopewell P. C. and Murray J. F. (1976) Effects of continuous positive pressure ventilation in experimental pulmonary oedema. *J. appl. Physiol.* **40**, 568.

James O., Quail A. and Gibbons J. (1974) Chest injury, the indications for artificial ventilation. *Anaesth. Intensive Care* **2**, 27.

Jesch F., Webber L. M., Dalton J. W. et al. (1975) Oxygen dissociation after transfusion of blood stored in ACD or CPD. *J. thorac. cardiovasc. Surg.* **70**, 35.

Johnson E. E. and Hedley-Whyte J. (1972) Continuous positive pressure ventilation and portal flow in dogs with pulmonary oedema. *J. appl. Physiol.* **33**, 385.

Kafer E. R. (1971) Pulmonary oxygen toxicity. A review of the evidence for acute and chronic oxygen toxicity in man. *Br. J. Anaesth.* **43**, 687.

Katz J. P. and Barash P. G. (1977) Positional hypoxaemia following post traumatic pulmonary insuffiency. *Can. Anaesth. Soc. J.* **24**, 346.

Kerry J. H. (1975) Pulmonary oxygen transfer during IPPV in man. *Br. J. Anaesth.* **47**, 695.

King E. G., Jones R. L. and Patakas D. A. (1973) Evaluation of positive end expiratory pressure therapy in the adult respiratory distress syndrome. *Canad. Anaesth. Soc. J.* **20**, 546.

Kirby R. R. (1978) Membrane oxygenators: what role (if any) in acute ventilatory insufficiency. *Crit. Care Med.* **6**, 19.

Kirby R. R., Downs J. B., Civetta J. M. et al (1975a) High level positive end expiratory pressure in acute respiratory insufficiency. *Chest.* **67**, 156.

Kirby R. R., Perry J. C., Calderwood H. W. et al. (1975b) Cardiorespiratory effects of high positive end expiratory pressure. *Anesthesiology* **43,** 533.

Kumar A., Falke K. J., Geffin B. et al. (1970) Continuous positive pressure breathing in acute respiratory failure. *N. Engl. J. Med.* **283,** 1430.

Ledingham I. McA. (1977) Factors influencing oxygen availability. *J. clin. Pathol. Suppl.* **30,**

Leigh J. M. (1973a) Towards the rational employment of dephlogisticated air described by Priestley. *Ann. R. Coll. Surg. Engl.* **52,** 234.

Leigh J. M. (1973b) Audible noise levels of oxygen masks operating on venturi principle. *Br. med. J.* **2,** 652.

Levine B. A., Petroff P. A., Slade C. L. et al. (1978) Prospective trials of dexamethasone and aerosolised gentamycin in the treatment of inhalation injury in the burned patient. *J. Trauma* **18,** 188.

Lindholm C. E., Ollman B., Snyder J. et al. (1976) Flexible fibreoptic bronchoscopy in critical care medicine. In Shoemaker W.C. (ed.) *The Lung in the Critically Ill Patient.* Baltimore, William & Wilkins, pp. 88–99.

Lloyd J. W., Crampton Smith A. and O'Connor B. T. (1965) Classification of chest injuries as an aid to treatment. *Br. med. J.* **1,** 1518.

Lowbury E. J. L., Thom B. T., Lilly H. A. et al. (1970) Sources of infection with Pseudomonas aeruginosa in patients with tracheostomy. *J. med. Microbiol.* **3,** 39.

Lowe R. J., Moss G. S., Jilek J. et al. (1977) Crystalloid versus colloid in the etiology of pulmonary failure after trauma: a randomised trial in man. *Surgery* **81,** 676.

McConn R. and Del Guercio R. M. (1971) Respiratory function of blood in the acutely ill patient and the effect of steroids. *Ann. Surg.* **174,** 436.

McDonald R. (1977) Red cell, 2,3 diphosphoglycerate and oxygen affinity. *Anaesthesia* **32,** 544.

MacKenzie C. F., Klose S. and Browne D. R. G. (1976) A study of inflatable cuffs on endotracheal tubes. Pressures exerted on the trachea. *Br. J. Anaesth.* **48,** 105.

Magovern G. J., Shively J. G., Fecht D. et al. (1972) Clinical and experimental evaluation of a controlled pressure intratracheal cuff. *J. thorac. cardiovasc. Surg.* **64,** 747.

Marshak A. and Marshak G. (1973) Zinc sulphate for vocal cord granulomas. *J. laryngol. otol.* **87,** 573.

Marty A. T. (1974) Hyperoncotic albumin therapy. *Surg. Gynecol. Obstet.* **139,** 105.

Mathias D. B. and Wedley J. R. (1974) The effects of cuffed endotracheal tubes on the tracheal wall. *Br. J. Anaesth.* **46,** 489.

Meers P. D., Foster C. S. and Churcher G. M. (1978) Cross infection with *Serratia marcescens. Br. med. J.* **1,** 237.

Milledge J. S. (1976) Therapeutic fibreoptic bronchoscopy in intensive care. *Br. med. J.* **2,** 1427.

Millen J. E., Vandree J. and Glauser F. L. (1978) Fibreoptic bronchoscopic balloon occlusion and re-expansion of refractory unilateral atelectasis. *Crit. Care Med.* **6,** 50.

Milligan G. F., MacDonald J. A. E., Mellon A. et al. (1974) Pulmonary and hematologic disturbances during septic shock. *Surg. Gynecol. Obstet.* **138,** 43.

Modell J. H., Calderwood H. W., Ruiz B. C. et al. (1974) Effects of ventilatory patterns on arterial oxygenation after near-drowning in sea water. *Anaesthesiology* **40,** 376.

Molnar I. and Refsum H. E. (1974) Influence of simultaneous and equal increase in external dead space and tidal volume on arterial blood gases in artificially ventilated patients. *Acta. anaesthiol. scand.* **18,** 161.

Morgan B. C., Crawford P. W. and Guntheroth W. G. (1969) The hemodynamic effects of changes in blood volume during intermittent positive pressure ventilation. *Anesthesiology* **30**, 297.

Morgan B. C., Martin W. E., Hornbein T. F. et al. (1966) Hemodynamic effects of intermittent positive pressure ventilation. *Anesthesiology* **27**, 584.

Nakahora H., Ishikawa T., Sarai Y. et al. (1977) Gentamicin resistance in Japan. *Lancet* **1**, 911.

Nicholl R. M., Holland E. L. and Brown S. S. (1967) Mendelson's syndrome; its treatment by tracheostomy and hydrocortisone. *Br. med. J.* **1**, 745.

Nylén A. and Sylvén C. (1976) Induced fat embolism in rabbits by means of radioactively labelled fat. Evaluation of different treatments. *Acta chir. scand.* **142**, 361.

Parker F. B. Jr., Racz G. B., Wax S. D. et al. (1974) The haemodynamics of experimental fat embolism and associated therapy. *Chest* **65**, Suppl. 54S–56S.

Pavlin E. G., van Nimwegan D. and Hornbein T. F. (1975) Failure of a high compliance low pressure cuff to prevent aspiration. *Anesthesiology* **42**, 216.

Pearson F. G. and Fairley H. B. (1970) Tracheal stenosis complicating tracheostomy with cuffed tubes. *Int. anaesthesiol. Clin.* **8**, 889.

Petty T. L. and Ashbaugh D. G. (1971) The adult respiratory distress syndrome. Clinical features, factors influencing prognosis and principles of management. *Chest* **60**, 233.

Philbin D. M., Patterson R. W. and Baratz R. A. (1972) Continuous positive pressure ventilation and oxygen delivery. *Br. J. Anaesth.* **44**, 667.

Phillips I., King A., Jenkins S. et al. (1974) Control of respirator associated infection due to *Pseudomonas aeruginosa*. *Lancet* **2**, 871.

Piehl M. A. and Brown R. S. (1976) Use of extreme position changes in acute respiratory failure. *Crit. Care Med.* **4**, 13.

Pilon R. N. and Bittar D. A. (1973) The effect of positive end-expiratory pressure on thoracic duct lymph flow during controlled ventilation in anaesthetised dogs. *Anesthesiology* **39**, 607.

Powers S. R. Jr., Shah D., Ryan D. et al. (1977) Hypertonic mannitol in the therapy of the acute respiratory distress syndrome. *Ann. Surg.* **185**, 619.

Powner D. J., Eroos B. and Grenvick A. (1977) Differential lung ventilation with PEEP in the treatment of unilateral pneumonia. *Crit. Care Med.* **5**, 170.

Pullen F. (1970) Post intubation tracheal granuloma. A preliminary report on the efficienty of zinc sulphate. *Arch. Otolaryngol.* **92**, 340.

Qvist J., Pontoppidan H., Wilson R. S. et al. (1975) Hemodynamic responses to mechanical ventilation with PEEP; the effect of hypervolaemia. *Anesthesiology* **42**, 45.

Reid J. M. and Baird W. L. M. (1965) Crushed chest injury: some physiological disturbances and their correction. *Br. med. J.* **1**, 1105.

Richardson J. D., Franz J. L., Grover F. L. et al. (1974) Pulmonary contusion and haemorrhage: crystalloid versus colloid replacement. *J. surg. Res.* **16**, 330.

Riedler G. F. and Scheitlin W. A. (1969) Hypophosphataemia in septicaemia: higher indicence in Gram-negative than in Gram-positive infections. *Br. med. J.* **1**, 753.

Rokkannen P., Alho A., Avikainen V. et al. (1974) The efficacy of corticosteroids in severe trauma. *Surg. Gynecol. Obstet.* **138**, 69.

Rooth G., Hedstrand V., Tyden H. et al. (1976) The validity of the transcutaneous oxygen tension method in adults. *Crit. Care Med.* **4**, 162.

Rosen M. and Hillard E. K. (1970) Aspects of tracheal suction. *Int. Anesthiol. Clin.* **8**, 935.

Roy R., Powers S. R., Fenstel P. J. et al. (1977) Pulmonary wedge catheterisation during positive end expiratory pressure ventilation in the dog. *Anesthesiology* **46**, 385.

Ruiz B. C., Calderwood H. W., Modell J. H. et al. (1975) Effect of ventilatory patterns on arterial oxygenation after near-drowning with freshwater. A comparative study in dogs. *Anesth. Analg. (Cleve)* **52,** 570.

Schimmel L., Civetta J. M. and Kirby R. R. (1977) A new mechanical method to influence pulmonary perfusion in critically ill patients. *Crit. Care Med.* **5,** 277.

Seinfeld H., Giuliani V. and Merzel D. (1975) Corticosteroid derivatives in the treatment of inhalation burns. *Burns* **1,** 261.

Shackford S. R., Smith D. E., Zarino C. K. et al. (1976) The management of flail chest: a comparison of ventilatory and non-ventilatory treatment. *Am. J. Surg.* **13,** 759.

Simmons R. L., Heisterhamp C. A. III, Collins J. et al. (1969) Respiratory insufficiency in combat casualities III. Arterial hypoxaemia after wounding. *Ann. Surg.* **170,** 45.

Singer M. M., Wright F., Stanley L. K. et al. (1970) Oxygen toxicity in man: a prospective study in patients after open heart surgery. *N. Engl. J. Med.* **283,** 1473.

Sladen A. (1976) Methylprednisolone: pharmacologic doses in shock lung syndrome. *J. thorac. cardiovasc. Surg.* **71,** 800.

Sladen A., Aldridge C. F. and Albarran R. (1973) PEEP versus ZEEP in the treatment of flail chest injuries. *Crit. Care Med.* **1,** 187.

Sladen A., Laver M. B. and Pontoppidan H. (1968) Pulmonary complications and water retention in prolonged mechanical ventilation. *N. Engl. M. Med.* **279,** 448.

Smith G., Cheney F. W. and Winter P. M. (1973) The contribution of mixed venous oxygenation to the change in Qs/Qt that occurs with change in cardiac output. *Br. J. Anaesth.* **45,** 1230.

Stein L., Beraud J. J., Cavanilles J. et al. (1974) Pulmonary oedema during fluid infusion in the absence of heart failure. *J. Am. med. Ass.* **229,** 65.

Suter P. M., Fairley H. B. and Isenberg M. D. (1975) Optimum end expiratory airway pressure in patients with acute pulmonary failure. *N. Engl. J. Med.* **292,** 284.

Szabö G. (1970) The syndrome of fat embolism and its origin. *J. clin. Pathol.* **23,** Suppl. 4, 123.

Tachakra S. S. and Sevitt S. (1975) Hypoxaemia after fractures. *J. Bone Joint Surg.* **57B,** 197.

Taylor G. and Prys-Davies J. (1968) Evaluation of endotracheal steroid therapy in acid pulmonary aspiration syndrome. *Anesthesiology* **29,** 19.

Taylor P. A. and Waters H. R. (1971) Arterial oxygen tensions following endotracheal suction on IPPV. *Anaesthesia* **26,** 289.

Thornton D., Penhold H., Butler J. et al. (1975) Effects of pattern of ventilation on pulmonary metabolism and mechanics. *Anesthesiology,* **42,** 4.

Tonneson A. S., Gabel J. C. and McLeavey C. A. (1977) Relation between lowered colloid osmotic pressure, respiratory failure and death. *Crit. Care Med.* **5,** 239.

Toung T. J., Bordes D., Benson D. W. et al. (1976) Aspiration pneumonia: experimental evaluation of albumin and steroid therapy. *Ann. Surg.* **183,** 179.

Travis S. F., Sugerman H. J., Ruberg R. L. et al. (1971) Alterations of red cell glycolytic intermediates and oxygen transport as a consequence of hypophosphataemia in patients receiving intravenous hyperalimentation. *N. Engl. J. Med.* **285,** 763.

Trinkle J. K., Bennett S. E., Furman R. W. et al. (1973) Pulmonary contusion, pathogenesis and current management. *Ann. thorac. Surg.* **16,** 568.

Trinkle J. K., Richardson J. D., Franz J. L. et al. (1975) Management of flail chest without mechinical ventilation. *Ann. thorac. Surg.* **19,** 355.

Vandam L. D. (1965) Aspiration of gastric contents in the operative period. *New. Engl. J. Med.* **273,** 1206.

Virgillio R. W., Rice C. L., Smith D. E. et al. (1972) Crystalloid versus colloid resuscitation: Is one better? *Intens. Care Med.* **3**, 113.

Visick W. D., Fairley H. B. and Hickey R. F. (1974) The effects of tidal volume and expiratory pressure on pulmonary gas exchange during anaesthesia. *Anesthesiology* **39**, 285.

Wennig C. S., Pietak S., Hickey R. F. et al. (1974) Relationship of preoperative closing volume to functional residual capacity and alveolar arterial oxygen difference during anesthesia with controlled ventilation. *Anesthesiology* **41**, 3.

Wertzburger J. J. and Peltier L. F. (1968) Fat embolism: the effect of corticosteroids on experimental fat embolism in the rat. *Surgery* **64**, 143.

West J. B. (1976) Pulmonary gas exchange in the critically ill patient. In Shoemaker W. C. (ed.) *The Lung in the Critically ill Patient.* Baltimore, Williams & Wilkins, pp. 3–12.

Winter P. M. and Smith G. (1972) The toxicity of oxygen. *Anesthesiology.* **37**, 210.

Young J. A., Lichtman M. A. and Cohen J. (1973) Reduced red cell 2,3 diphosphoglycerate and adenosine triphosphate, hypophosphatemia and increased haemoglobin, oxygen affinity after cardiac surgery. *Circulation* **47**, 1313.

Young R. K. B., Campbell D., Reid J. H. et al. (1974) Respiratory intensive care: a 10 year survey. *Br. med. J.* **1**, 307.

Zimmerman J. E. (1971) Respiratory failure complicating post traumatic acute renal failure. Etiology, clinical features and management. *Ann. Surg.* **174**, 12.

E. Truman Mays

4 Injuries of the Liver

THE PROBLEM

Half the patients admitted to UK hospitals for abdominal injuries have suffered damage to the liver (Blumgart and Vajrabukka, 1972; Bolton et al., 1973). Half of these hepatic injuries are minor wounds and require little or no corrective operative treatment (Balasegaram, 1976; Lucas and Ledgerwood, 1976). Minor wounds of the liver almost never cause death; mortality is nearly always due to associated injuries or pre-existing diseases.

But fifty per cent of patients have hepatic injuries which are crucial wounds. In these persons, associated injuries and pre-existing disease almost never cause death; mortality in this group is nearly always directly related to injury of the liver.

The greatest number of survivors occurs in people with minor lacerations or penetrations of the liver. When such individuals are included in surveys of patients with injury of the liver, the overall death rate is reduced significantly. But this kind of statistical integration is deceptive. Despite a favourable decrease in overall mortality, the disheartening fact remains that bursting injuries of the liver frequently cause death and there has been little decrease in the death rate from acute rupture of the liver during the last century. Edler (1886–7) reported a 78 per cent mortality in the nineteenth century and Mikesky et al. (1956) noted a 71 per cent mortality in this century.

The truth about mortality and injuries of the liver emerges when the two groups are separated. By selecting only patients with penetrating hepatic injuries, Grahame (1958) could report a record low death rate of 2 per cent, while Mays (1966) excluded patients with minor wounds and focused on patients with bursting injuries; the mortality rate here was 92 per cent.

A poignant fact about treating persons with injury to the liver is that avoidance of detrimental treatment yields increased survival and better quality of life. During the last half of World War II the death rate from hepatic injuries dropped from 30 per cent to 17 per cent (Madding et al., 1942–3; Tanphiphat, 1976). This encouraging progress came about mostly by abandoning gauze packs for primary treatment of hepatic wounds. Despite a chronicle of harmful effects, gauze packing continues to be used (in some institutions it is one of the most common treatments) with disastrous results.

In patients with crucial wounds of the liver, resuscitation must be prompt. Immediate blood volume and extracellular fluid replacement are paramount. There is burgeoning evidence that crystalloid promotes a more benign recovery for seriously injured victims than copious transfusions with stored blood. Fresh whole blood is the most desirable replacement fluid but is rarely available. Sequestered components of whole blood are better than stored whole blood with its many drawbacks. When fresh whole blood is not readily available, packed cells, platelets and fresh frozen plasma should be used as indicated. Massive transfusion of stored blood causes serious coagulopathy and non-mechanical bleeding after injury of the liver. Clagett and Olsen (1978) reported that profuse hepatic haemorrhage complicated the operative course of 17 of 33 (51·5 per cent) patients suffering severe injury to the liver. They found no convincing evidence of disseminated intravascular coagulation nor abnormal fibrinolysis in their patients. They concluded that copious transfusions with stored blood was likely to be the culprit. Finally, under certain conditions it may be impossible to obtain an effective circulating blood volume; in such situations, coeliotomy is an integral part of resuscitation. In urgent circumstances, a specific diagnosis of hepatic injury is unimportant. Operation should accompany rather than follow restoration of blood volume.

CAUSE OF DEATH

Any worthwhile discussion of hepatic trauma must begin by scrutinizing the cause of death in patients with hepatic fatalities. Haemorrhage is the main cause of death. A compilation of over 2 000 patients treated in various medical centres throughout the USA makes this fact incontrovertible (Mikesky et al., 1956; Lucas, 1971; Defore et al., 1976). Exsanguination may be acute or it may be delayed. In addition to the large group of people dying from primary or secondary haemorrhage, there is an equally large number of patients who die from renal failure and pulmonary insufficiency. These two complications must be included under the general category of haemorrhage because they arise directly out of clumsy attempts to stop bleeding from the liver. This ineptitude to staunch quickly the flow of blood from the injured liver creates extended periods of poor tissue perfusion and requires copious amounts of stored blood; both are progenitors of renal failure and respiratory distress syndromes.

Sepsis is the second most common cause of death in patients with injury of the liver. The infection is about evenly distributed between superinfections in the perihepatic spaces and in the lungs. Sepsis below the diaphragm is usually in the form of subphrenic or subhepatic abscesses. Occasionally the sepsis results from intrahepatic cavities produced by surgeons closing over deep crevasses with sutures. The tightly closed space undergoes necrosis and forms an abscess cavity inside the liver. Haemorrhage and sepsis together or separately are also the most common cause of re-operation in patients with hepatic trauma. Such second or third operations are often lethal in already seriously ill patients.

Associated injuries are the third most common cause of death. The undisputed influence of associated injuries in the death of patients with wounds of the liver evokes a concept known as 'multiplicity factor'. The scheme directly relates the number of additional organs injured to the mortality rate.

Such 'multiplicity factors' are one of the most important predictions of outcome. Under combat conditions four or more organs injured as well as the liver resulted in 80 per cent mortality (Wallace, 1918; Madding et al., 1942). In civilian practice four or more associated organ injuries has a mortality of 40 per cent (Defore et al., 1976). Multiple injuries to the same organ are counted as a single organ injury. For example, perforations of the caecum, transverse and sigmoid colon are counted as a single organ injured plus the liver. But perforation of the caecum and a cerebral haematoma count as two system injuries added to the hepatic injury and increase the mortality rate appreciably. Of all the solitary organ injuries associated with hepatic wounds, colonic injuries are the deadliest.

MINOR INJURIES

Low-velocity missiles and stab wounds of the liver usually cause minimal bleeding and almost no disruption of the surrounding hepatic parenchyma. Such wounds nearly always undergo spontaneous haemostasis and require no corrective operative procedure. Occasionally blunt trauma causes only a superficial tear in Glisson's capsule without tearing the main blood vessels or bile ducts. Wounds of the thin parts of the liver whether caused by knife, gun or blunt trauma are also minor and usually do not involve the important scaffolding of the liver. These kinds of wounds do not bleed threateningly and usually do not sequester parenchymal tissue nor drain significant amounts of bile.

For many years surgeons treated such minor hepatic wounds with simple drainage alone, now advancing technology requires us to reassess this practice. Carnevale et al. (1977) used the peritoneoscope to evaluate patients with suspected intra-abdominal injuries. They reported five patients in whom they found minor wounds of the liver. None of these hepatic injuries were drained. They had no complications and an average hospital stay of 3–4 days. But much greater clinical experience must be gained before such treatment can be recommended for general use. An overlooked colon injury or underestimation of an injury to the liver followed by bile peritonitis can mean death for an unfortunate patient. But their results present cogent reasons to question the dogma that all hepatic wounds need drainage. The extensive drainage procedures described later for serious hepatic wounds certainly are unthinkable in persons with only minor wounds.

COMPLEX PENETRATING WOUNDS

The nature of hepatic wounds is changing as wounding forces change from decade to decade. Technology, life style, even the affluence of society have a distinct part in this. Penetrating wounds of the liver have always been most frequent but have changed greatly. Magnum handguns have become generally available to an affluent populace. The human liver struck by a bullet from one of these guns bursts with violence. Great commotion and disruption of architecture occurs over a wide region. Such penetrating wounds of the liver have become in most respects equal to bursting wounds of the liver produced by blunt trauma.

While by far the greatest number of penetrating hepatic wounds are made by low velocity missiles or stilleto punctures, about twenty per cent of hepatic wounds are complex (Mays, 1971a). They involve the scaffolding parts of the liver, the bile ducts, the veins and arteries. Such complex penetrating wounds are characterized by profound shock, profuse haemorrhage, clotting deficiencies, metabolic derangements, sepsis and often death.

The principles involved in diagnosing and treating complex penetrating hepatic wounds are the same as those used to treat injury of the liver produced by blunt trauma.

DIAGNOSIS

Clinical features and diagnostic aids helpful in detecting acute damage to the liver are pain, peritoneal irritation, rib fractures, peritoneal lavage and laparoscopy. Sophisticated evaluation with sonography, computerized axial tomography and angiography have no place in the treatment of patients with acute injuries accompanied by profound shock and copious haemorrhage. London (1978) stated that a distended belly in a completely relaxed and exsanguinated patient usually means severe rupture of the liver. Delay for elaborate diagnostic tests in these patients may lead to multiple organ failure. There is no place for diagnostic tests which might delay coeliotomy.

Pain

In alert, conscious patients, pain in the right upper quadrant is the most consistent diagnostic sign of hepatic damage. The pain is sharp and aggravated by motion or deep breathing. Irritation of the diaphragm by blood and bile often produces pain referred to the right shoulder (Kehr's sign).

It is postulated that if the convex surface of the right liver is ruptured, the pain is referred to the subscapular region on the right, while rupture of the concave surface of the liver causes pain in the anterior abdominal region at the waist-line. These attempts to determine the part of the liver injured by patterns of pain distribution are not reliable. Pain is most frequently due to blood and bile. Since both are liquid, they obey the laws of gravity, and they seek the lowest level causing pain by irritation of the peritoneum remote from the site of actual rupture. Attempts at diagnosing the specific part of the liver ruptured may delay operation.

Peritoneal Irritation

Bursting of the liver pours out bile and blood onto the peritoneum. The peritoneum responds almost immediately with classical signs of varying degrees. In the most keen response muscles of the abdominal parieties contract with spasm, giving board-like rigidity. Less severe injuries may cause only a localized reaction limited to the right upper quadrant of the abdomen. The patient voluntarily splints and guards this area from further hurt. Segmental spasm of one rectus can usually be detected by careful examination. It is important not to hurt the patient; palpation should be gentle and the hands of the examiner should be warm.

Irritation of the peritoneum can also be detected by rebound tenderness and referred rebound from the left abdomen to the right upper quadrant. If the patient is alert and cooperative a good way to detect peritoneal irritation is by pain related to cough. The patient is asked to cough. In the presence of acute peritoneal irritation the sudden bouncing and stretching of the peritoneum elicits sharp pain localized to the site of peritoneal irritation. Patients can then point to the region where they feel pain. Cough-related signs of peritoneal irritation are helpful but in confused, intoxicated or uncooperative patients they are useless.

Rib Fractures

A reliable diagnostic sign of hepatic rupture is fracture of one or more ribs over the right lower thoracic cage. This is especially true of the posterior segments of ribs nine to twelve. When the victim has sustained blunt forces great enough to fracture those ribs it is nearly always sufficient to rupture the liver. While this is true in adults, it is not a helpful aid in children whose elastic rib cage does not break easily. Children can have significant damage to the liver without rib fractures.

Blunders arise because some physicians rely solely on the chest roentgenogram to detect fractured ribs. Most accident surgeons know that roentgenography is not entirely reliable for this purpose and that the detection of rib fractures is best done by palpating each rib individually. While doing so, the examiner checks meticulously for false motion, crepitus, pain on pressure, and other signs of a broken rib. An excellent method is to ask the patient to inspire deeply while inward pressure is placed on the rib with a finger. The two forces acting in different directions will nearly always produce clear signs of rib fracture.

Peritoneal Lavage

The best method for detecting haemoperitoneum is catheter lavage of the peritoneal cavity, but the discovery of a haemoperitoneum is not diagnostic of hepatic rupture; however the presence of blood in the effluent makes coeliotomy mandatory. At laparotomy rupture of the liver can be recognized. Several years ago abdominal paracentesis was advocated as an aid in detecting intraperitoneal haemorrhage, but negative paracentesis continued to plague this method of detecting intraperitoneal haemorrhage.

Poor results with needle aspiration of the peritoneal cavity encouraged physicians to develop better technique of detecting blood in the peritoneal spaces. Root and Hauser (1965) advocated lavaging the peritoneal spaces with balanced salt solutions. The method varies from one hospital to another and is constantly undergoing modification, but the essentials have been described by Perry (1970). Some physicians place a sample of the effluent from the peritoneal lavage into a centrifuge and spin it down to obtain a haematocrit while others do cell counts on the returned fluid and examine it with a microscope to look for intestinal contents. These and other refinements are relevant for injuries other than the liver, but in most patients with hepatic rupture the aspirate from the peritoneal spaces will be clearly stained with blood indicating a haemoperitoneum and the need for laparotomy.

The tendency to disclose intraperitoneal bleeding from lesions not requiring operation means that surgeons must use their clinical judgement more shrewdly. Many patients with serious hepatic rupture do not need a peritoneal lavage to coax their surgeon into doing coeliotomy. The clinical pattern is clear, and a decision to operate is not difficult. But in unconscious patients or in those whose states of consciousness are altered by alcohol or other drugs the usual physical signs are masked. In these patients peritoneal lavage can uncover an otherwise unsuspected hepatic injury.

Diagnostic Aids in Subacute Damage

Not all injuries of the liver result in immediate operation. There are some injuries which have none of the above diagnostic findings. Such injuries fracture the hepatic parenchyma but fail to disrupt Glisson's capsule. The haemorrhage resulting from this injury is contained beneath the capsule of the liver resulting in a subcapsular haematoma. Sometimes the damage and haemorrhage are deep inside the liver resulting in an intrahepatic haematoma or contusion. Because acute signs of shock are absent such hepatic ruptures may pass unnoticed during the initial evaluation especially if there are co-existing injuries to distract the examiner.

To detect such damage to the liver evaluating tests inappropriate to obvious bursting injuries are helpful. These diagnostic aids are hepatic gammascans, hepatic arteriography, sonography, computerized axial tomography, biochemical tests of liver function and peritoneoscopy.

Little et al. (1967) used colloidal [198]Au to photoscan the liver and spleen in patients with abdominal trauma. They reported that this technique was helpful in the preoperative diagnosis, postoperative assessment and monitoring repair and regeneration of the liver. After reviewing their experience at the Royal Albert Hospital Lancaster they stated that absolute reliance cannot be placed on hepatic scans alone. Newer radionuclides such as $^{99}Tc^m$, colloid sulphur and improvements in scanning instruments can probably prevent some of the false-positive and false-negative scans which misled Little and his colleagues.

Freeark et al. (1968) used aortography to assess obscure injuries after blunt trauma. Since then angiographic techniques have been refined so that with more modern catheters and image intensification it is now possible to selectively catheterize various hepatic arteries, hepatic veins and the portal vein. These roentgenographic diagnostic tests are not universally available, but when accessible they are helpful, especially in detecting intrahepatic contusions, haematomas and subcapsular haematomas. Selective hepatic arteriography is also an extremely helpful method of evaluating late complications of hepatic trauma and complications emanating from certain kinds of treatments (*see* Detrimental Methods, p. 83).

The damaged liver overlooked by a cursory evaluation on the day of injury can be discovered by sequential measurement of biochemical variables. Advancing technology has made such clinical appraisals practical. Multi-channel autoanalysers display day-to-day changes in important functions of the liver. A decreasing serum albumin concentration and an increasing bilirubin value are two frequent concomitants of intrahepatic contusions and haematomas. There is an accompanying hyperenzyme-anaemia including lactic dehydrogenase, serum glutamic oxalacetic transaminase, serum glutamic pyruvic transaminase, and serum alkaline phosphatase. The number of enzymes increased in the serum and degree of their elevation varies depending upon the extent of damage to the liver.

The inherent ability of the liver to regenerate means that most minor injuries heal spontaneously and patients with minimal intrahepatic contusion rarely require operative treatment. The healing of such lesions can be followed by hepatic scintiscans and hepatic function tests. Only a progressive deterioration of the patient's clinical condition and a worsening of hepatic function should prompt the surgeon to operate.

A subcapsular haematoma, however, requires laparotomy, not because of blood beneath Glisson's capsule but because it nearly always accompanies a grave central rupture of the liver. Such a complex of central anatomic disruption beneath an intact Glisson's capsule (subcapsular haematoma) is frequently complicated by haemobilia.

Peritoneoscopy
The development of safe methods of viewing intra-abdominal organs with a laparoscope makes it possible nowadays to assess wounds of the liver but this is not appropriate in patients with shock and severe blood loss.

INCISIONS

For elective operations on the liver and biliary tract there is no best incision but when operating on critically injured patients a generous mid-line incision from the tip of the xiphoid cartilage to beyond the umbilicus is best. It can be accomplished quickly with little bleeding because the linea alba is almost avascular. If injuries of pelvic viscera are discovered the mid-line incision can be rapidly extended to the pubis. The mid-line incision permits inspection and exposure of the extreme lateral parts of the abdominal cavities. Finally, the mid-line incision can be extended cranially when needed. The conversion of the mid-line abdominal incision into median sternotomy may occasionally be necessary.

Various para-rectus, para-median and lateral rectus incisions permit adequate exposure on one side of the abdomen only. Exposure of the other side requires vigorous retraction, and if an injury is uncovered here, operative repair is difficult. In muscular men or obese people sufficient retraction for adequate exposure and treatment of injuries in the contra-lateral gutter is nearly impossible.

Some surgeons have advocated using a combined thoraco-abdominal incision for treating the ruptured liver, especially to expose and suture the inaccessible dome of the liver. This incision is accomplished by extending the original abdominal incision into the pleural space via the seventh or eight intercostal space. After the thoracic extension is completed the diaphragm is sharply divided in a ventral to dorsal direction. This combined thoracic and abdominal incision always produces a large triangle shaped bulk of tissue containing ribs, cartilages, and upper abdominal wall. The composition of this flap makes it extremely elastic and since it contains several ribs with their accompanying cartilages it snaps back into position whenever retraction fails. A slip of the retractor and the rib-containing section comes flying back into place completely obstructing the view of the surgeon. This elastic recoil always happens just when the surgeon is about to cut or suture a critically important structure.

The thoraco-abdominal incision is not only frustrating to the surgeon it is also detrimental to the patient's recovery because atelectasis and pneumonia of the right lower lung nearly always follow. In the immediate postoperative period this incision causes severe pain as when the patient attempts to cough the two edges of cut cartilage rub against each other causing excruciating pain and discouraging further coughing. Voluntary splinting and a reluctance to cough enhance accumulation of pulmonary secretions and aggravate the already present atelectasis.

When access to the right side of the chest is deemed necessary a sternal split is better than the classic thoraco-abdominal incision. Postoperative pain, atelectasis and other pulmonary complications are less after the median sternotomy than after a combined thoraco-abdominal incision. But nearly all operations used to treat the ruptured liver can be done through a simple mid-line abdominal incision. Only a small number of patients will need either kind of thoracic extension.

HEPATIC HAEMOSTASIS

Haemorrhage has always been the prime cause of death in hepatic trauma. This fact makes hepatic haemostatsis the most important goal of any surgeon treating patients with ruptured livers. While some hepatic injuries are minor and require nothing more than simple drainage, the ruptured liver bleeds profusely and the patient enters the accident ward in profound shock. Such patients die from haemorrhage.

In addition to those patients who die on the operating table from exsanguination and those who die in the first few days of secondary or recurrent bleeding, there are a considerable number of late deaths resulting from the physiologic consequences of severe haemorrhage and shock. Under listings of causes of death, these appear as renal failure, pulmonary insufficiency, and septic shock. We know that renal failure is related to flux of nephrotoxins associated with prolonged reductions in renal blood flow. In other words, multiple transfusions of stored blood are given because of delays in controlling bleeding from the liver. Pulmonary insufficiency has been similarly linked to prolonged states of catecholamine stress resulting from failure to stop haemorrhage quickly. Even septic shock is related to the amount of haemorrhage, degree of shock and delay in controlling haemorrhage.

A few simple facts are clear. The quicker haemorrhage is controlled the less blood transfusions required, the shorter the duration of shock the fewer patients develop renal failure, pulmonary insufficiency and sepsis. Whatever method the surgeon uses to stop bleeding from the liver it must be quick, simple and effective. Methods that can be used only in large regional medical centres or special casualty hospitals defeat the prime axiom of treatment: immediate control of haemorrhage. If patients with ruptured livers are allowed to continue bleeding while being transported to centralized hospitals for care, we can anticipate postoperative renal failure, pulmonary insufficiency and sepsis.

Many methods of obtaining hepatic haemostasis have been abandoned and are of historical interest only. Others have been used in experimental animals and never applied in humans. A partial list includes thermic methods (cautery or cryogenic), tourniquets and clamps, packing, suture techniques, topical agents, absorbable haemostatic agents and hepatic lobectomy. Some methods, such as application of microcrystalline collagen or the rapidly polymerizing adhesive resins require a dry field to be effective. This presupposition of a dry surface does not exist in ruptured livers.

The numerous traditional methods of hepatic haemostasis have had ample opportunity to prove their effectiveness, but the failure of all these conventional methods to successfully stop bleeding from the liver is attested by persistence of haemorrhage as the prime cause of death in reports from numerous medical centres around the world. Better methods of stopping bleeding from the human liver must be used.

ARTERIAL BLEEDING

The most recalcitrant bleeding from the ruptured liver is arterial, as has been displayed in experimental cadaver livers and injured persons. I perfused the arterial tree of cadaver livers with barium sulphate and subjected them to blunt forces sufficient to produce rupture (Mays, 1966). After the injury roentgenographic assessment of the extent of intrahepatic arterial injury showed multiple disruptions in the tertiary rami of the hepatic arteries. But there remained the question of how much these experimental results could be transposed to clinical medicine. Now, selective hepatic arteriography has shown such defects can also occur in patients with trauma to the liver (*Fig. 4.1*). This is the kind of arterial disruption causing persistent bleeding, secondary haemorrhage and haemobilia.

Such arterial tears deep within the interior of the liver do not lend themselves to control by suture techniques as to dissect into the depths of the liver in search of bleeding vessels, proposed by some, is dangerous. This so-called 'tractotomy' can cause increased bleeding and destruction of parenchymal tissue beyond that done by the original accident.

After completing studies on cadaver livers, I started using hepatic artery

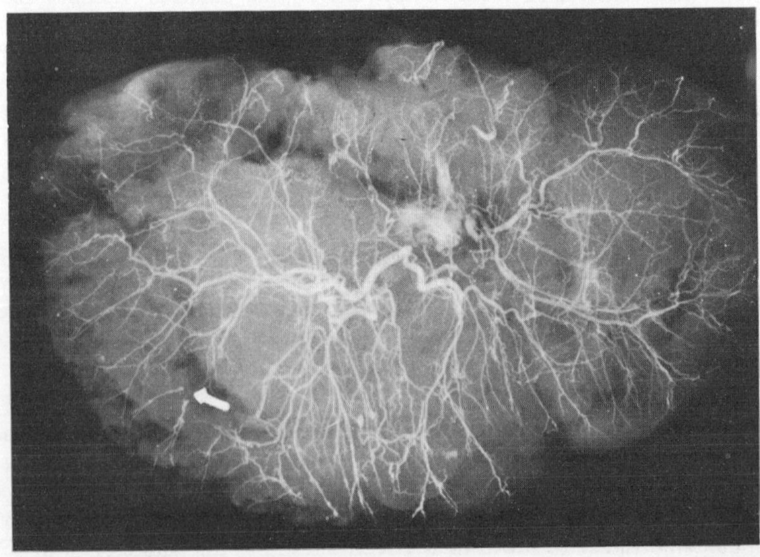

a

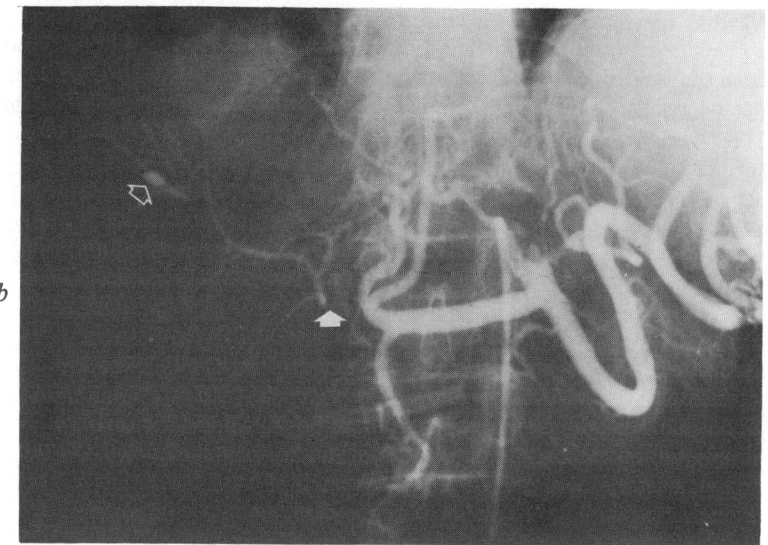

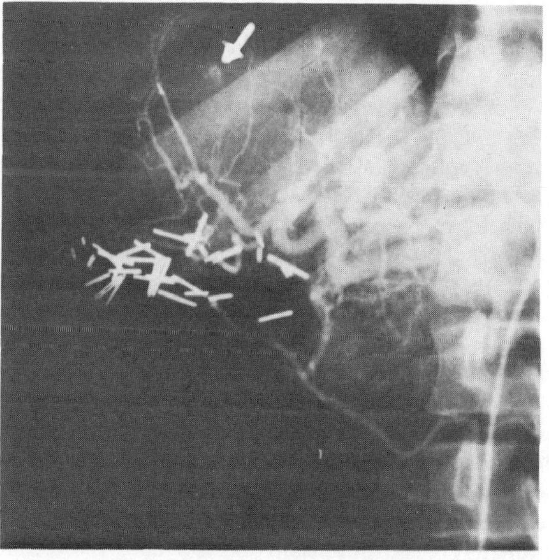

Fig. 4.1. This series of arteriograms made after injury of the liver displays the kinds of arterial defects producing recalcitrant bleeding (see also *Fig. 4.7*). *a,* Cadaver liver — experimental trauma. Arrows denote disruption of tertiary hepatic arteries. *b,* Disruption of tertiary ramus of right hepatic artery (open arrow) after motor vehicle accident. The ramus of the right hepatic artery has been ligated (solid arrow). *c,* The white arrow denotes site of extravasation of contrast from a tertiary branch of the right hepatic artery. This man developed haemobilia after a crevasse in his right liver was sutured.

ligation to stop arterial bleeding from ruptured livers. Because tradition condemned intentional interruption of the hepatic artery in humans, our first trials were done only in desperate situations (Mays, 1972a). As expected many of these patients died, but not from hepatic haemorrhage! They died from associated injuries such as transection of cervical spinal cord, extensive cranio-cerebral trauma, etc. The total absence of septic hepatic necrosis in these patients attracted our attention. More importantly hepatic artery ligation stopped hepatic haemorrhage. Encouraged, we began to use hepatic artery ligation more often. Our initial treatment programme included plans to return the patient to the operating theatre 48–72 hours after hepatic artery ligation if the lobe should necrose. But these patients recovered rapidly and uneventfully thereby preventing secondary operations. Our experiences with hepatic artery ligation over the past ten years proves it to be a quick, simple, highly effective means of stopping haemorrhage from the ruptured liver (Mays, 1972a, 1973, 1974; Aaron et al., 1975). Other surgeons are now reporting the efficacy and safety of hepatic artery ligation for hepatic haemostasis (Lewis et al., 1974; Canty, 1975; Tanphiphat, 1976).

In 1943 Sir Gordon Gordon-Taylor told the British Medical Association 'it is an unpalatable truth that, in man, ligature of the hepatic artery or its main branches is an operation fraught with peril to life' (Gordon-Taylor, 1943). These and numerous other admonitions against ligating the hepatic artery were based on two facts: (1) the belief that hepatic arteries were end-arteries and (2) the fact that ligating the hepatic artery in dogs and rabbits caused septic hepatic necrosis.

Each of these foundations supporting the teachings about hepatic arteries must be re-examined in the light of new knowledge. First, hepatic arteries are not end-arteries. While Michels (1960) had shown 26 collateral pathways outside the surface of the liver, arteries within the interior appeared to be end-arteries. In 1923 a Canadian, Segall (1923), said '. . . smaller vessels which terminate within the liver do not participate in subcapsular anastomoses and are therefore end-arteries'. Sir Gordon Gordon-Taylor (1943) concurred, 'There can be no manner of doubt that anastomosis between the arterioles in the interior of the liver is infrequent and at best scanty'. Michels (1960) said 'each hepatic artery is an end-artery with a selective distribution to a definite area of the liver and therefore cannot be sacrificed without resultant necrosis of liver'.

Unfortunately these physicians did not have the technology to study intrahepatic arteries in living subjects and thus to learn about the place of neuro-humoral controls in living persons. Using selective catheterization of the hepatic artery and image intensifiers, the intrahepatic blood flow was studied in humans after ligating various hepatic arteries (Mays and Wheeler, 1974) which were found not to be end-arteries, as previously taught. Our investigations delineated translobar and subcapsular collaterals capable of reconstituting blood flow in a ligated hepatic artery within 24 hours

(*Fig. 4.2*). Extrahepatic collaterals also contribute to reconstitution of flow within the liver.

Secondly, in humans, unlike animals used for experiments, the portal vein blood and the liver are sterile (From and Alli, 1956; Orloff et al., 1958), which is the main reason why septic hepatic necrosis does not occur after ligating the human hepatic artery. Hepatic artery ligation has proved extremely effective in stopping haemorrhage from the ruptured

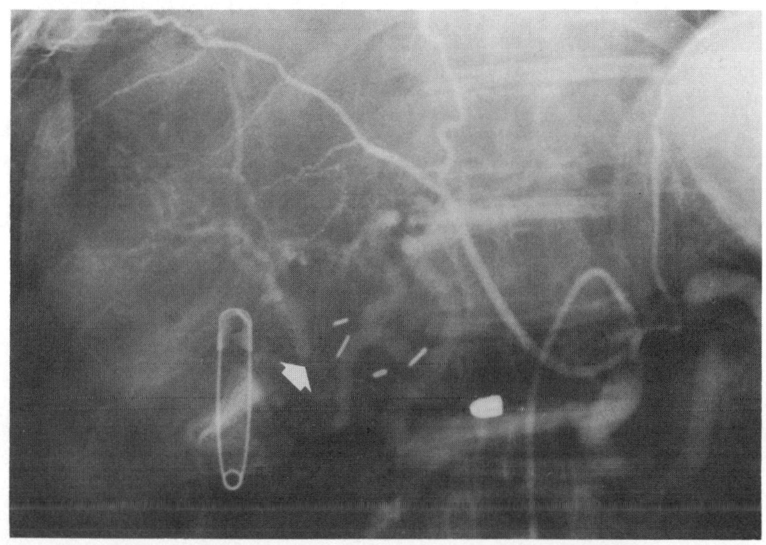

Fig. 4.2. Hepatic arteries are not end-arteries. This arteriogram shows filling of a ligated right hepatic artery by collaterals. Solid arrow shows site of ligature.

livers (Mays, 1973) and the operative technique is simpler than any other. It requires no special instruments and any qualified surgeon can do this procedure in any operating theatre, which is its greatest advantage.

Procedure

The abdomen is opened in the midline. If the liver is ruptured, the common hepatic artery should be identified in the hepatoduodenal ligament. When both lobes are involved or when there is a large deep crevasse along the lobar fissure, no further dissection is needed. If only the right lobe is injured additional dissection must be done. The common hepatic artery is traced to its bifurcation, from which the right ramus is traced to its entrance into the substance of the liver, where a ligature or clip is applied. If the injury is confined to the left lobe, the left hepatic artery should be dissected and occluded with a ligature or metal clip. The gall bladder should also be removed whenever hepatic arteries are interrupted.

Ligation of an hepatic artery causes definite biochemical consequences. The hepatic enzymes are increased in the serum and there is hyperbilirubinemia; hepatic synthesis is reduced and blood protein and cholesterol are decreased, but similar changes occur in patients with hepatic injury treated by other methods. However, if bleeding has been controlled before massive blood transfusions are needed these biochemical changes return to normal within seven to fourteen days. The restoration of flow through collateral vessels can be displayed by selective hepatic arteriograms (*Fig. 4.3*) but these are necessary only if bleeding has not stopped; in this case it is essential to know whether the appropriate artery has been ligated. Tying the wrong artery probably accounts for reports of persistent bleeding even after ligation of an artery.

After ligation of the hepatic artery the liver begins to extract additional oxygen from the portal venous blood. This means oxygenation and blood flow in the portal vein must be well sustained throughout the operative and postoperative periods. This is achieved by starving the patient for

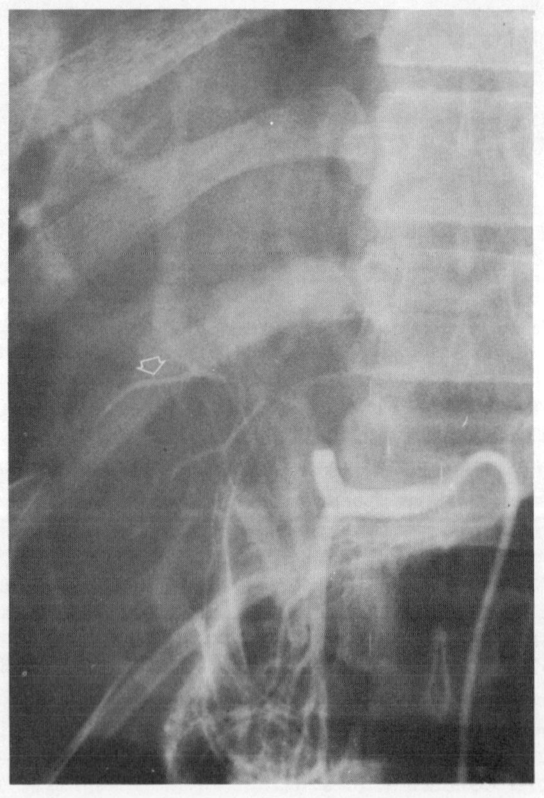

a

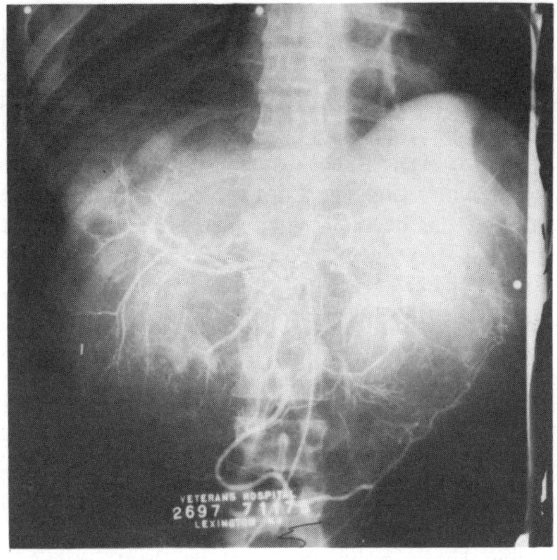

b

Fig. 4.3. a, Early intrahepatic blood flow can be seen in this arteriogram after ligation of the common hepatic artery. *b,* Reconstitution of intrahepatic arterial blood flow after ligation of right hepatic artery.

seven to ten days. Portal venous blood flow must be maintained by replacing extracellular liquids as well as blood.

If cardiac action is reduced, portal venous flow should be enhanced by giving cardiotonic drugs. Atelectasis, pneumonia, inadequate gaseous exchange and other complications that reduce the oxygenation of blood must be prevented or, if they occur, treated vigorously and early. Regular recording of the arterial blood gases can be very helpful in guiding treatment.

VENOUS BLEEDING

Haemorrhage from disrupted veins within the liver is not a great obstacle to recovery but bleeding from the great veins outside Glisson's capsule (major hepatic veins, portal vein and retrohepatic vena cava) is often lethal. The tendency of venous bleeding inside the substance of the liver is to stop spontaneously but we can assist the thrombogenic powers of the liver by ligating the hepatic artery and then temporarily inserting packs while attending to other operative necessities. If venous oozing from the interior of the liver continues, the hepatoduodenal ligament must be re-examined to ascertain whether the appropriate hepatic artery has been occluded. It is important to remember that in 12 per cent of patients the right hepatic artery comes off the superior mesenteric as a separate trunk.

Avulsion of the main hepatic veins from the vena cava is a rare injury and usually is due to an extreme and sudden deceleration injury (Burns and Dritt, 1975). Such injuries are lethal and extremely difficult to treat. Several kinds of intracaval shunts have been devised to treat them (Aaron and Mays, 1975). Some surgeons advocate inserting the shunt through the right atrial appendage after doing a median sternotomy (Schrock et al., 1968). Others prefer inserting the shunt into the inferior vena cava below the liver. A catheter has been designed specially to be threaded through the common femoral vein and placed by fluroscopic control in the retro-hepatic vena cava (Pelcher et al., 1977). The reason for all these different operations is to isolate the liver from the circulation while repair of the hepatic vein is done. These are dangerous and difficult operations and there have been few reported survivors.

A better method of treating avulsion of the hepatic vein is direct ligation of the vein and suture repair of the vena cava. Surgical dogma says it is necessary to resect hepatic tissue acutely deprived of venous outflow. But studies using porcine livers, which are similar to the vascular anatomy of the human liver, disclose intercommunications between the left and right hepatic veins when one or the other has been ligated (Kaman and Cerveny, 1971).

Corrosion casts of human livers have displayed hepatic vein collaterals like those present in pigs. Compulsory hepatic resection after venous ligation is not necessary in humans. This new concept has been shown by Feldman (1966) who reported a patient with a tear of the left hepatic vein. Feldman repaired the inferior vena cava and ligated the left hepatic vein without doing an hepatic resection; his patient survived and had no adverse sequelae. Depinto et al. (1976) ligated the middle and left hepatic vein in a 19-year-old male who sustained blunt avulsion in an automobile accident. The patient's postoperative course was uncomplicated and ten months later the patient's hepatic scan was normal except for a small wedge-shaped defect. Ligation of the torn hepatic vein and repair of the vena cava do not require the special shunts or instruments available only in large medical centres. This operation can be done in most hospitals set up to care for accident victims.

HEPATIC RESECTION

Surgical ablation of parts of the liver is not new, although many are inclined to think so because of a recent surge of interest for treating injuries of the liver (Mays, 1971b). Another peak of interest in hepatic resection burgeoned in 1897; fourteen cases of partial hepatectomy were reported in that year alone.

There are two major difficulties in successfully using hepatic resection to treat patients with ruptured livers. Firstly, there are no clear criteria for deciding which patients need this fashionable but formidable operation. Secondly, the mortality rate for major hepatic resections done in hypovolemic, acutely injured patients is high. Most university medical centres in the USA and the UK are reporting 43–59 per cent death rates. Occasionally, an initial report of a mortality of 20 per cent has been followed by a second report from the same institution admitting to a greater death rate. After publishing a report advocating hepatic resection in 1972 (Mays, 1972b) I have had to change my thinking on the matter because whereas I found hepatic resection to be effective in lowering the mortality rate in our university medical centre, it proved dangerous when used in community hospitals.

Terminology is confused, misleading and therefore dangerous. One group will remove the lateral segment of the left lobe and report this as a left lobectomy. Such a segmental resection has almost no morbidity and mortality. Others read this report and attempt a true left lobectomy and find the death rate outrageous. The main reason for this is a failure to discern the intrahepatic anatomy. An hepatic lobectomy has not been done until the liver is transected through the main lobar fissure, first described by Cantlie (1897) and such lobectomies should not be done in acute injuries. The place for hepatic lobectomy is in treating late complications of hepatic injury, in which conditions the mortality rate of an anatomical lobectomy is much less than that following resections while the patient is in varying degrees of shock before the operation begins.

There are five different kind of hepatic resections used to treat ruptured livers: (1) resectional debridement; (2) right lobectomy; (3) left lobectomy; (4) segmental (sublobar resections); (5) trisegmentectomy (right hepatic lobectomy extended to include the medial segment of the left lobe).

Resectional 'Debridement'
Of the five, resectional 'debridement' is the only logical treatment for the acutely injured patient. It is simply resection of hepatic tissue already separated from the liver by the initial accident. Resectional debridement certainly should not be used in central ruptures of the liver and it is inappropriate in the large stellate ruptures of the right lobe and large subcapsular haematomas with an underlying, deep rupture of the liver. The technique is straightforward. The handle of the scalpel is used to dissect through the remaining tissue and one teases out the vascular and biliary elements between the thumb and index finger before ligating or clipping them. Because this resection is not an anatomical resection it should be accompanied by ligation of the hepatic artery supplying the injured lobe. However, it must be emphasized that there are hazards because more or less of the liver is deprived of its vascular and biliary connections and infarction, venous congestion and biliary obstruction occur in such segments. This may delay recovery or cause death from sepsis.

Hepatic Lobectomy
Hepatic lobectomy is a formidable operation and mortality rates are 43–50 per cent. It should rarely be used in acutely hypovolemic patients.

The reduction of a single lobe to complete pulp is one indication. Another is to expose and repair the retrohepatic vena cava when exposure cannot be obtained by other simpler methods.

The third use of hepatic lobectomy is for treating the late complications of rupture. The operative technique of hepatic lobectomy has been described in detail (Mays, 1978).

PERIHEPATIC DRAINAGE

As the second most common cause of death, sepsis is nearly always related to inadequate drainage of the ruptured liver. The perihepatic spaces are notoriously difficult to drain (Mays, 1977). They have a remarkable propensity to collect bile, blood, serum and sequestered parenchymal tissue. One reason why these spaces are so difficult to drain is the juxta-position of the rigid thoracic cage, against which the liver becomes tightly jammed by swelling so that flexible rubber drains are useless. A second reason why these perihepatic spaces are troublesome is the prolonged time

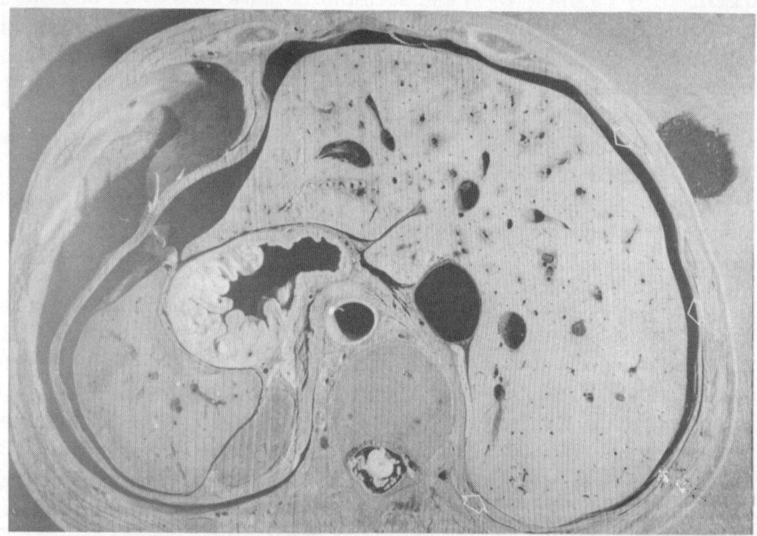

Fig. 4.4. A cross-section at the level of the liver shows the large potential spaces that must be adequately drained.

most injured patients spend in the supine position. A cross-section of the human cadaver shows the extreme dependency of these spaces and their large capacity (*Fig. 4.4*).

While many patients with minor uncomplicated wounds of the liver recover promptly with only rubber drains brought out through the ventral abdominal wall, patients with complex wounds of the liver do not. When only soft rubber drains are used, subphrenic and subhepatic collections and consequent sepsis nearly always occur and impede recovery. Second and third operations are necessary and a number of unfortunate patients die. It is incumbent upon the surgeon, therefore, to drain adequately at the first operation.

To drain the perihepatic spaces effectively requires several suction catheters spread out fan-like over the dome of the liver, dorsal to the liver and below it. They should be brought out through a stab wound in the right flank for right lobar injuries or a stab wound in the left upper quadrant for left lobar ruptures. Suction should be gentle otherwise hollow viscera may be caught against the holes. Intestinal fistulae can result from suction injuries of the bowel wall.

Resection of the Twelfth Rib

Most hepatic injuries involve the right lobe and for adequate drainage of the subdiaphragmatic space the twelfth rib is resected and a large drainage hole is made in the back and extended ventrally into the right flank. In thin or normal sized patients this can be done through the mid-line incision at the initial laparotomy (*Fig. 4.5*). In obese and very muscular individuals the rib cannot be removed easily from the ventral approach and the patient has to be turned onto the left side. The twelfth rib is removed after the abdominal incision is closed. After the rib has been removed the incision is continued through the periosteal bed of the rib. Since the pleural reflexion is attached to the most medial part of the twelfth rib it is best to avoid this area and to extend the incision into the flank and subcostally onto the ventral surface of the abdomen. As the incision is deepened it should be large enough for the surgeon to insert his hand up to the wrist.

Such a large defect causes a grave problem with postoperative bleeding and it cannot be packed because this prevents the drainage for which the defect was made. The best method of arresting bleeding from this large wound while leaving it open for drainage is to encircle the entire wound with a haemostatic stitch; this should include all layers of the parieties and each loop should be locked to achieve haemostasis (*Fig. 4.6*). If the patient is so large that one stitch cannot go through all layers of the parieties, two interlocking rows of a running haemostatic stitch must be terraced one upon the other.

Drainage by this route is extremely effective in preventing collections around the ruptured liver. When not used as primary treatment of the ruptured liver, it frequently has to be done some days or weeks later to drain subphrenic and subhepatic abscesses.

Hepatostomy

Some surgeons have advocated the insertion of a large rubber catheter into intrahepatic cavities to achieve drainage. This treatment is hazardous

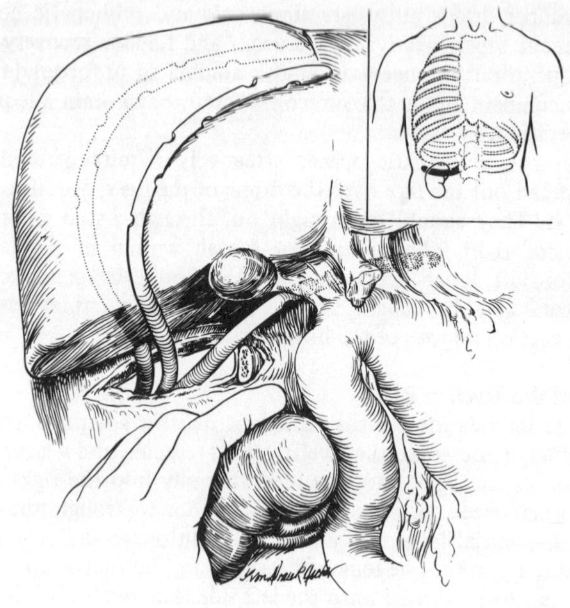

a

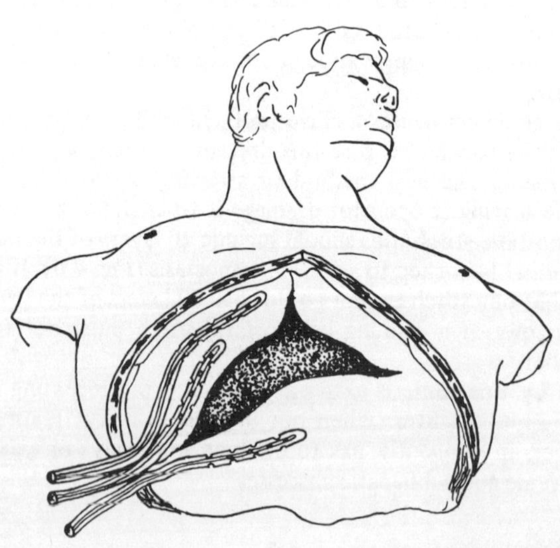

b

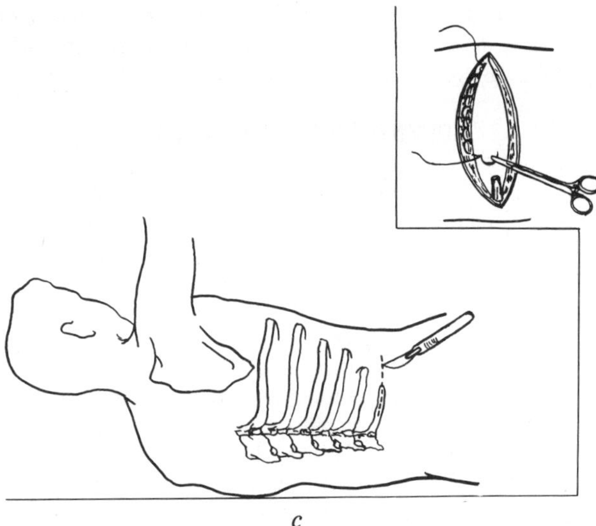

Fig. 4.5. Method of resecting twelfth rib and draining perihepatic spaces: *a*, anterior approach; *b*, suction catheters used to drain perihepatic spaces; *c*, external approach to twelfth rib must be used in obese people.

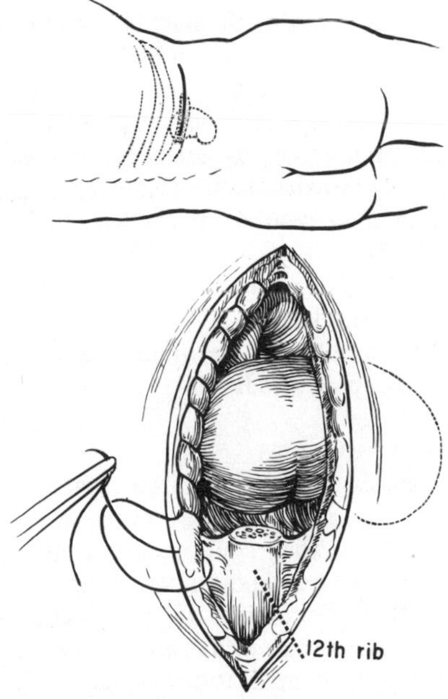

Fig. 4.6. Haemostatic suture is used to stop bleeding from wound edges while leaving hole open for dependent drainage.

because of the risk of uncontrolled haemorrhage and damage to adjacent uninjured hepatic tissue. These cavities are frequently infected and the presence of a foreign body in infection is unwise.

DETRIMENTAL METHODS

Packing

Boljarski (1910) recommended treating fractures of the liver with an isolated pack of omentum sutured into the hepatic wound. Halstead used an omental pack to treat a large perforating wound of the liver. Mikulicz recommended use of a free gauze pack for control of bleeding. Packing the liver was the main method of treating ruptured livers in the years following World War I. It was recommended in all surgical texts at that time. In World War II surgeons adopted this method and between 1942 and 1943 used gauze packs instead of omentum to pack ruptured livers. Madding et al. (1942–3) noted serious complications; disastrous haemorrhage frequently followed the removal of packs, abscesses occurred within the liver or in the perihepatic spaces, hepatic necrosis was observed in areas that had been packed. Peritonitis, hepatitis, fistulae and numerous other complications followed this method of treatment. Such complications led to abandonment of packing as primary treatment of ruptured livers in the last years of the war. There followed an immediate reduction in the death rate from 30 to 17 per cent.

Despite these vivid lessons, packing the liver has been revived. In 1975 a university group reported their revival of Boljarski's (1910) technique of isolating a section of the omentum and suturing it into the ruptured liver. A modest number of patients are still being treated with gauze packing despite its universal condemnation by experienced surgeons. As recently as 1976 packs were second only to absorbable haemostatic agents as the most frequent method used to treat wounds of the liver in 1 590 consecutive patients (Defore et al., 1976).

Some patients in whom packs have been used as primary treatment survive but recovery has been delayed and survival is in spite of and not because of packs, which do not promote drainage and are less successful than arterial ligation for stopping bleeding.

Absorbable Haemostatic Agents

Gelatin sponges and fabrics prepared by the controlled oxidation of regenerated cellulose have been credited with avoiding the dangers associated with gauze packs. Because they could be dissolved and 'absorbed' by the body they did not have to be removed, which appeared to be a great advantage since many of the shortcomings of gauze packing coincided with their removal, but after clinical trials using various absorbable haemostatic agents in and about the liver, complications similar to those noted from gauze packs became evident. In small amounts these synthetic materials are absorbed by human tissue but in the amounts required to control hepatic haemorrhage they remain as foreign bodies and should not be used.

Suturing Crevasses

After strong condemnation of packing, suturing the liver became the next most widely used method but suturing deep cracks in the liver is hazardous and frequently followed by haemobilia, traumatic sequestra, secondary haemorrhage and intrahepatic cavitation, with subsequent sepsis and hepatic failure. Establishing better drainage of the injured liver may account for the survival of some of the patients and there are no facts available to suggest that such patients would have died if they had not been treated by extensive drainage without suture.

A search for evidence to support suturing of the liver as a primary method of treatment yields none, whereas evidence that hepatic wounds can be left unsutured comes from both animal experiments and human clinical trials. Shires (1966) reported 78 patients from Parkland Memorial Hospital in Dallas, Texas, whose torn livers were left unsutured. None of these patients had any episode of rebleeding, biliary fistula, biliary peritonitis or excessive drainage of bile. On the basis of his experience Little (1971) also advocates leaving wounds of the liver unsutured. Patients who have recovered rapidly after suturing of the liver could have probably recovered with drainage alone.

The main reason proclaimed for using sutures as primary treatment is to stop haemorrhage but most recalcitrant bleeding is from tertiary rami of intrahepatic arteries deep within the liver. In severely burst livers there are too many arterial and venous disruptions to find and suture individually and they are nearly always too deep to be reached with sutures. There are better and simpler methods of achieving hepatic haemostatsis.

Another reason many surgeons suture hepatic wounds is to control bile leakage but except for injury to a large extrahepatic bile duct, there is no evidence that sutures have at any time stopped bile leakage. In fact, Glenn et al. (1966) found that there is more bile leaked from hepatic wounds after they had been sutured than before.

Finger Exploration of Wounds

The digital exploration of wounds of the liver to identify 'soft spots' is extremely hazardous. Exploration of cracks and crevasses in the liver is also dangerous, having on occasion increased bleeding and caused death from haemorrhage. An organ with potential for profuse haemorrhage should not be provoked by unnecessary interference.

Haemobilia

Bleeding into the biliary system after hepatic trauma was reported as early as 1848. Sandblom (1948) suggested the term 'traumatic haemobilia' and elucidated the anatomical and pathological mechanisms. Haemobilia has been linked to primary suture of deep liver ruptures (Aronsen et al., 1970; Mays, 1976) and the majority of reported cases of traumatic haemobilia have occurred in patients treated by either packing or suturing. Both techniques produce the same anatomical derangement. A deep crevasse in the liver occluded either by packing or sutures prevents the escape of bile, blood and sequestered liver from the bottom of such cavities. Subsequent bleeding from hepatic arteries exerts pressure in this closed space. Pressure necrosis eventually makes a large cavity containing macerated liver. Such an intrahepatic cavity can cause sepsis and liver failure or in other instances it can erode bile ducts and establish a false track between artery and bile duct, producing haemobilia, or erode into the portal vein and produce an arteriovenous fistula, as illustrated in *Fig. 4.7*. Each of these complications was preceded by suturing a wound in the liver.

The treatment of such complications is frustrating to the surgeon and dangerous to the patient. MacVaugh et al. (1966) surveyed the reported cases of haemobilia and noted that resection of the liver containing the necrotic cavity in seven of forty patients resulted in only one death, whereas in thirty-three patients treated without hepatic resection there

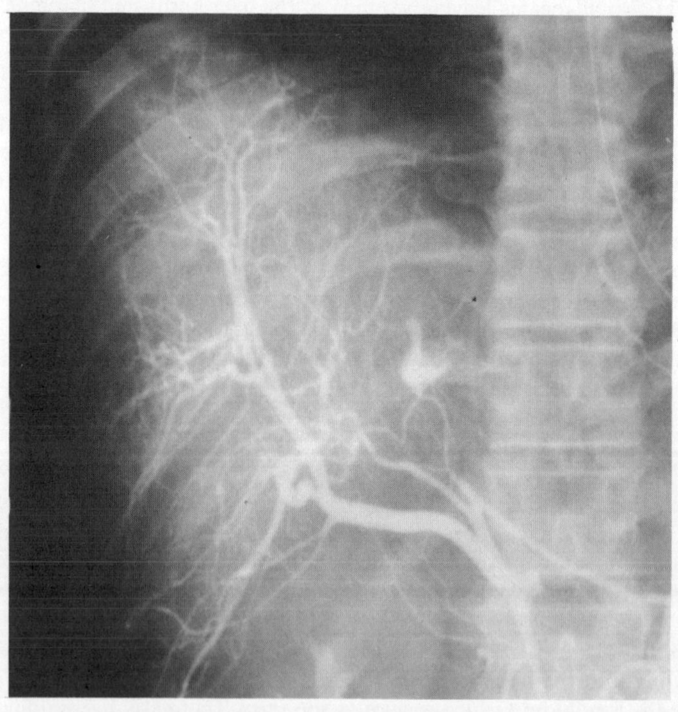

a

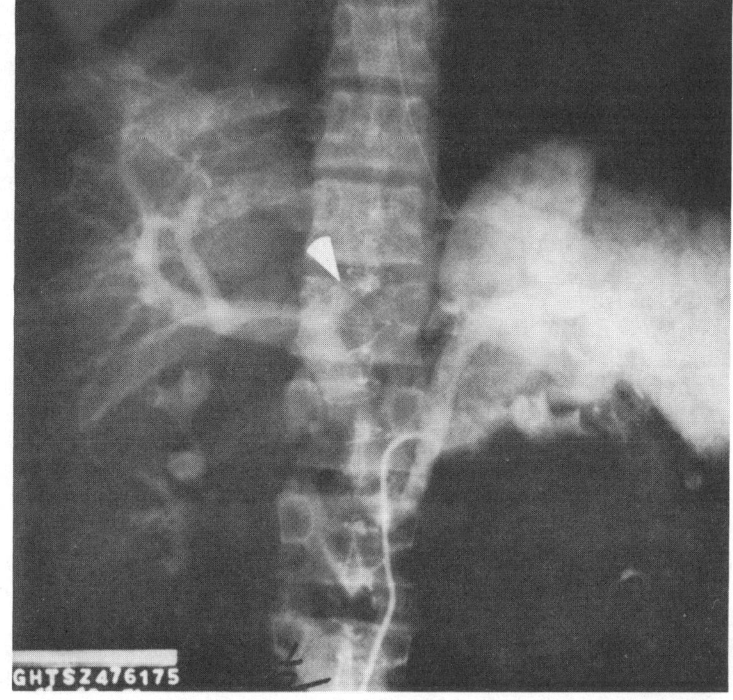

b

Fig. 4.7. This arteriogram displays a fistula between the hepatic artery and portal vein in the liver after a motor vehicle accident: *a*, defect in tertiary branch of left ramus of the hepatic artery; *b*, immediate filling of the portal vein from the hepatic arterial fistula.

were twelve deaths. Such results led to the agreement that hepatic resection is the treatment of choice when haemobilia springs from a traumatic intrahepatic cavity produced by suturing or packing. But, as always, prevention is more important than treatment, especially when that treatment happens to be a risky, formidable operation such as hepatic resection. When there is no sign of intrahepatic cavitation, by hepatic scans or by hepatic arteriography, ligation of the hepatic artery is better and safer than lobectomy. Deliberate embolism of the hepatic artery aided by arteriography has also been reported to correct haemobilia (Heimback et al., 1978).

Clamping the Porta Hepatis

In 1908 J. H. Pringle proposed arresting hepatic haemorrhage by clamping the afferent blood supply in the hepatoduodenal ligament (Pringle, 1908). This method became instantly popular and widely used. Now referred to as the Pringle manoeuvre, it is said to be safe for period of 10—15 minutes in normothermic patients, but as with other detrimental methods this technique is based not upon sound physiology but upon tradition and desperation.

All hepatologists know that the liver is exquisitely sensitive to hypoxia. An organ with responsibility for homeostasis should not have hypoxia imposed upon it and then be expected to re-establish homeostasis. Most ruptures of the liver involve a single lobe and it is unreasonable to subject the entire liver to anoxia when only one lobe has been injured.

Choledochal Tubes

It has been said that the insertion of a T-tube into the common duct, can decompress the intrahepatic biliary tree and should reduce the incidence of biliary fistulae and decrease extravasation of bile after rupture of the liver (Merendino et al., 1963). There were other theoretical advantages. Bile has a fibrinolytic effect on blood clots and any method of reducing biliary stasis should counteract the breakdown of clots. The T-tube could also act to detect haemobilia and evaluate the biliary tract with roentgenograms in the postoperative period.

Such bonuses never materialized in prospective clinical trials conducted by Lucas (1971) and the consequences of surgical decompression of the biliary passages or the gall bladder by tube were alarming. There was a notable increase in intra-abdominal abscesses, stress gastric haemorrhage and ascending cholangitis. Dilatation of the hepatic duct as compared with the common bile duct occurred in 13 patients of the 107 studied.

Glucagon

Any method of improving blood flow and oxygenation of an ischaemic liver should benefit the patient. It is easy to understand why a polypeptide such as glucagon, which increases portal venous blood flow by as much as 100 per cent, won immediate praise (Shoemaker et al., 1959). The enhancement of splanchnic blood flow by infusions of glucagon is said by many to justify its routine use in patients with injured livers. When splanchnic blood flow is reduced by bleeding, injection of glucagon restores it approximately to previous levels; the main cause of this restoration is vasodilatation of the splanchnic vascular bed, but increased cardiac output also occurs.

Glucagon causes glycogenolysis in hepatocytes and so increases their need for oxygen. Whereas the haemodynamic effects of intravenous glucagon are desirable in patients with ruptured livers, the glycogenolytic response is not, unless the necessary increase in oxygen can be made available.

The curtailment by glucagon of hepatocyte respiration in the ischaemic liver has been proven by the studies of Fredlund et al. (1972) who observed an accelerated liberation of lysosomal enzymes, reflecting accentuated hepatocyte damage after glucagon. A combination of glucagon and arterial ligation produced widespread necrosis of the hepatic parenchyma in those animals given glucagon. Witte et al. (1978) found that glucagon did not increase the PaO_2 in hepatic tissue even though it did cause increased oxygenation and blood flow in the portal vein.

REFERENCES

Aaron W. S., Fulton R. L. and Mays E. T. (1975) Selective ligation of the hepatic artery. *Surg. Gynecol. Obstet.* **141**, 187.

Aaron W. S. and Mays E. T. (1975) Isolation of the retrohepatic vena cava by balloon catheter: An experimental assessment. *Rev. Surg.* **32**, 222.

Aronsen K. F. and Ericsson B. (1970) Haemobilia after primary suture of deep liver rupture. *Acta Chir. Scand.* **136**, 517.

Balasegaram M. (1976) The surgical management of hepatic trauma. *J. Trauma* **16**, 141.

Blumgart L. H. and Vajabukka T. (1972) Injuries to the liver. *Br. Med. J.* **1**, 158.

Boljarski N. (1910) Uber Leberverletzungen Klinischer and experimenteller Hinsicht untes besonderer Berucksichtigung der isolierten Netzpkstik. *Arch. Klin. Chir.* **93**, 507.

Bolton P. M., Wood C. B., Quartey-Papafio J. B. et al. (1973) Blunt abdominal injury: A review of 59 consecutive cases undergoing surgery. *Br. J. Surg.* **60**, 657.

Burns R. P. and Britt L. G. (1975) Massive venous injuries associated with penetrating wounds of the liver. *J. Trauma* **15**, 757.

Cantlie J. (1897) On a new arrangement of the right and left lobes of the liver. *Proc. Anat. Soc. Great Britain, Ireland* **32**, 4.

Canty T. G. and Aaron W. S. (1975) Hepatic artery ligation for exsanguinating liver injuries in children. *J. Pediatr. Surg.* **10**, 693.

Carnevale N., Baron N. and Delaney H. M. (1977) Peritoneoscopy as an aid in the diagnosis of abdominal trauma: a preliminary report. *J. Trauma* **17**, 634.

Claget G. P. and Olsen W. R. (1978) Non-mechanical haemorrhage in severe liver injury. *Ann. Surg.* **187**.

Defore W. W., Mattox K. L., Jorden G. L. et al. (1976) Management of 1590 consecutive cases of liver trauma. *Arch. Surg.* **111**, 493.

Depinto D. J., Mucha S. J. and Powers P. C. (1976) Major hepatic vein ligation necessitated by blunt abdominal trauma. *Ann. Surg.* **183**, 243.

Edler L. (1886–7) Die traumatischen Verletzungen der parenchymatosen Uferleigsorgane. *Arch. Klin. Chir.* **34**, 343, 573, 738.

Feldman E. A. (1966) Injury to the hepatic vein. *Am. J. Surg.* **111**, 244.

Fredlund P. E., Callum B. and Tibblin S. (1972) Influence of glucagon on the ischaemia liver in the pig. *Arch. Surg.* **105**, 615.

Freeark R. J., Shoemaker W. C. and Baker R. J. (1968) Aortography in blunt abdominal trauma. *Arch. Surg.* **96**, 705.

From P. and Alli J. H. (1956) Bacteriologic study of the human liver. *Gastroenterology* **31**, 33.

Glenn F., Mujahed Z. and Grafe W. R. (1966) Graded trauma in liver injury. *J. Trauma* **6**, 133.

Gordon-Taylor G. (1943) A rare cause of gastrointestinal haemorrhage. *Br. Med. J.* **1**, 504.

Grahame E. W. (1958) The management of civilian liver injuries. *Lancet* 727:1295.

Heimbach D. M., Ferguson G. S. and Harley J. D. (1978) Treatment of traumatic haemobilia. *J. Trauma* **18**, 221.

Kaman J. and Cerveny C. (1971) Formation of intrahepatic collaterals after obstruction of hepatic veins in pigs. *Acta Anat.* **80**, 481.

Lewis F. R., Lim R. C. and Blaisdell F. W. (1974) Hepatic artery ligation: adjunct in the management of massive haemorrhage from the liver. *J. Trauma* **14**, 743.
Little J. M. (1971) *Management of Liver Injuries*. Edinburgh, Livingstone.
Little J. M., McRae J. and Smitanada N. et al. (1967) Radioisotope scanning of liver and spleen in upper abdominal trauma. *Surg. Gynecol. Obstet.* **125**, 725.
London P. S. (1978) Personal communication.
Lucas C. E. (1971) Prospective clinical evaluation of biliary drainage in hepatic trauma. *Ann. Surg.* **174**, 830.
Lucas C. E. and Ledgerwood A. M. (1976) Prospective evaluation of hemostatic techniques for liver injuries. *J. Trauma* **16**, 442.
MacVaugh H., Hacept G. S. and Myers R. N. et al. (1966) Traumatic haemobilia. *Surgery* **60**, 547.
Madding G. F., Lawrence K. B. and Kennedy P. A. (1942–3) Forward surgery of the severely injured. Second Aux Surgical Group **1**, 307.
Mays E. T. (1966) Bursting injuries of the liver. *Arch. Surg.* **93**, 92.
Mays E. T. (1971a) Complex penetrating hepatic wounds. *Ann. Surg.* **173**, 421.
Mays E. T. (1971b) Hepatic lobectomy. *Arch. Surg.* **103**, 216.
Mays E. T. (1972a) Lobar dearterialization for exsanguinating wounds of the liver. *J. Trauma* **12**, 397.
Mays E. T. (1972b) Lobectomy, sublobar resections and resectional debridement for severe liver injury. *J. Trauma* **12**, 309.
Mays E. T. (1973) Hepatic trauma *N. Engl. J. Med.* **288**, 402.
Mays E. T. (1974) The hepatic artery. *Surg. Gynecol. Obstet.* **139**, 595.
Mays E. T. (1976) The hazards of suturing certain wounds of the liver. *Surg. Gynecol. Obstet.* **143**, 201.
Mays E. T. (1977) Critical wounds of the liver and juxtahepatic veins. *Am. Surg.* **43**, 635.
Mays E. T. (1978) Rupture of the Liver in Operative Surgery. In: London P. S. (ed.) *Operative Surgery*. London, Butterworth.
Mays E. T. and Wheeler C. S. (1974) Demonstration of collateral arterial flow after interruption of hepatic arteries in man. *N. Engl. J. Med.* **290**, 993.
Merendino K. A., Dillard D. H. and Cammock E. E. (1963) The concept of surgical biliary decompression in the management of liver trauma. *Surg. Gynecol. Obstet.* **117**, 285.
Michels N. A. (1960) New anatomy of liver – Variant blood supply and collateral circulation. *J. Am. Med. Ass.* **172**, 125.
Mikesky W. E., Howard J. M. and DeBakey M. E. (1956) Injuries of the liver in 300 consecutive patients. *Surg. Gynecol. Obstet.* **103**, 323.
Orloff M. J., Peskin G. W. and Ellis H. L. (1958) A bacteriologic study of human portal blood: implications regarding hepatic ischaemia in man. *Ann. Surg.* **148**, 738.
Pelcher D. B., Harman P. K. and Moore E. E. (1977) Retrohepatic vena cava balloon shunt introduced via the sapheno-femoral junction. *J. Trauma* **17**, 837.
Perry J. F. (1970) Blunt and Penetrating Abdominal Injuries. In: *Current Problems in Surgery*. Chicago, Year Book. Med. Pub. Chicago May.
Pringle J. H. (1908) Notes on the arrest of hepatic haemorrhage. *Ann. Surg.* **48**, 451.
Root H. D. and Hauser C. W. (1965) Diagnostic peritoneal lavage. *Surgery* **57**, 633.
Sandblom P. (1948) Haemorrhage into the biliary tract following trauma – Traumatic haemobilia. *Surgery* **24**, 571.
Schrock T. F., Blaisdell F. W. and Matherson C. (1968) Management of blunt trauma to the liver and hepatic veins. *Arch. Surg.* **96**, 698.
Segall H. N. (1923) An experimental anatomical investigation of the blood and bile channels of the liver. *Surg. Gynecol. Obstet.* **37**, 156.
Shires G. T. (1966) *Care of the Trauma Patient*. McGraw-Hill, New York, p. 374.

Shoemaker W. C., van Itallie T. B. and Walker W. G. (1959) Measurement of hepatic glucose output and hepatic blood flow in response to glucagon. *Am. J. Physiol.* **192**, 315.
Tanphiphat C. (1976) Lobar dearterialization in liver trauma. *Br. J. Surg.* **63**, 213.
Wallace C. (1918) *War Surgery of the Abdomen.* London, Churchill.
Witte C. L., Witte M. H. and Kintner K. (1978) Effect of glucagon on hepatic lymph (tissue) PO_2 and after ligation of the hepatic artery: an experimental study. *J. Trauma* **18**, 27.

Graham Teasdale

5 Monitoring of Head Injuries

INTRODUCTION

Each year thousands of patients with head injuries are admitted to hospital. The majority have been only slightly injured and are discharged after a brief period of observation, but others have injuries so overwhelming that from the start their survival seems unlikely. Between these extremes are those patients for whom treatment is a crucial matter: patients with severe, but recoverable injuries, and patients developing life-threatening complications after what initially apppeared to be a minor injury. The initial assessment of a head injured patient can provide only a provisional guide to treatment. It is the monitoring of the subsequent course of events which discloses the true pattern of brain damage and so determines a patient's management.

Brain Damage after Head Injury

Damage to the brain, rather than the scalp or skull, is the most serious aspect of head injury. Brain damage after head injury may be focal or diffuse and may occur either as a primary event or develop as a secondary complication (Adams, 1975). Primary damage, sustained at the time of the injury, includes obvious focal macroscopic contusions and lacerations on the brain surface. These are probably overshadowed in importance by the diffuse destruction and distortion of nerve fibres and connections, which are visible only with the electron microscope. Focal secondary damage results from complications such as traumatic intracranial haematomas, cerebral oedema and abscesses. It is associated with shift of the brain and, eventually, with herniation and haemorrhagic infarction of the midbrain or medulla. Diffuse secondary brain damage from oxygen lack is a common finding in the brains of patients who die after head injury. Such hypoxic brain damage is often due to a drop in cerebral blood flow, brought about by raised intracranial pressure but cerebral oxygenation can also be threatened by many of the extracranial complications associated with head injury.

What Can be Monitored?

It is helpful to distinguish the two main purposes for which monitoring is performed. The first, which is the main concern of this review, is to determine changes in the functional state of the brain; improvement indicates that recovery is taking place, deteriorating responsiveness makes a secondary complication likely. The second purpose of assessments is to provide information about the integrity of a number of physiological processes upon which the brain's vitality depends. There are many different ways in which either the extent of brain damage, or the factors responsible for it, might be assessed (*Fig. 5.1*). In practice, the methods employed can be broadly divided into clinical and investigative.

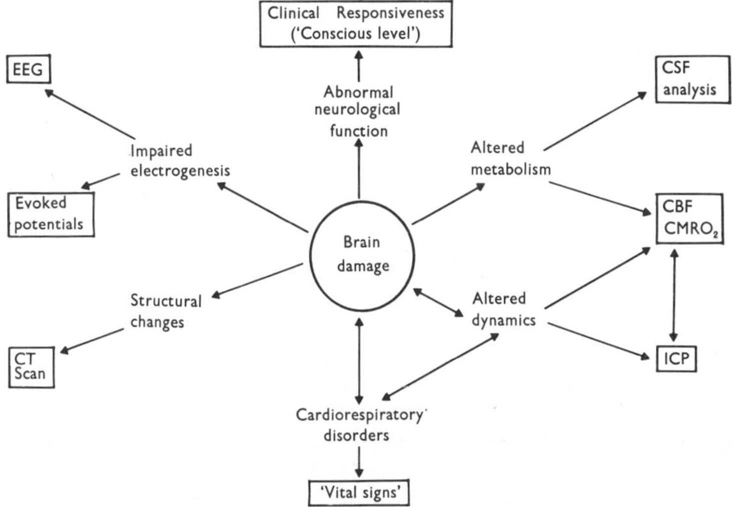

Fig. 5.1. The various effects of brain damage and the ways in which they may be monitored. [(EEG = electroencephalogram: CT = computer tomography: CSF = cerebrospinal fluid: CBF = cerebral blood flow: CMRO₂ = cerebral metabolic rate for oxygen: ICP = intracranial pressure).]

Clinical Assessment for Responsiveness
Traditionally, much of head injury management has been based on repeated assessment of the patient's clinical responsiveness – the so-called 'conscious level'. This is still true for the majority of head injured patients. Improvements in methods of assessing patients have enhanced the value of clinical observation and these will be described in detail.

Investigations
Computer Tomography
Computer tomography of the brain is a recent development. Already its importance in head injury management is unquestioned and investigations of head injured patients can disclose intracranial complications in advance of obvious clinical signs of deterioration. Thus the scan can provide warning of complications, and one definition of monitoring is 'giving warning'.

Intracranial Pressure

The technology of monitoring cardiovascular or respiratory disorders will not be described here despite their influence in producing secondary hypoxic brain damage. Instead, I have concentrated upon those intracranial factors which can impair cerebral blood flow, and hence oxygenation, and amongst these I have focused upon the measurement of intracranial pressure because its value is still debated after many years of clinical use.

Electrophysiological Techniques

Finally, the EEG and certain methods for assessing brain function electrophysiologically also merit discussion, although their role is likely to be restricted to selected cases in certain units.

CLINICAL ASSESSMENT

The Conscious Level

Diffuse brain damage and dysfunction are reflected in impairment of consciousness. The importance attached to the monitoring of conscious level is reflected in the wide variety of systems for assessment which have been described. Additional scales have been described recently from Munich (Brinkman et al., 1976), Leeds (Price, 1976) and Glasgow (Teasdale and Jennett, 1974) and the latter seems to be gaining wide acceptance (Plum, 1975; Langfitt, 1978). In contrast with most previous systems, the Glasgow scale does not depend upon the existence of a natural hierarchy of discrete, overall 'levels' of coma, nor does it presume distinctive anatomical—clinical syndromes, as neither of these exists in practice. Instead, it is based on observing three aspects of responsiveness, each of which is described according to simple well-defined criteria.

The Glasgow scale is composed of eye opening, motor and verbal responses (Table 5.1).

Eye Opening

Is eye opening spontaneous, induced by command, only after painful stimulation, or not at all? Standardization of the degree of painful stimulus is important in ensuring consistent observations; we have found pressure upon the fingernail the most useful form. Opening of the eyes does not necessarily indicate awareness but can be taken as an indication that the arousal mechanisms in the brainstem are active. Once a maximum level of arousal has been obtained the integrity of verbal and motor performance is assessed.

Verbal Response

If speech is present this indicates a high degree of cerebral functioning even if the response is confused or restricted to non-conversational words or expletives. A non-verbalizing patient may moan or groan in response to stimulation and this is the lowest level of response.

Table 5.1 The Glasgow Coma Scale

	Score
Eye Opening	
Spontaneous	4
To sound	3
To pain	2
Never	1
Best Verbal Response	
Orientated	5
Confused	4
Inappropriate words	3
Incomprehensible sounds	2
None	1
Best Motor Response	
Obey commands	6
Localize pain	5
Flexion normal	4
Flexion abnormal	3
Extension	2
None	1
Possible overall highest score	15

Motor Response

Motor responses are particularly useful in a patient who is not talking. When testing for the ability to obey commands it is important that the instruction is sufficiently specific and complex to avoid misinterpreting reflex responses. When an examiner's fingers are placed in a patient's hand a reflex grasp response is sometimes obtained; this should not be regarded as obeying commands. Localizing movements occur when the patient clearly attempts to remove the source of a painful stimulus.

If a patient flexes only to pain this is an indication of an impairment of integration between stimulus and response. This reaches its most extreme form when abnormal stereotyped responses are present. These are sometimes difficult to classify and some patients may show both flexion and extension movements during the same examination. 'Decorticate' and 'decerebrate' states have been traditional diagnoses but should not be used to describe head injured patients. These terms are inadequate to describe the changing patterns seen either during one examination or evolving over a period of time, and the assumption that they might reflect exact underlying anatomical localizations is invalid (Feldman, 1971a, b). Extension responses may occur as a manifestation of acute lesions anywhere between the cerebral cortex and cervical spinal cord (Fisher, 1969); moreover, in severe head injury a diffuse pattern of damage is to be expected (Adams et al., 1977).

A Bedside Chart

The Glasgow scale has been incorporated into a bedside chart (*Fig. 5.2*) which is simple to complete (*Fig. 5.3*) and easy to review (Teasdale et al., 1975). Many units do not favour such a formal system for assessing

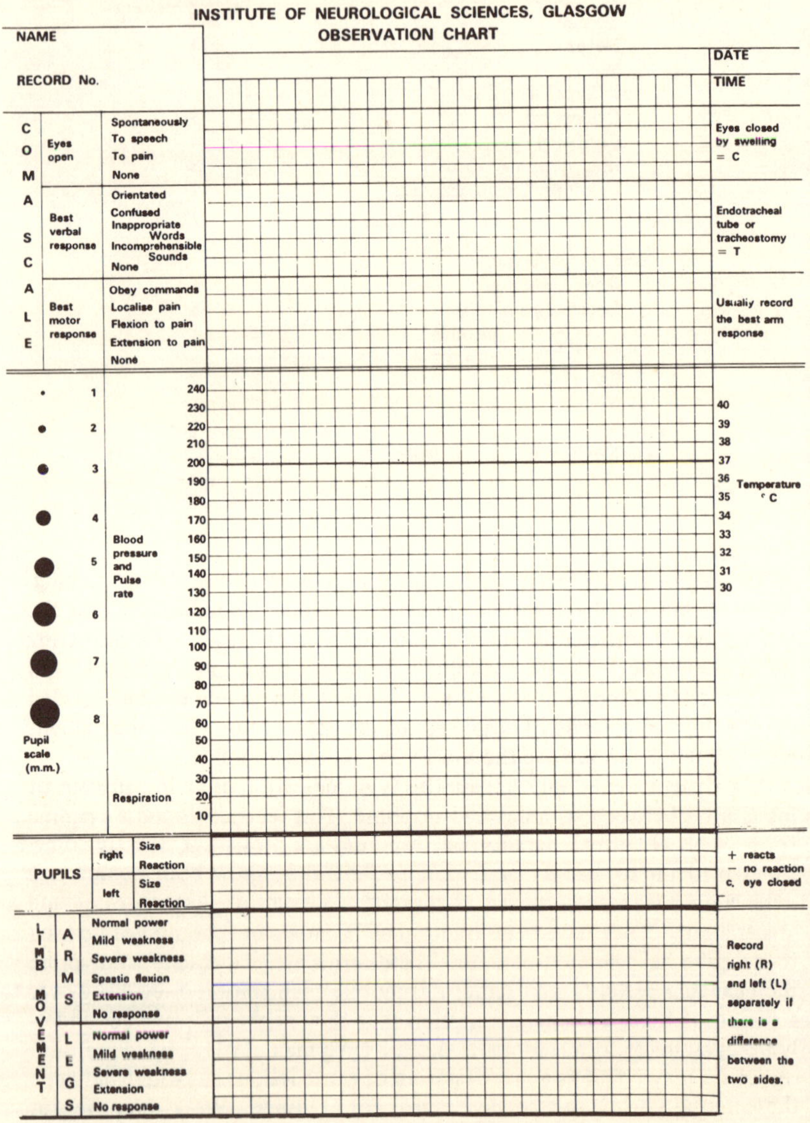

INSTITUTE OF NEUROLOGICAL SCIENCES, GLASGOW
OBSERVATION CHART

Fig. 5.2. The Glasgow chart for recording observations on patients with head injury. (*Figs. 5.2. and 5.3. are reproduced from 'Nursing Times'.*)

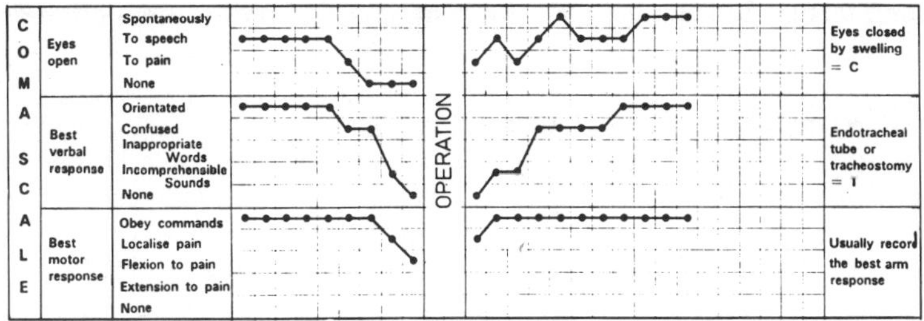

Fig. 5.3. A patient with an intracerebral haematoma; record shows progressive impairment of responses, despite treatment to reduce intracranial pressure, and recovery after surgery.

consciousness, preferring to have longhand descriptions of a patient's state at each observation. Such records are often of doubtful legibility and reliability, and nurses have welcomed the more formal scale and chart as a means of saving time. Also, because their records are so clear, and thus readily reviewed, nurses become stimulated to make observations frequently and reliably. The use of the scale does not preclude writing a more complete description of the patient at less frequent intervals, for example, once per nursing shift. Its use also encourages a consistent attitude towards observing and recording, an advantage as the personnel caring for a patient changes throughout the day.

Reliability of Observations

When observations are made by different people it is important to take into account the possibility of inter-observer variability. This can arise from a number of sources: differences in methods of examining patients; differences in interpretation of terms; as well as being due to a real change in the state of the patient. We have carried out studies in which groups of observers examined the same patients and recorded their findings (Teasdale et al., 1978). We found that the Glasgow scale was more reliable than a simple, hierarchical division of consciousness into different levels and also when compared with such traditional terms as 'decerebrate' and 'decorticate'. What was also important was that junior doctors and nurses were as reliable as experienced neurosurgeons in using the scale. These studies showed that, if the single observations of two different observers are compared and there is a difference of one point on any part of the scale, there can be a 30 per cent chance of this being due merely to inter-observer variability. However, if the discrepancy between observations is by 2 or more points, the likelihood of there being a real difference is then increased and the chance of its being due to variability is only 12 per cent. When the same observer re-examines a patient, or when consistent recordings are made by different observers, the 'significance' attached to any change is even greater. The Glasgow scale has been widely adopted and has been found to be a reliable method of detecting deterioration after head injury and of identifying the onset of complications.

'Best' Response versus Focal Neurological Signs

The use of the best verbal response and best motor response in the scale for conscious level has a double significance. If a patient's performance varies during an examination, improving as stimulation is continued or repeated, it is the optimum level of performance which is recorded. This is important in achieving consistent assessments. The second point is that assessments are made as far as possible excluding the effects of focal neurological damage. Of course any of the responses may be affected by focal neurological injury rather than being depressed because of an overall impairment of brain function. Thus the eyes may be closed by swelling or by a third nerve palsy, speech may be lost as a consequence of dominant hemisphere damage and dysphasia, and focal hemisphere damage may impair the motor response on one side or the other. These can be important features, particularly in localizing the site of an intracranial complication or in indicating its expansion, but such 'focal' signs should be seen separately from the assessment of the overall level of cerebral function. A note should be made of any complicating local factors and also whether there is an iatrogenic cause for the assessment being clouded, e.g. intubation, tracheostomy or even paralysis for the purpose of artificial ventilation.

The extent of examination for possible focal signs depends upon the degree of co-operation from the patient. In the unconscious patient, assessment may be largely limited to comparing the responses of the two sides of the body and eliciting pupillary and other brainstem reflexes (Plum and Posner, 1972). The information derived from focal neurological signs is of two kinds. The first relates to the specific part of the brain which is damaged. Thus the early signs of a developing supratentorial haematoma are usually weakness in the contralateral limbs, and dysphasia if the dominant hemisphere is involved; characteristic localizing signs are unusual with a clot in the posterior fossa, unless evolution is prolonged, e.g. over several days. Secondly, focal neurological signs may be produced also as a non-specific consequence of shift of the brain. This causes focal compression and ischaemia at the sites of herniation. Herniation through the tentorium cerebelli is characterized by changes in the pupils which almost always occur first on the same side as the developing haematoma. A hemiplegia may develop as a result of compression of the brainstem against the tentorium but the side on which this occurs may be the opposite to the haematoma (Kernohan's notch). Impaired eye movements can be a useful sign of herniation at the tentorium and also of brainstem damage; they can be detected in the unconscious patient by making use of oculo-cephalic or oculo-vestibular reflexes. A sixth nerve palsy, so well described as a false localizing sign in raised intracranial pressure due to cerebral tumour, is hardly even seen as such after head injuries. When, very occasionally, bilateral sixth nerve palsies are seen they are usually the result of damage to the nerves at the time of injury.

Assessment of Vital Signs

Observations of such features as pulse, blood pressure, respiration and temperature, have been given undue prominence in the past. One reason for this may have been the failure to appreciate that in clinical practice, cardiovascular abnormalities appear only very late in the course of an expanding intracranial lesion. It cannot be overemphasized that the bradycardia and elevation of blood pressure described by Cushing (1902) as a response to increased intracranial pressure are seen clinically only when brain damage is extremely severe. Sometimes the explanation for a delay in seeking neurosurgical advice about a deteriorating patient was that there had been no change in blood pressure! Troupp (1975) in a series of 50 patients, noted that changes in cardiovascular function preceded changes in consciousness on only one occasion and then only by 15 minutes. Progressive hypotension after head injury is rarely a reflection of brain damage, except at a terminal stage when all vital functions are failing. The presence of hypotension is a signal to seek for the site of bleeding elsewhere in the body (Illingworth and Jennett, 1965). Similarly, disorders of respiratory pattern are common in head injured patients but are most often a reflection of pulmonary abnormalities and thus a response to hypoxic drive, rather than being useful indications of brain function.

The main reason that observing cardiovascular and respiratory function is important is the brain's extreme vulnerability to ischaemia and hypoxia. Clinical observations of 'vital signs' is sufficient to detect abnormalities in more patients. Heart rate can be obtained from monitoring the ECG, and respiratory rate from impedance recording as used for apnoea monitors. But even when these provide a digital reading there is still a need for some form of data recording and summarization, and there is evidence that nursing records can be more sensitive to important changes in a patient's condition than those derived entirely mechanically (Taylor, 1975). Nurses exercise their judgement when making records and filter out some of the background 'noise' which results from insignificant fluctuations in a patient's condition. Routine monitoring of intra-arterial pressure and central venous pressure cannot be justified alone by their contributions to the management of the injured brain, unless major extracranial injuries have compromised cardiovascular function.

Frequency of Observation

A question often raised concerns the frequency with which observations should be made. The answer clearly varies from patient to patient and from time to time. In the first few hours after injury observations may be needed several times in any hour. This is particularly so if the patient already had evidence of impaired consciousness when first seen because this substantially increases the risk of a haematoma developing within the subsequent 48 hours (Galbraith and Smith, 1976). A report from Birmingham (Buxton, 1978) discusses 86 patients who underwent craniotomy for a suspected intracranial haematoma and came to similar conclusions. The majority of patients were in coma when admitted and surgery was performed within a short time. Also, in the 30 cases where the indication for surgery was progressive deterioration in conscious level, none of the patients had a normal conscious level at the time of admission.

Some have questioned whether patients with slight head injuries involving no skull fracture or alteration in conscious level need to be admitted to hospital for observation (Galbraith et al., 1977). When the policy of a unit is to admit such people, it seems unnecessary to insist upon wakening them unduly frequently.

Analysing Clinical Records: Comparing Patients
There is often a need to compress the mass of data accumulated in the course of routine clinical management. This may be for the purpose of reviewing a single case or for comparing the results of treatment of series of head injuries.

The coding of data from the clinical records is simplified by allocating each component of the coma scale a number, successively higher for more normal responses. The scores for each of the three responses can then be summed into an overall score, which ranges from 3 (no eye, verbal or motor responses) to 15 (spontaneous eye opening, orientated and obeying commands). This has proved a useful device in comparing and contrasting groups of patients even though there are theoretical reservations about its validity. We do not recommend using a 'coma score' as a means of exchanging information about the progress of an individual clinical case. The state of a head injured patient is an evolving one and we have found it useful to record the extent of change which takes place in successive epochs. Thus we note both the best and worst states exhibited in the first day; in the second and third days; in the remainder of the first week; and so on.

The course of recovery can be plotted using the best coma score in successive epochs (*Fig. 5.4*). This method is more useful and practicable than recording the state at any given time, e.g. on admission, or 24 hours after injury, or the average over a given period.

In one large study coma was defined using the Glasgow scale, as no eye opening, no verbal response and not obeying commands. A severe head injury was described as one followed by coma for six hours (Jennett et al., 1977). As well as demonstrating that the characteristics of severely head injured patients were very similar in different centres, this study also showed that it was possible to predict the outcome of individual patients on the basis of their clinical features within the first few days of injury (Jennett et al., 1976).

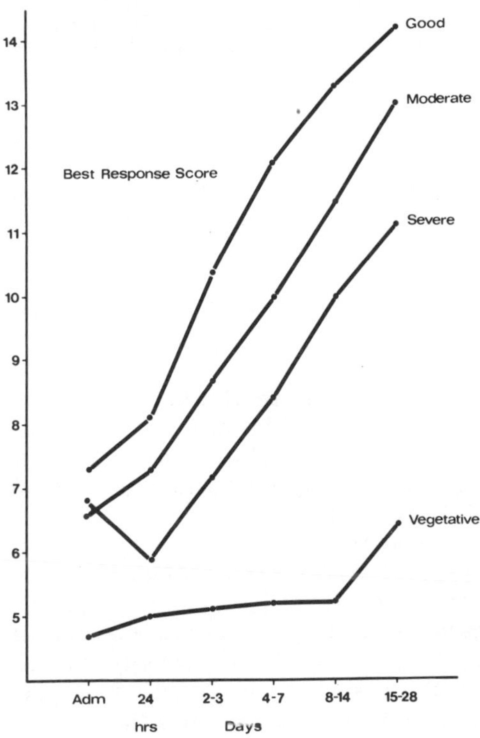

Fig. 5.4. The rate of recovery in head injury survivors with different outcomes. The mean score for responsiveness, on the Glasgow scale, in each group is shown for successive epochs.

INVESTIGATIONS

Computerized Tomography after Head Injury

Hounsfield, working at EMI, developed a method of analysing data regarding the amount an X-ray beam becomes attenuated in its passage across the head, to produce cross-sectional pictures of the brain and skull. The technique is known as computerized tomography (CT scan), and was introduced into clinical practice by Ambrose (1973) and Hounsfield (1973). Its value in detecting intracranial haematomas was soon recognized.

An acute intracranial haematoma usually shows as an area of abnormally increased density in the scan, accompanied by shift of the mid-line. Doubt about the presence of a haematoma is extremely rare (Galbraith et al., 1976). Extradural, subdural and intracerebral haematomas have characteristic patterns and in more than 80 per cent of patients an accurate diagnosis of the type of haematoma present can be made before operation. A restless patient presents difficulties because good quality scans cannot be obtained if a patient moves during scanning. With the early models we found it necessary to anaesthetize the majority of severely head injured patients but find this is required much less now that technical developments have reduced the scanning time for a single slice to as little as one minute.

It may seem difficult to regard the performance of an elaborate and expensive radiological investigation in the same light as making repeated observations of simple clinical features. Yet one of the advantages of computer tomography is that its lack of invasiveness makes it much more feasible to repeat than was the case with angiography. Also it has become feasible to advise investigation in patients who are not deteriorating, and it has become clear that in some of these patients it will show an intracranial haematoma.

Although many such patients are able to compensate for the presence of the lesion, others deteriorate and require surgery. In these latter patients therefore, the early identification of the presence of the clot, by means of a CT scan, offers the best opportunity for minimizing secondary brain damage resulting from the clot. Neurosurgeons are not yet agreed whether this is done by operating upon all patients in whom a haematoma is detected, or only upon cases in whom subsequent clinical events declare the need for surgery.

We have explored an expectant policy in a series of patients in Glasgow (Teasdale et al., 1978). Surgery became necessary in only 40 per cent but the management of the whole group was difficult and not without morbidity. At present we believe that a conservative approach is justified in the presence of a CT scan diagnosis of an intracranial haematoma if the patient has never shown signs of deterioration. In these cases we monitor intracranial pressure and, if this is high, advise early surgery. Although it is not clear yet whether the results of this approach will prove to be an improvement upon the past, we now have to face the possibility that selected groups of head injured patients will have to undergo CT scanning on a more or less routine basis. French and Dublin (1977) have already shown that simple clinical criteria can be used to indicate the likelihood of a patient having an abnormal CT scan (Table 5.2). Several other studies have also shown that between a third to a half of all head injured patients in coma have an intracranial haematoma whatever method of investigation is employed (Pagni, 1973; Becker et al., 1977). The number of patients to be scanned, and whether scanning is best done in the accident departments of the general hospitals to which the patient is first admitted, or after transfer to the regional neurosurgical unit are questions which will have to be answered in future.

It seems likely that for some time to come the expense and scarcity of facilities will mean that scanning will be carried out largely within regional neurosurgical centres. These may now have to accept a greater number of

Table 5.2. Incidence of Abnormalities in Computer Tomographic Scans of Head Injured Patients (French and Dublin, 1977)

Clinical Findings		Abnormal scans (per cent)
Impaired consciousness	Focal deficit	
—	—	13
Present	—	35
—	Present	50
Present	Present	85

head injuries than in the past, even if only for a short period for the purposes of scanning, returning the patient to the referring unit if the investigation is negative.

Monitoring Intracranial Pressure
Physiopathology
Cerebral perfusion pressure (CPP) is defined as the difference between cerebral arterial pressure and intracranial venous pressure. For practical purposes a close approximation is the difference between systemic arterial pressure (SAP) and intracranial pressure (ICP).

$$CPP = SAP - ICP$$

The level of cerebral blood flow (CBF) also depends upon the resistance of the cerebral vasculature (CVR).

$$CBF \, \alpha \, CPP/CVR$$

Normally, the brain's resistance vessels dilate and constrict to maintain a constant blood flow over a wide range of changes in cerebral perfusion pressure. After head injury these adaptive changes are usually impaired, rendering the brain vulnerable to ischaemic damage from any drop in perfusion pressure, whether as a result of systemic hypotension or raised intracranial pressure.

Recent interest in intracranial pressure is charted in the Proceedings of a series of International Symposia (Brock and Dietz, 1972; Lundberg et al., 1975; Beks et al., 1976) and references to monitoring after head injury are frequent.

Intracranial pressure may be measured at several points. It is the local pressure within the cerebral tissue which is important in determining perfusion, but, in practice this is almost the same as the pressure within the cerebrospinal fluid (CSF), at least within the same intracranial compartment. The rate at which CSF is formed (approximately 0·3 ml/min in man) is relatively constant, irrespective of changes in pressure. The level of intracranial pressure is thus determined by a hydraulic component: the degree of resistance to the egress of CSF from the intracranial cavity, and by a visco-elastic component; the distensibility of the walls of the CSF pathways and also by volume of the CSF. The visco-elastic component is altered by changes in blood volume, blood pressure and brain water content and is reflected by the compliance of the CSF pathways, often called the 'stiffness' of the brain. In explaining raised ICP, the biophysical balance sheet is still incomplete and there is evidence that both increased resistance to flow and absorption and increased brain 'stiffness' can be involved after head injury (Marmarou et al., 1976).

One important factor determining the level of intracranial pressure is the balance between the size of an expanding lesion and the volume of the other intracranial contents; as a lesion expands there is a compensatory reduction in the volume of other intracranial constituents, particularly the CSF. A rise in intracranial pressure may therefore be because the lesion has increased in size or it may be due to a relative reduction in the capacity for compensatory changes. Conversely, a reduction of intracranial pressure may be achieved by evacuating the offending lesion or by enhancing

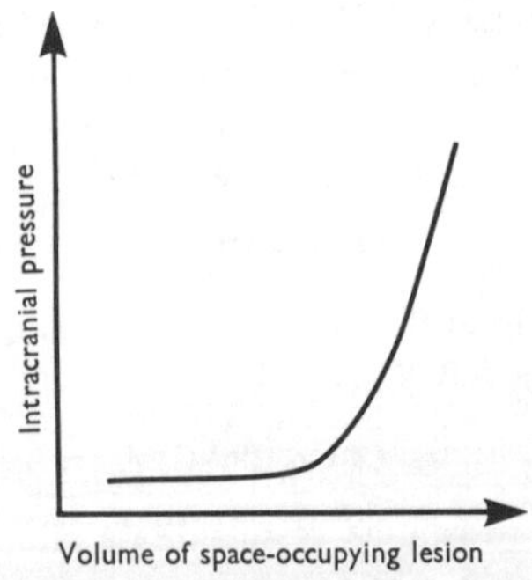

Fig. 5.5. Progressive increase in intracranial pressure during expansion of an intracranial lesion.

compensatory reserve. Experimentally, as an intracranial lesion is expanded there is an initial phase when pressure rises only slightly but then, as compensation becomes exhausted, the increase becomes exponential (Langfitt, 1969) (*Fig. 5.5*). The increase in pressure per unit volume change is a measure of the overall compliance or its inverse, the elastance of the system and this indicates the 'tightness' of the brain. The 'tighter' the brain the more likely is a precipitous rise in intracranial pressure from any additional stress. This is the basis of clinical testing of volume/pressure relationships (Miller, 1975).

If the exact mechanisms responsible for bringing about elevations of intracranial pressure, whether continuous or intermittent, are still arguable, it is relatively easy to list the factors which can be responsible for raised intracranial pressure, and the corresponding ways in which it may be lowered (Table 5.3).

Table 5.3. Causes of Raised Intracranial Pressure and methods of treatment

Cause of raised intracranial pressure	Mechanism	Specific treatment
Intracranial Mass		
Haematoma	Space-occupation	Evacuate
Abscess		Drain
Cerebral Engorgement		
Hypoxia	Increased	Oxygenate
Hypercarbia	CBF	Ensure Ventilation
Halogenated Anaesthetics	or	Avoid
Cerebral Activity	CBV	Sedate?
Coughing	Impaired	
Head down tilt	Venous	Avoid or
Neck compression	Drainage,	Correct
Physiotherapy	Increased	
Badly adjusted ventilator	CBV	
Cerebral Oedema		
Hypoxia/ischaemia		
Hyperthermia	Increased	Prevent or
Hypertension	Tissue	Correct
Status epilepticus	Water	
Associated with haematomas		? Steroids
'Traumatic oedema'		mannitol
Hydrocephalus		
Posterior fossa clot	Increased	Drain
Arachnoidal fibrosis	CSF volume	Shunt

Also irrespective of the specific cause, intracranial pressure can be lowered even if only temporarily, by any measure which affects a relative reduction in the volume of any component of the intracranial contents (James et al., 1977) (Table 5.4).

Continuous Monitoring of Intracranial Pressure

There are many different methods for measuring intracranial pressure. The main variations are in the site where intracranial pressure is sensed and the location of the device by which pressure is transduced to provide electrical

Table 5.4 General Methods for Lowering Intracranial Pressure

Reduce volume of CSF	Ventricular drain / Inhibit CSF production
Reduced cerebral blood volume	Hyperventilation / Depress metabolism
Reduce brain water content	Osmotics (e.g. mannitol) / Diuretics (e.g. frusemide)
Increase effective size of cranial cavity	Decompressive Craniectomy

signals. Brain tissue measurements are of experimental interest only and clinically intracranial pressure has been measured from the ventricles, and from the subarachnoid, subdural and extradural spaces. The use of intraventricular pressure measurements in head injury was popularized by Lundberg (1965) and this method is widely regarded as being the most reliable for routine use. A burr hole or twist drill hole is made in the right frontal region, anterior to the coronal suture and in the line of the pupil. A plastic catheter is directed perpendicularly downwards towards the bridge of the nose; penetration of the ventricle is signalled by a sudden increase then drop in resistance. The catheter is then connected to a pressure transducer. Recording over a pressure range of 0–100 mmHg is most useful, greater ranges very rarely being required. If intracranial pressure is not high an ability to record a lower range can be useful in increasing the sensitivity. Systems providing only the choice of venous (0–30 mmHg) or arterial ranges (0–300 mmHg) of pressure are not convenient.

An alternative method of obtaining ventricular pressure measurements is to connect the catheter to a subcutaneous reservoir. This is then punctured percutaneously. This method may have some advantages when measurements are being made intermittently over a long period but we have not found that it reduces complications or confers advantages for acute monitoring.

The pressure from cortical subarachnoid or subdural space can be measured simply by means of a rigid but hollow device which fits into a precisely matched hole in the skull. In the most commonly used form, this is a hollow metal screw (Vries et al., 1973). This screw is then connected to a pressure transducer in the same way as for a ventricular catheter. Another simple alternative is to introduce a semi-rigid plastic catheter, as used for ventricular measuring, into the subdural space.

The advantages of intraventricular measurements lie in their accuracy and the possibility of either withdrawing CSF to reduce pressure or making minute additions in order to assess elasticity (Miller et al., 1973). Among the disadvantages are the occasional difficulty in locating the ventricle in a head injured patient and rare examples of haemorrhage along the catheter track. The most serious risk is of infection; although this has been reported in only 1 per cent of cases (Sundbärg et al., 1972) most experienced users admit to a rate of 3–5 per cent (Rosner and Becker, 1976; Jennett, 1976). The chance of infection seems to increase with the number of times the system is manipulated and the duration of monitoring. It may also be increased by concurrent administration of steroids. Monitoring subarachnoid or subdural pressure avoids the risks of brain puncture but, if intracranial pressure is high, and the system not completely watertight, brain may be extruded into the screw and the consequent blockage results in loss of the tracings. Another disadvantage is the inability to withdraw CSF. The risks of infection appear to be similar with both methods and this has led some workers to favour measurements of pressure from the extradural space.

Extradural pressure measurements are usually made by inserting a transducer so that the diaphragm is applied to the dura. Measurements made this way have been shown to approximate to intradural pressure but there may be a time lag before this is achieved. It is also important that the transducer lies absolutely flat on the dura (Dorsch and Symon, 1975) otherwise stresses and strains in the dura can distort the measurements. Perhaps the major problem with extradural pressure measurements, as with all implanted pressure-sensitive devices, is electronic; i.e. the possibility of a drift from the base-line. Unless this can be checked and recalibration carried out, erroneous readings may be obtained.

Recording and Display

A continuous record is important and is most easily obtained by means of a calibrated chart recorder. This should be run sufficiently rapidly to detect and analyse transient changes in pressure but not so fast that an indigestible mountain of paper results. Most of the useful information can be obtained by rapid visual review of the tracing. Some workers record the data electronically and process it to produce frequency distributions showing the proportion of any period during which intracranial pressure lay in any particular range.

Normal intracranial pressure is about 10 mmHg. It has pulsatile components reflecting heart beat and respiration and may show transient increases to extremely high levels as when intrathoracic pressure changes in coughing and in straining. A high level of intracranial pressure may occur as a sustained phenomenon but wave-like elevations are also common. The most sinister of these is the so-called 'plateau wave' (Lundberg, 1960), but these are relatively uncommon after head injury. It is the intermittent wave-like way in which intracranial pressure may be elevated which makes continuous monitoring imperative.

Raised Intracranial Pressure after Head Injury

Definition

Johnston et al. (1970) suggested that intracranial pressure levels above 20 mmHg could be regarded as moderately elevated, and sustained levels above 40 mmHg as severely elevated. This view is supported by Miller (1978b) but the levels quoted have varied in different series, making comparisons difficult (Langfitt, 1976).

Incidence

So numerous are the factors which can raise intracranial pressure after head injury that its presence is not surprising when severely injured patients are monitored. In one study, more than 75 per cent of patients in coma at the time of admission to hospital had raised intracranial pressure (defined as over 15 mmHg) (Miller et al., 1977). In this study elevation of pressure was almost invariable amongst patients who had space-occupying intracranial complications, the only exceptions being patients who had CSF leaks through basal skull fractures. Even after the intracranial haematoma was evacuated, raised intracranial pressure continued to be a problem in 50 per cent of these patients. In the absence of an intracranial haematoma, raised intracranial pressure is uncommon; even among patients in coma it is present in only a third and the level is rarely more than moderately elevated (Fleischer et al., 1976; Miller et al., 1977).

Significance

Despite its frequency, the meaning of raised intracranial pressure after head injury is much debated; does brain damage cause raised intracranial pressure, or does raised intracranial pressure cause brain damage? Miller (1978b) concluded that the answer, unsatisfactorily, to both questions, was 'yes'. Sometimes raised intracranial pressure may merely reflect the swelling of an already damaged brain. Moreover, although raised intracranial pressure can certainly sometimes reduce, even halt, cerebral perfusion and so damage the brain by ischaemia, it is the belief of most investigators that the rate of cerebral blood flow in head injured patients does *not* show a close relationship to the level of intracranial pressure (Langfitt, 1976).

In head injured patients who have only diffuse brain damage (i.e. no intracranial mass or haematoma) raised intracranial pressure may be mostly a reflection of the severity of the brain damage. Certainly some studies (Fleischer et al., 1976; Miller et al., 1977) have shown that both the incidence and the level of raised intracranial pressure correlate with such patients' clinical state. An elevated pressure is associated with clinical evidence of more profound damage to the brain in the early stages, and with a worse eventual outcome. Yet it is possible for a very severe degree of diffuse white matter damage to be sustained without any evidence of raised intracranial pressure, either during the course of clinical monitoring (Johnston et al., 1970), or when the brain is examined at autopsy (Adams et al., 1977). The reasons for this discrepancy are not clear.

In some patients there is little doubt that a rise in intracranial pressure is associated with or even precedes evidence of clinical deterioration and intracranial herniation. But it can be questioned again whether the change of intracranial pressure is just another sign, although an early one, of a worsening intracranial situation.

Perhaps the patients in whom there might be least doubt that raised intracranial pressure can be a mechanism resulting in brain damage, are those with intracranial haematomas. The effect of intracranial pressure on blood flow will depend upon the simultaneous level of systemic arterial pressure (and thus the cerebral perfusion pressure) and upon whether the mechanisms of autoregulation have been disturbed. When systemic arterial pressure is in the normal range an increase of intracranial pressure above 40 mmHg is usually associated with decline in blood flow, even in a previously normal brain. It is interesting that an intracranial pressure above this threshold was associated with an increasingly severe clinical state in a series of patients with intracranial mass lesions (Miller et al., 1977). But even in patients with an intracranial haematoma there is no level of intracranial pressure which can be regarded as always being significant, either from the point of view of causing a reduction in cerebral blood flow or as an indication of a particular degree of brain shift (Miller and Pickard, 1974). It may be that the overall level of cerebral blood flow falls only at a very advanced stage of cerebral compression and that before this stage has been reached, distortion and shift of the brain are the most significant mechanisms. At an early stage compensatory mechanisms may prevent more than a minimal rise in intracranial pressure and it is here that measures of brain 'tightness' can help. Miller and Pickard (1974) found a correlation between an abnormal volume/pressure response and mid-line shift in head injured patients.

Value of Measuring Intracranial Pressure after Head Injury
Jennett (1972) defined three roles for intracranial pressure measurements: (1) in diagnosis; (2) in prognosis; and (3) in determining the treatment and subsequently its effectiveness.

After head injury, intracranial pressure measurements have, at the most, a subsidiary part in the diagnosis of complications such as an intracranial haematoma. This is especially so when CT scanning is available and used routinely. After initial negative studies, the development of a space-occupying lesion is uncommon, but a rise of intracranial pressure in a patient made inaccessible to clinical examination by reason of sedation or relexants can indicate the need for repeated studies. Prognostically a high intracranial pressure is bad. Yet only at very extreme levels, found in a minority of patients, does it reliably indicate irretrievable brain damage. Moreover, about a third of the mortality and severe morbidity after head injury is amongst patients with little or no increase in pressure (Langfitt, 1976).

The contribution of continuous intracranial pressure measurements to clinical practice must be judged by the difference it makes to the treatment and the outcome of the monitored patient, and it is here that evidence is least conclusive and opinions most conflicting. It is necessary to make a distinction between the undoubted contribution of intracranial pressure measurements to our concepts and understanding of brain damage; once a particular measure has been shown to promote, or conversely to reduce, raised intracranial pressure it may not be necessary to continue demonstrating the effect, before taking appropriate action. Intracranial haematomas can be evacuated, abscesses can be drained, and hypoxia, hypercarbia, hypotension and other causes of cerebral engorgement can be prevented or specifically remedied without ever having to demonstrate that the patient has raised intracranial pressure. It has even been suggested that the early administration of high doses of steroids ($>$ 100 mg dexamethasone in the first day) can prevent increases in intracranial pressure due to oedema in the damaged brain (Reulen et al., 1975; Gobiet, 1977) but more recent evidence is against this being true.

Much of the debate centres upon the value of non-specific treatment aimed at reducing raised intracranial pressure, rather than eliminating its origin: profound hyperventilation; osmotics (e.g. mannitol) and other diuretics; or the use of barbiturate-induced cerebral depression. There are hazards with each of these methods and they should be considered only if intracranial pressure measurements are being used to show that the level is indeed high and continued only if measurements show it has responded to treatment. However, in a large collaborative study of head injury (Jennett et al., 1977), intracranial pressure measurements were recorded in 21 per cent of patients in one centre; in the other centres they were performed in only 5 per cent. There is no evidence that the increased use of intra-cranial measurements, or the additional use of steroids, ventilation and diuretics in the first centre, led to patients having better prognoses. Apparently at variance with this observation are reports from other centres of intensive management regimens which may improve upon the overall results of the collaborative study (Becker et al., 1977). The criteria for inclusion in each study and the basis for such comparisons need careful scrutiny. Moreover, measurement of intracranial pressure on a routine basis has been only one component of the 'intensive' regimens. Studies of head injured children (Gobiet et al., 1976) have attributed improved outcomes to the measurement of intracranial pressure and the treatment of abnormalities, but the events taking place in the brain of a head injured child may be at variance with those in the adult. There is no conclusive evidence that, by itself, intracranial pressure measurement can substantially affect the outcome of a head injured patient. It would probably be un-realistic to expect so.

In whom then, might intracranial pressure measurements be useful? Amongst patients who do not have impaired consciousness, the risk of a haematoma or other intracranial complication is small. Even enthusiasts monitor only as a routine patients who are not obeying commands, and some monitor only those not localizing painful stimuli. In contrast, because of the frequency of raised intracranial pressure after evacuation of an intradural haematoma (subdural or intracerebral) this may prove to be the circumstance where measurements are of greatest value, provided that effective treatments can be based upon their findings. In the absence of a haematoma the return from pressure measurement is debatable and Fleischer et al. (1976) considered that there might be no reason to monitor a head injured patient once the presence of an intracranial mass had been excluded.

In deciding whether to recommend that a particular unit should be monitoring intracranial pressure, its own particular circumstances, the personnel available and the sort of patient encountered will usually indicate what is appropriate. The degree of expertise needed to manage intracranial pressure monitoring and especially to interpret and to act upon its results should not be underestimated. Experienced users share reservations about recommending that intracranial pressure is instituted either solely for use in head injured patients or in a unit in which the necessary neurosurgical and neuroanaesthetic expertise are not immediately available throughout the day and the night. Even those enthusiastic about its use believe that it should probably be restricted to neurosurgical centres (Miller et al., 1977) where many other reasons for monitoring and treating intracranial pressure will be found.

Electrophysiological Assessment of Brain Function

The development of computerized methods for processing electro-physiological data has given new impetus to the study of cerebral electrical potentials. Interest in investigating the electrical activity of the brain after head injury has been stimulated by the hope that the results might prove more 'objective', more sensitive and thus more reliable than clinical examination. It has yet to be shown that this is true. There are two main alternatives: recording the spontaneous electroencephalogram or eliciting evoked electrocerebral responses.

Electroencephalography

Standard electroencephalographic (EEG) methods have been used in head injured patients for many years and the results of serial observations were reported nearly thirty years ago (Dawson et al., 1951). Slowing in the EEG in general correlated with severity of injury, but individual patterns are extremely varied. A developing intracranial haematoma can show increased unilateral slow wave activity; suppression of amplitude or increased generalized slow waves, which may be rhythmic or arrhythmic. Intra-cerebral haematomas may produce few specific EEG features. The EEG changes may result from the pressure of the haematoma on the adjacent cortex but rhythmic slow waves can also be a feature of brainstem compression. Unfortunately, changes due to a haematoma are often masked by non-specific effects resulting from the impairment of consciousness.

Practical considerations impose severe limitations: recording is difficult in the restless patient; scalp lacerations may require unconventional electrode replacement, and this can suggest a spurious asymmetry; scalp oedema or haematoma may reduce the voltage of the records; and pulsations in the scalp can produce artefactual slow waves. For these reasons alone an experienced technician should be present during the recording as the interpretation of the record also requires expertise.

It is now possible, by means of a computer, to analyse the spectrum of frequencies within the EEG and also to integrate the voltage within a record. These may provide a quantitative index of electrocortical activity but the acquisition of the original data is subject to the same problems as in the ordinary EEG; as yet there is no report which would indicate that these methods are of value in head injury care. The development of an intracranial haematoma is often associated on the one hand with slowing of the EEG, and on the other hand with an increase in amplitude of individual waves, therefore it is important that these aspects are studied separately. Integration of the two components to an overall index of cerebral function could obscure changes.

The standard EEG has found little place in the routine care of head injuries other than in the hands of a few devotees, and recent interest has centred upon the electrocerebral events which occur in response to specific sensory stimuli.

Evoked Cerebral Potentials
Potentials evoked by Sensory Stimuli

Applying a suitable stimulus to a sensory peripheral or cranial nerve results in changes in cerebral electrical potential. These can be detected by means of scalp electrodes. The potential changes produced by a single stimulus are obscured in the background EEG, but the potentials resulting from a sequence of stimuli can be stored and averaged by computer. The resulting waveforms usually consist of a number of peaks of characteristic height and latency. Evoked responses currently employed include visual, auditory and somatosensory responses.

The same technical factors need to be taken account of as for the EEG. Also it is necessary to establish that the peripheral sensory organ is intact before assuming that abnormal potentials are a reflection of central nervous system damage.

Larson et al. (1973) demonstrated the feasibility of studying evoked responses in head injured patients and Greenberg et al. (1977) have reported the findings in 51 patients with severe head injury. Abnormalities in evoked potentials were frequent and correlated with the presence of clinical abnormalities and also with outcome. Abnormalities in those components of the responses which reflect the function of cerebral hemispheres were found more often than were abnormalities indicative of brainstem dysfunction. This is consistent with current views that the cerebral hemispheres are more vulnerable to damage than the brainstem, whether from diffuse impact forces or secondary hypoxia.

An important question, as yet unresolved, concerns the ability of electrophysiological studies to provide warning, as distinct from providing an indication that brain damage has become established. Symon et al. (1977) has shown that change in the amplitude of the somatosensory evoked response (SER) is maintained until cerebral blood flow falls to a critical threshold level, beyond which there is an abrupt loss of potential. Although this is somewhat above the level necessary to produce ischaemic damage, the absence of premonitory changes limits the use of the SER as an index of the adequacy of cerebral perfusion.

Sensory evoked electrocortical responses offer a non-invasive method of assessing the integrity of central nervous system pathways in a more direct way than clinical observations. Aside from their practical limitations, which may be lessened by technical developments, a number of questions need to be answered before they can be recommended for routine use. Do they afford any more information that can be obtained by clinical methods? Will they show progressive changes, either during deterioration or recovery? Will they ever be more than a research procedure or will they be sufficiently reliable for use in selected patients? One instance when they may be useful is when muscle relaxants and central nervous system depressants have been given and the patient has been rendered inaccessible to clinical examination.

We find it impossible, with present techniques, to carry out a comprehensive examination of the full range of potentials in less than two hours. Technical developments may improve upon this and reduce the cost, which at present is several thousand pounds for the equipment to have the capacity to monitor even a single patient.

Direct Cortical Response

A progressive change, over a wider range of blood flow than that over which the SER is lost, is seen in the responsiveness of the cerebral cortex to an electrical stimulus applied directly to its surface. This direct electro-cortical response is obtained by stimulating one point on the cortex and recording a few millimetres away on the same gyrus. Its disappearance occurs at levels of blood flow similar to those at which the SER and EEG disappear but studies in animals have shown that this is preceded by a progressive decline in the amplitude of the response as cerebral blood flow falls below normal (Teasdale et al., 1977). The need to stimulate the cortex means that the direct response is likely to be useful only in limited circumstances, for example, after the evacuation of an intracranial haematoma. The use of the response after head injury has not been reported but its decline and subsequent recovery has been observed when cerebral blood flow has been altered by hypotension during the course of surgery for intracranial aneurysms (*Fig. 5.6*).

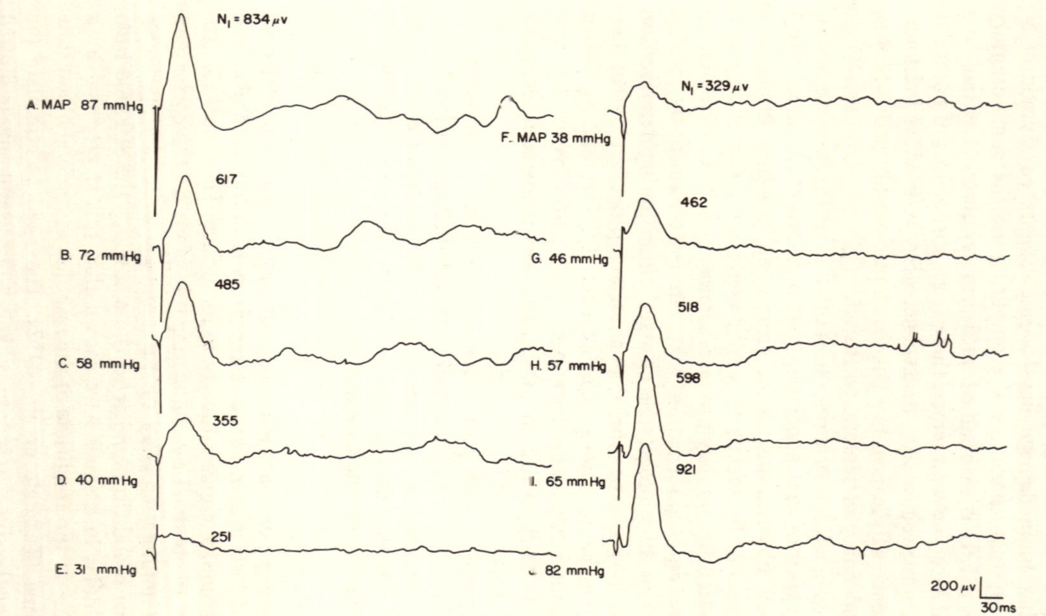

Fig. 5.6. Decline in direct electrical response of human cerebral cortex during hypotension. The patient was undergoing surgery for an intracranial aneurysm. Traces A—E show reduction in the amplitude of the response when cerebral pressure was lowered from a mean of 87 mmHg to a mean of 31 mmHg. Traces F—J show the subsequent recovery of the response when blood pressure, and presumably cerebral blood flow, were restored. (*By kind permission of the 'Journal of Neurosurgery'.*)

CONCLUSIONS

Head injury management still depends largely upon the clinical assessment of changes in conscious level and other aspects of responsiveness. The observations made by nurses and junior medical staff remain the cheapest, simplest and perhaps the most reliable way of monitoring head injured patients. The investment of both financial resources and personnel associated with some of the recent technological approaches to monitoring the function of the brain are such that their contribution needs to be better defined before they are widely adopted. At present the value of intracranial pressure measurement is still controversial, and there are formidable barriers to the use of evoked potentials to monitor all but a few patients in a few extremely specialized units. By contrast, the value of CT scanning of head injured patients is so clear that it is necessary to reappraise the means by which patients with an intracranial haematoma are identified.

When the detection of the presence of an intracranial haematoma depends solely upon clinical evidence of deteriorating responsiveness there is a danger that some patients may deteriorate so far that irretrievable secondary brain damage can ensue. The relative safety, simplicity and reliability of CT scanning raises the possibility that it might be used to screen large numbers of head injured patients in a way which was never practical nor even justifiable with angiography. By giving warning of the presence of the haematoma, before deterioration has occurred, screening by means of CT scanning might improve outcome. It is clearly not feasible to screen each of the many thousands of head injuries at present admitted to hospital. Fortunately, it is possible to select groups of patients for scanning, on the basis of simple clinical criteria to increase the yield of positive scans. The group of patients who seem to be most at risk of harbouring an intracranial haematoma are those with impaired consciousness; about 50 per cent of patients in coma after head injury have a significant intracranial haematoma.

Questions such as who should care for head injuries? (Jennett, 1975), What is an appropriate number of scanners? and Where should they be sited? (Bartlett and Neil-Dwyer, 1978; Bartlett et al., 1978) raised broad issues. But it seems likely that to attempt to manage large numbers of head injured patients without rapid access to CT scanning will come to be regarded as less than adequate provision of care.

REFERENCES

Adams H. (1975) The neuropathology of head injury. In: Vinken P. J. and Bruyn G. W. (eds.), *Handbook of Clinical Neurology*, Vol. 23. Amsterdam, North Holland, pp. 35–65.

Adams H., Mitchell Dorothy E., Graham D. I. et al. (1977) Diffuse brain damage of immediate impact type. Its relationship to 'primary brainstem damage' in head injuries. *Brain* **100**, 489.

Ambrose J. (1973) Computerised transverse axial scanning (tomography). II. Clinical Application. *Br. J. Radiol.* **46**, 1023.

Bartlett J. R. and Neil-Dwyer G. (1978) Clinical study of the EMI scanner: implications for provision of neuroradiological services. *Br. Med. J.* **2**, 813.

Bartlett J. R., Neil-Dwyer G., Banham J. M. M. et al. (1978) Evaluating cost effectiveness of diagnostic equipment: the brain scanner case. *Br. Med. J.* **2**, 815.

Becker D. P., Miller J. D., Ward J. D. et al. (1977) The outcome from severe head injury with early diagnosis and intensive management. *J. Neurosurg.* **47**, 491.

Beks J. W. F., Bosch D. A. and Brock M. (1976) *Intracranial Pressure III.* Berlin, Springer.

Brinkman R., von Cramon D. and Schultz H. (1976) The Munich coma scale. *J. Neurol. Neurosurg. Psychiat.* **39**, 788.

Brock M. and Deitz H. (1972) *Intracranial Pressure.* Berlin, Springer.

Buxton R. A. (1978) Management of the patient with a head injury. *Br. J. Clin. Pract.* **32**, 103.

Cushing H. (1902) Some experimental and clinical observations concerning states of increased intracranial pressure. *Am. J. Med. Sci.* **124**, 375.

Dawson R. E., Webster J. E. and Gurdjian E. S. (1951) Serial electroencephalography in acute head injuries. *J. Neurosurg.* **8**, 613.

Dorsch N. W. C. and Symon L. (1975) The validity of extradural measurements of the intracranial pressure. In: Lundberg N., Ponten U. and Brock M. (ed.), *Intracranial Pressure II.* Berlin, Springer, pp. 403–408.

Feldman M. H. (1971a) The decerebrate study in the primate. I: Studies in the monkeys. *Arch. Neurol.* **25**, 501.

Feldman M. H. (1971b) The decerebrate study in the primate. II: Studies in man. *Arch. Neurol.* **25**, 517.

Fisher C. M. (1969) Neurological examination of the comatose patient. *Acta Neurol. Scand.* **45**, Suppl. 36.

Fleischer A. S., Nettleton S. P. and Tindall G. T. (1976) Continuous monitoring of intracranial pressure in severe closed head injury without mass lesions. *Surg. Neurol.* **6**, 31.

French B. N. and Dublin A. B. (1977). The value of computerised tomography in 1000 consecutive head injuries. *Surg. Neurol.* **7**, 171.

Galbraith S., Murray W. R. and Patel A. R. (1977) Head injury admissions to a teaching hospital. *Scott. Med. J.* **22**, 129.

Galbraith S. and Smith J. (1976) Acute traumatic intracranial haematoma without skull fracture. *Lancet* **1**, 501.

Galbraith S., Teasdale G. and Blaiklock C. (1976) Computerised tomography of acute traumatic intracranial haematomas: reliability of neurosurgeons' interpretations. *Br. Med. J.* **2**, 1371.

Gobiet W., Brock W. J., Liesegang J. et al. (1976) Treatment of acute cerebral oedema with high dose dexamethasone. In: Beks J. W. F., Bosch D. A. and Brock M. (eds.), *Intracranial Pressure III.* Berlin, Springer, pp. 231–325.

Gobiet W. (1977) Advances in management of severe head injury in children. *Acta Neurochir.* **39**, 207.

Greenberg R. P., Becker D. P., Miller J. D. et al. (1977) Evaluation of brain function in severe human head trauma with multimodality evoked potentials. II: Localisation of brain dysfunction and correlation with post-traumatic neurological conditions. *J. Neurosurg.* **47**, 173.

Hounsfield G. N. (1973) Computerised transverse axial scanning (tomography). I: Description of the system. *Br. J. Radiol.* **46**, 1016.

Illingworth C. and Jennett B. (1965) The shocked head injury. *Lancet* **2**, 511.

James H. E., Langfitt T. W., Kumar V. S. et al. (1977) Treatment of intracranial hypertension. Analysis of 105 consecutive continuous records of intracranial pressure. *Acta Neurochir.* **36**, 189.

Jennett B. (1972) Techniques for measuring intracranial pressure. In: Brock M. and Dietz H. (ed.), *Intracranial Pressure*. Berlin, Springer, pp. 365–371.

Jennett B. (1975) Who cares for head injuries? *Br. Med. J.* **3**, 267.

Jennett B. (1976) Closing comments. In: Beks J. W. F., Bosch D. A. and Brock M. (ed.), *Intracranial Pressure III*. Berlin, Springer, pp. 343–346.

Jennett B., Teasdale G., Braakman R. et al. (1976) Predicting outcome in individual patients after severe head injury. *Lancet* **1**, 1031.

Jennett B., Teasdale G., Galbraith S. et al. (1977) Severe head injuries in three countries. *J. Neurol. Neurosurg. Psychiat.* **40**, 291.

Johnston I. H., Johnston J. A. and Jennett B. (1970) Intracranial pressure changes following head injury. *Lancet* **2**, 433.

Langfitt T. W. (1969) Increased intracranial pressure. *Clin. Neurosurg.* **16**, 436.

Langfitt T. W. (1976) The incidence and importance of intracranial hypertension in head injury patients. In: Beks J. W. F., Bosch D. A. and Brock M. (ed.) *Intracranial Pressure III*. Berlin, Springer, pp. 67–72.

Langfitt T. W. (1978) Measuring the outcome from head injuries. *J. Neurosurg.* **48**, 673.

Larson S. J., Sances A., Ackmann J. J. et al. (1972) Non invasive evaluation of head trauma patients. *Surgery* **74**, 34.

Lundberg N. (1960) Continuous recording and control of ventricular fluid pressure in neurosurgical practice. *Acta Psychiat. Scand.* **36**, Suppl. 149.

Lundberg N., Ponten U. and Brock M. (1975) *Intracranial Pressure II*. Berlin, Springer.

Lundberg N., Troupp H. and Lorin H. (1965) Continuous recording of ventricular fluid pressure in patients with severe acute traumatic brain injury. A Preliminary Report. *J. Neurosurg.* **22**, 581.

Marmarou A., Shapiro K. and Shulman K. (1976) Isolation factors leading to sustained elevations of the ICP. In: Beks J. W. F., Bosch D. A. and Brock M. (ed.) *Intracranial Pressure III*. Berlin, Springer. pp. 33–36.

Miller J. D. (1975) Volume and pressure in the craniospinal axis. *Clin. Neurosurg.* **22**, 76.

Miller J. D. (1978a) Personal communication

Miller J. D. (1978b) Intracranial pressure monitoring. *Br. J. Hosp. Med.* **19**, 497.

Miller J. D., Becker D. P., Ward J. D. et al. (1977) Significance of intracranial hypertension in severe head injury. *J. Neurosurg.* **47**, 501.

Miller J. D., Garibi J. and Pickard J. D. (1973) Induced changes of cerebrospinal fluid volume. *Arch. Neurol.* **28**, 265.

Miller J. D. and Pickard J. D. (1974) Intracranial volume/pressure studies in patients with head injury. *Injury* **5**, 265.

Pagni C. A. (1973) The prognosis of head injured patients in a state of coma with decerebrated posture. Analysis of 471 cases. *J. Neurosurg. Sci.* **17**, 4.

Plum F. (1975) State of consciousness scoring system. Comment. *J. Neurosurg.* **43**, 251.

Plum F. and Posner J. B. (1972) *Diagnosis of Stupor and Coma*. 2nd ed. Davis, Philadelphia.

Price D. J. (1976) Analogue to digital conversion of consciousness. *J. Neurol. Neurosurg. Psychiat.* **39**, 919.

Reulen H. J., Graham R. and Klatzo I. (1975) Brain oedema. In: Lundberg N., Ponten U. and Brock M. (ed.), *Intracranial Pressure II*. Berlin, Springer, pp. 233–238.

Rosner M. J. and Becker D. P. (1976) Intracranial Pressure Monitoring: Complications and Associated Factors. In: Keener E. (ed.), *Clinical Neurosurgery*. Baltimore, Williams and Wilkins, pp. 494–519.

Sundbärg G., Kjallquist A., Lundberg N. et al. (1972) Complications due to Prolonged Ventricular Fluid Pressure Recording in Clinical Practice. In: Brock M. and Dietz H. (ed.), *Intracranial Pressure*. Berlin, Springer, pp. 348–352.

Symon L., Branston N. M. and Strong A. J. (1977) Extracellular Potassium Activity, Evoked Potential and rCBF during Experimental Cerebral Ischaemia in the Baboon. In: Ingvar and Lassen. (ed.), *Cerebral Function. Metabolism and Circulation.* Copenhagen, Munksgaard, p. 5.

Taylor D. E. M. (1975) Interaction of Men and Machines in Intensive Care Units. In: Walker A. E. and Taylor D. E. M. (ed.), *Intensive Care.* Churchill Livingstone, Edinburgh, pp. 219–227.

Teasdale G., Galbraith S. and Clarke K. (1975) Acute impairment of brain function. 2. Observation record chart. *Nurs. Times* 71, 972.

Teasdale G., Galbraith S. and Jennett B. (1979) Operate or observe? ICP and the management of the 'silent' traumatic intracranial haematoma. In: Schurmann K., Miller J. D., Hochwald G. and Becker D. (eds.), *Proceedings of the IVth International Symposium on Intracranial Pressure.* New York, Springer Verlag. In the press.

Teasdale G. and Jennett B. (1974) Assessment of coma and impaired consciousness. *Lancet* 2, 81.

Teasdale G., Knill-Jones R. and van der Sande J. (1978) Observer variability in assessing impaired consciousness and coma. *J. Neurol. Neurosurg. Psychiat.* 41, 603.

Teasdale G., Rowan J. O., Turner J. et al. (1977) Cerebral perfusion failure and cortical electrical activity. In: Ingvar D. H. and Lassen N. A. (ed.), *Cerebral Function, Metabolism and Circulation.* Copenhagen, pub. pp. 23.14–23.15.

Troupp H. (1975) Neurological Problems in Trauma: Development of Resources. In: Walker and Taylor (ed.), *Intensive Care.* Churchill Livingstone, Edinburgh, pp. 199–206.

Vries J. K., Becker D. P. and Young H. F. (1973) A subarachnoid screw for monitoring intracranial pressure. *J. Neurosurg.* 39, 416.

T. R. Fisher

6 Microsurgery in the Injured

INTRODUCTION

In 1960 Jacobsen and Suarez wrote an article entitled 'Microsurgery in the anastomosis of small vessels' in which they stated 'Results of arterial surgery have been uniformly poor in vessels below 4 mm in diameter. The reason, it seems to us, is purely technical.' So began the era of microvascular and microneural surgery, with subsequent reports of limb and digit replantation, the free transfer of skin flaps, and free flaps containing composite tissues of skin, muscle, bone and nerve, and fascicular nerve repairs, and interfascicular nerve grafts.

1960–70

The pioneer work on microsurgical techniques undertaken by surgeons and research workers during the decade 1960–70 demonstrated the feasibility of performing the successful anastomosis of small vessels of less than 1 mm in diameter and of repairing injured peripheral nerves by a perineurial suture. The monograph by O'Brien (1977) and the review by Ostrup and Fredrickson (1976) on microvascular surgery have described the work of this period and they have indicated with clinical reports the application of these microsurgical techniques to acutely injured tissues and their use in secondary reconstructive procedures.

1970–78

The last eight years have revealed the relevance of that initial observation. Hayhurst and O'Brien (1975) reporting on an experimental study of the patency rates after microvascular surgery concluded that technical adequacy was the most important factor in ensuring final patency of the vessels. Concurrent with greater surgical expertise has been the improvement in instruments, with the availability of finer needles and suture material (*Fig. 6.1*) and more versatile operating microscopes that allow one or more assistants to view the same operating field as the surgeon (O'Brien, 1977). Experimentally it has been shown that vessels of 0·4–0·5 mm diameter can be anastomosed with an 85–90 per cent patency rate (Fujimaki et al., 1977). Recent reports on the survival rates of replanted hands and digits vary between 76 per cent and 93 per cent (Tamai et al., 1977; Urbaniak, 1977; Weilland et al., 1977). Reliability through improved surgical technique has encouraged the evolution of more sophisticated free transfers of single tissues such as the fibula (Taylor et al., 1975), rib

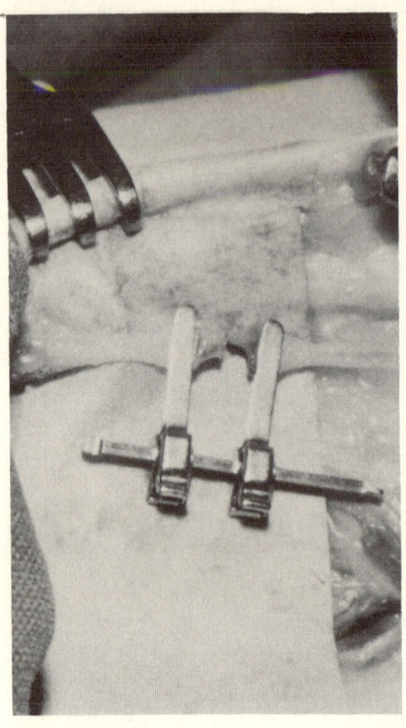
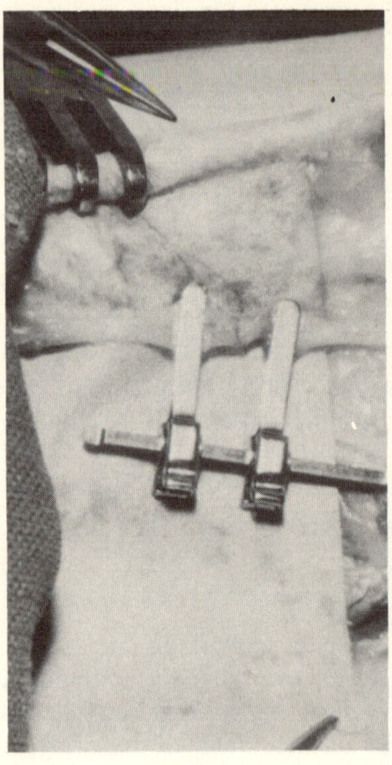

a   b

Fig. 6.1. a, Double clamp with bar to allow approximation of vessel ends without tension. *b,* Anastomosis of vessel with interrupted 10/0 nylon suture.

(Bunche et al., 1977), muscle (Terzis et al., 1978; Schenk, 1978) and nerve (Taylor and Ham, 1976) and in certain situations the big toe or adjacent two toes can be transferred *in toto* to the hand (Ohtsuka et al., 1977).

In massive trauma of the lower limbs major skin loss has been successfully replaced by the free transfer of the groin flap and this has been shown to halve the immobilization and in-patient time (Serafin et al., 1977). Taylor and Watson (1978) have successfully used a free groin flap containing iliac crest to reconstruct severe compound fractures of the tibia with bone and skin loss.

However, the most significant development has been the extension of teaching and training facilities between major centres and microsurgical groups, particularly in the USA, Austria and Australia. Microsurgery has lent itself to practical workshops, combining closed circuit television of operative methods, both in theatre and in the experimental situation and to guided practical instruction in the laboratory. The skill gained by surgeons in these training sessions has taken microsurgery into many centres throughout the world so that the dominant trend in the 1960s for specialized microsurgical units has been radically altered in recent years.

Future
It is likely that all major accident units in the UK will in time have the availability of surgeons interested in microsurgical techniques. In these accident departments treating all forms of injury such skills will be more commonly used in the repair of injured peripheral nerves than in the repair of small vessels, as complete amputations of limbs and digits are uncommon even in large industrial centres. However, the increasing awareness of the importance of repairing divided vessels in incomplete amputations or where two vessels have been severed, despite the distal part of the limb having an obvious blood flow, might redress the balance.

ORGANIZATION OF AN ACCIDENT DEPARTMENT

The skills needed in microvascular and microneural surgery are similar although each has its own procedure. They have the following fundamental needs:
 (1) Patience, motivation to learn and the availability of the surgeon.
 (2) A suitable operating microscope with supporting instrumentation.
 (3) Adequate theatre operating time, and anaesthetic support.
 (4) A laboratory for the training of assistants, including medical and nursing staff.
 (5) Research facility.

Instrumentation
In selecting an operating microscope it is important that it is seen to be effective in the operating room. It has to be more manoeuvrable than in the laboratory as human wounds are longer and microsurgical repairs are often performed in deep tissue layers. For ease of operating it is required that the microscope shall have a magnification of at least 25x. The microscope frequently has to be angled, particularly when operating on the neurovascular bundle in the axilla, or in the supraclavicular fossa while repairing brachial plexus injuries. A foot-pedal control for magnification change and altering the focus is essential to allow undisturbed use of the hands for operating. The more recent Zeiss operating microscopes have an additional binocular system for the assistants which allows them to view the same operating field as the surgeon. The operating time can be considerably reduced, an important factor as the operating time has often been a point of criticism of the technique.
 The choice of scissor or needle holder has to be a personal decision made at the moment of handling that particular instrument. The instruments are varied in their size, in the power that is required to open and close them and in their shape. It has been found to be inadvisable to order them from a catalogue. In general terms an optimum length is between 8–10 cm, and the handle of the needle holder and forceps should be textured and cylindrical to allow rotation of the instrument, as when holding a pencil. There has always been difficulty in holding the round-

bodied needle with the flat surfaces of the needle holder tips, but further developments should overcome this difficulty. Microdissection of the scarred peripheral nerve has often required more robust scissors than those required for freeing or dissecting a small vessel.

The operating table should allow the surgeon to rest his elbows and wrists to obtain maximum stability while working. For operating on distally placed wounds, below the knee or the elbow, a simple half moon cut-out on the two sides of the table has been found to be satisfactory. Gordon and Bunche (1978) have reported their own design of a universally adaptable table allowing microsurgical repairs on the length of the limbs, as well as on the head and neck.

Anaesthesia

In many upper limb injuries where direct anastomosis by primary repair has been undertaken, regional anaesthesia has overcome the need for general anaesthesia. The main disadvantage of regional anaesthesia has occurred when nerve grafts have been needed. The sural nerve has been the most advantageous donor graft and its removal is difficult without a general anaesthetic.

Trained Assistants

Experienced surgeons with well trained assistants have been able to accomplish microsurgical techniques with great rapidity. It has been reported that digit replants have been accomplished within two hours. The laboratory training of theatre staff has allowed them to become familiar with the instruments and with the demands of the technique. This has also been associated with an increase in morale and motivation within the team. A parallel experience has been noticed in the similar approach used by the AO specialists for their technique for the internal fixation of fractures.

MICROSURGERY

In accident surgery microsurgical techniques are limited to the anastomosis of small vessels and nerves either at the time of injury or later when tissues are transferred on their vascular pedicle. These latter reconstructive procedures are perhaps more in the province of the plastic surgeon than the accident surgeon.

Greater emphasis will be directed at microneural surgery for in comparison to microvascular techniques this subject has had less discussion. In microneural surgery the emphasis has been more on the change of approach to the management of peripheral nerve injuries. Unlike vascular repairs the results of nerve repair are not immediately dramatic and self-evident. Further, there has been difficulty in evaluating the results, partly due to the long period of follow-up required until final recovery has been realized, and partly due to the complex interaction of the central nervous system on sensory recovery. This has made the accurate assessment of recovery elusive. In addition, there have been no tightly controlled prospective studies on the various methods of nerve repair. It has been perhaps this lack of definition which has subdued the interest and lessened the impact of microsurgical techniques on peripheral nerve injury. But the opportunity which these techniques have given us for studying further the biological behaviour of peripheral nerves after injury has been very important.

Seddon (1975) in his classic review of his own extensive experience on peripheral nerve injuries advocated secondary epineurial repair of the injured nerve in preference to a primary epineurial repair for the following reasons:

(1) Unless the nerve had a clean division without epineurial tears he felt adequate assessment of intraneural damage was not possible.

(2) The tissues after epineurial suture would not have sufficient tensile strength to prevent separation of the nerve ends on mobilization of the joints of the limb.

(3) Trained surgeons with the necessary facilities and equipment were not often available.

In contrast, each of these disadvantages could be overcome at secondary exploration.

An alternative argument has now been made on the following basis. As a result of the development of training in hand surgery in the UK, many centres now have suitably trained surgeons with the requisite facilities for undertaking primary nerve repair. Also, the improvement in design and manufacture of fine instruments, needles and suture material, and access to the use of an operating microscope, which provides higher optical magnification, has challenged the validity of Seddon's points (1) and (2). For instance, the epineurial tear which was a definitive contraindication to primary repair can, with the aid of the operating microscope, be explored and the edges debrided and excised. The underlying fasciculi can be inspected and damaged fasciculi can be resected to normal tissue. An epineurial and, where applicable, a perineurial suture can be used for closure of the division. With the insertion of multiple 8/0 and 10/0 sutures sufficient strength at the suture line can be achieved to prevent later separation of the nerve ends.

Primary Nerve Repair

If the outer surface of the nerve, the epineurium, is sutured, it is not possible to see the alignment of the fasciculi within the nerve. As a result of too much tension, twisting or poor adaptation of the nerve stumps, the fasciculi at the suture line may be overlapping, buckled or turned back upon themselves. This inevitably leads to wastage of regenerating nerve axons into the surrounding epineurium and they do not find their way in to the fasciculi of the distal stump. However, as Edshage (1964) has shown, the more exact the epineurial suture achieved by suturing under minimum tension and more accurate matching of the surface vessels of the stumps, then the better will be the approximation of the fasciculi within the nerve.

Primary Epineurial Suture (*Fig. 6.2*)

There are certain conditions which favour primary epineurial suture.

(1) In children, up to the age of 14 years (the propensity for nerve regeneration is so good that other more time-consuming procedures such as a fascicular suture do not appear justified).

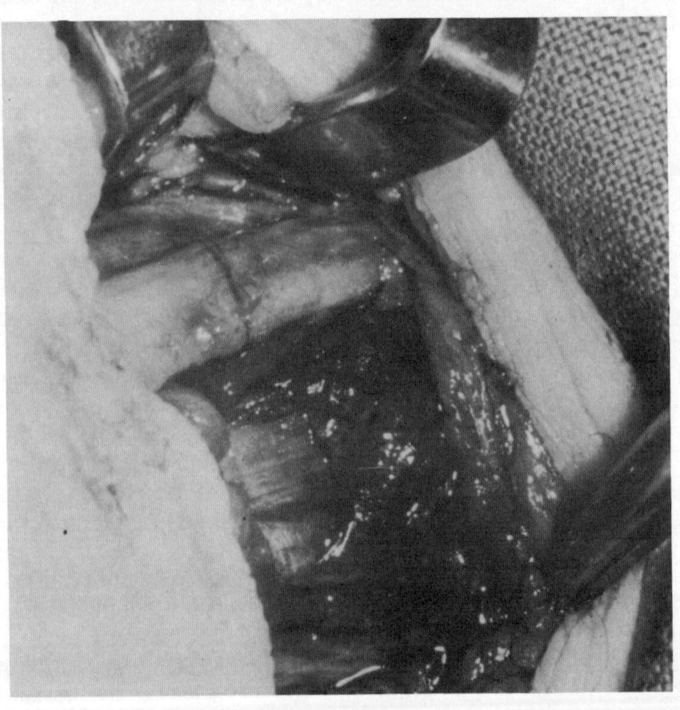

Fig. 6.2. Primary epineurial suture of median nerve with interrupted 10/0 nylon suture.

(2) In clean, incised wounds from a scalpel or a piece of glass, where there is minimal loss of nerve substance.

(3) In digit or limb amputations. In these cases there may be loss of nerve substance and further loss may have to be incurred through further excision of the damaged nerve ends. But, due to the necessary shortening of bone to achieve end-to-end vascular anastomosis, primary nerve suture

can be performed without tension, as the nerve gap will have been eliminated.

(4) Where there is loss of some nerve substance. When the nerve gap is 2 cm or less some joint flexion will allow satisfactory suture with 8/0 suture material. If the tension does not allow an 8/0 suture to be tied without tearing the epineurium then primary epineurial suture should be abandoned.

Primary Fascicular Suture (*Fig. 6.3*)

With the availability of microsurgical techniques Smith (1964) and Bora (1967) demonstrated that it was possible in animal experiments to resect part of the epineurium from the nerve stump ends to expose the fasciculi

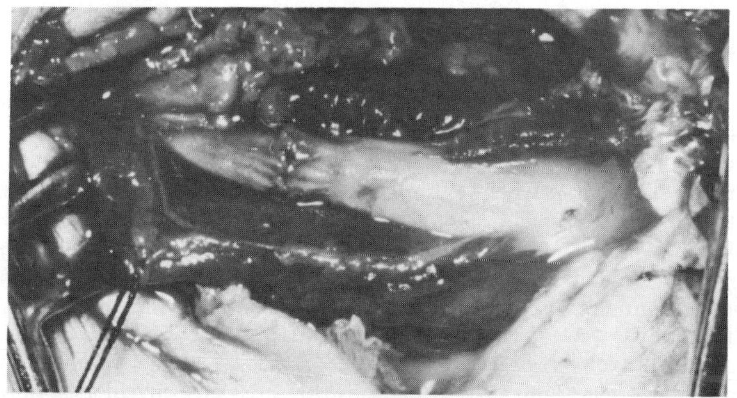

Fig. 6.3. Primary fascicular suture with 10/0 nylon suture, showing resection of epineurium.

with their ensheathing perineurium. The perineurium is a laminated, cellular layer which they found had the tensile strength to hold a micro-suture in conditions of low-tension. It was evident that nerve axons could regenerate across the fascicular suture line. There have since followed a number of research studies comparing primary epineurial versus primary fascicular suture in rabbits, cats and monkeys on the sciatic, median and ulnar nerves (Goto, 1967; Wise et al., 1969; Grabb et al., 1970; Yamamoto, 1974; Cabaud et al., 1976; Bora et al., 1976; Orgel and Terzis, 1977). Bora in 1967 compared the results of perineurial and epineurial sutures in 20 cat sciatic nerves and assessed results on the return of function by 'push-off' gait and sensation by withdrawal after pin prick, concluded that muscles were reinnervated more rapidly after a perineurial suture. But in 1976, studying the sciatic nerve in rabbits after perineurial and epineurial suture, and by using a biochemical assay of collagen and estimating the myelin content distal to the suture line, they concluded, on the basis of the myelin content, that nerve regeneration was more rapid in the epineurial repair if performed directly after division. Wise et al. (1969) studying similar repairs in the sciatic nerve of cats showed no statistical difference between an epineurial repair with magnification and a fascicular repair with magnification. Cabaud et al. (1976) studying the ulnar nerve in 20 cats and comparing the two techniques also concluded that 'following acute lacerations of peripheral nerves, epineurial repair with 8/0 nylon and some magnification is as satisfactory as is perineurial repair with 10/0 and higher magnification.'

Orgel and Terzis (1977) have published the most recent comparative study using the divided sciatic nerve in rabbits as the model to evaluate recovery after epineurial and perineurial repair; 10/0 nylon sutures were used in both groups and recovery was assessed on a histological and neurophysiological basis. There was a combined light and electron-microscopy assessment. The light microscopy evaluation of the distal stump included the measurement of myelinated fibre diameters, the area of each fascicle occupied by myelinated fibres, and the calculation of the number of myelinated fibres per square millimetre. Using the electron microscope non-myelinated fibres were studied for fibre diameters and the number of axons per Schwann cell unit. The neurophysiological examination included the measurement of the amplitude of nerve action potentials, expressed as a percentage of the proximal stump values, and nerve conduction studies proximal to and across the neuroma and over the distal stump. This excellent study came to the following conclusions. The authors were unable to detect any significant differences in the patterns of axonal regrowth in the nerves sutured by either technique. The perineurial repairs revealed a tendency towards large myelinated fibres with a greater area of coverage across the bundles and also a greater density of fibres. This improved histological picture was associated in the perineurial repairs by a greater amplitude of the action potentials and faster conduction velocities. However, the conclusion of this study could not show a statistical advantage of one method over another.

Conclusion

The conclusion drawn from the research studies reported to date is that none of the studies has shown that primary fascicular repair is statistically better, in terms of the parameters so far studied, than primary epineurial repair. But there appears to be agreement that either repair done with 8/0 or 10/0 nylon sutures with magnification is preferable to a repair with thicker suture material and done under normal vision. It is important to remember that in the animals studied the number of fasciculi within a given nerve is much fewer than in the human equivalent. It is perhaps the fewer number of fasciculi in an animal nerve (for instance three in the cat sciatic nerve) which has made it difficult to produce an obvious difference between the methods of repair — an epineurial suture if performed carefully will produce minimum distortion at the suture line. By contrast in the human median nerve at the wrist there may be twenty or more fasciculi. There is therefore a theoretical case for fascicular repair in this situation because there may be much greater chance for malalignment of the fasciculi.

The results of clinical studies have not contributed significantly to answering this question. Salvi (1973) compared 8 epineurial repairs to 16 perineurial repairs, and felt that in general the perineurial repairs recovered more quickly and were more likely to give better results. Jabaley (1976) looked for a possible correlation between regenerated nerve plexuses (specifically Meissner's corpuscles) and clinical recovery in a group of patients whose nerves had either been repaired by a standard epineurial repair or repaired by fascicular suture with an operating microscope. His study re-affirmed the great difficulty of assessing the results of nerve repair in humans. Jabaley concluded that the degree of quality of reinnervation did not correlate with clinical testing or the subjective impression of the result. A hand with an excellent histological recovery might have a poor functional return or, alternatively, skin with scarce evidence of rein-nervation could be associated with a good clinical recovery.

What then is the place for primary fascicular repair? On the evidence available so far its use appears to be restricted to a few select situations. An example has been stated (*see above*) where on exploration of a divided nerve the stump ends are seen to have been left with a ragged edge and with tears in the epineurium, and a haematoma within the epineurium. This suggests a poor prognosis. However, if the epineurium is examined under the microscope it can be shown that the damage is more apparent than real for the fasciculi are frequently less damaged than the surrounding epineurium. By resecting the torn epineurium 1 cm away from the nerve ends, a clean wound can be obtained. This procedure does prevent an epineurial repair but due to the preservation of length of the fasciculi these can now be repaired by a perineurial suture.

There has been some controversy over the definition of the fascicular or perineurial repair. The fasciculus is the smallest unit within the nerve. In a digital nerve with a small number of fasciculi these could be sutured individually. The suture has to be placed only into the covering fascicular sheath, the perineurium, but avoiding penetration into the endoneurium. This is the fascicular repair using a perineurial suture. Foreign suture material taken into the substance of the fasciculus containing the nerve axons would cause a mechanical obstruction to the regenerating axons and disturb their pathway to the distal stump. The needle also would take epineurial cells into the endoneurium to produce additional and thicker collagen fibrils that would cause further obstruction (Morris et al., 1972). In other nerves, particularly the median nerve, it would be impractical although not impossible to suture the twenty or more fasciculi. Instead a group of fasciculi held together by a thin covering of epineurium can be sutured to a corresponding group in the opposite nerve stump. This suture would more accurately be described as an 'epi-perineurial suture', as the fasciculi comprising the group would still be held together by the inter-fascicular epineurial tissue. It is this method which would be commonly used.

We have reached a time in microneural surgery where the technical facilities for nerve repair have begun to match the theoretical conclusions advanced by anatomists, as to the correct aims of nerve repair that would allow the best chance for nerve axons to advance across the nerve division into the distal stump. There is growing appreciation of the great plasticity of the cellular and structural details at the nerve ends and the extent of the remodelling that occurs during regeneration at the site of nerve repair. The remodelling occurs on at least two anatomical levels; the structural and the ultrastructural as the basic architecture of the nerve end changes as well as an interconversion between the Schwann cells, endoneurial fibroblasts and perineurial cells (Morris et al., 1972).

Ramon y Cajal (1928), in his beautifully illustrated monograph, described with light-microscopy studies the manner in which a simple regenerating axon produced numerous collateral and terminal sprouts. These sprouts ran in the same pathway as the parent nerve fibre and remained together in a group. They crossed the nerve gap with each nerve sprout often dividing into one or more branches either to by-pass an obstruction or to penetrate a number of separate Schwann tubes in the distal stump. However only a proportion of these sprouts survived and matured depending upon whether they developed a functioning capacity. Morris et al. (1972) in an ultra-structural study confirmed this concept and observed that a group of axonal sprouts was enveloped by a basal lamina. They described this structure as a 'regenerating unit'. Ramon y Cajal (1928) also noted that in the proximal stump of a divided nerve the fascicular pattern would be altered from a few large fasciculi into many small fasciculi as they crossed the nerve gap. This remodelling of the nerve structure was confirmed by Morris et al. (1972) who observed that this phenomenon occurred within the proximal nerve stump and only occurred in the distal stump when it contained regenerating axons. Then, with time and healing, restructuring occurred with the normal pattern (of a few major fasciculi) reasserting itself. Morris and his colleagues described this as 'compartmentation'.

We have therefore a process whereby there is an enormous increase in regenerating and sub-dividing axonal sprouts contained in the 'regenerating unit' which themselves are enclosed in multiple small fascicular 'compart-ments'. They have suggested that the remodelling is to protect the endoneurial environment by reconstructing a new perineurial sheath. It acts as a barrier separating the endoneurium both structurally and functionally from the outer epineurial environment. The perineurial suture is attempting to produce a surgical 'compartmentation'. The emphasis and aim of nerve surgery is therefore to protect the endoneurial space. The perineurial suture ensures closer adaptation of the fascicular interface and is as helpful in preventing nerve axons from escaping as in preventing obstructive elements from the epineurium entering the endoneurial space. The limited excision of the epineurium from the fascicular suture line might also be important in this respect. The disadvantage is the proximity of foreign suture material and the local tissue damage done by the needle at the fascicular junction.

Despite these considerations the surgeon must be aware that other factors such as variations in local vascularity, the degree of proximal retrograde degeneration of the nerve to the spinal cord, and the subsequent distortion of afferent responses to the cerebral cortex (Paul et al., 1972) may be the final arbiters in the ultimate functional recovery.

The timing of either a primary epineurial or primary fascicular suture can be adjusted to suit the available facilities. Either suture is ideally performed within 6 hours of the injury to prevent the possibility of infection. However, if the wound is clean and there has been no vascular impairment, the wound can be lavaged, covered with a sterile dressing and the limb splinted to await definitive surgery. A delay of up to 72 hours is possible without apparent ill effect. It is observed that with the absorption of the haematoma and the reduction in soft tissue swelling at that time, surgical repair has been found to be easier. After 72 hours connective tissue healing has begun to alter tissue planes; they have been seen not to separate as easily, and to have lost their elasticity. If these events have occurred it seems preferable to delay surgical repair 4–6 weeks when the wound has soundly healed.

Nerve Approximation

Nerve approximation is used predominantly where there has been associated damage to surrounding tissues, e.g. vessels, tendons and skin, but where the amount of nerve loss has been relatively small so that approximation of the nerve ends can still be done. With major loss of nerve substance the nerve ends are left lying in situ, with no attempt to mobilize and draw them together. In these complicated soft tissue injuries it has been common practice to leave the nerve suture and to concentrate on tendon and skin repair. It is now appreciated that there is a need to undertake micro-vascular repair of any associated vascular injuries as it is felt that full re-vascularization of the tissues will influence the final quality of the nerve recovery. The decision to delay formal repair has to be made on the basis of whether it is possible to achieve the best repair using 8/0 or 10/0 nylon suture with magnification. In many instances the shortage of time rather than the degree of nerve damage has dictated the decision.

The manner in which the approximation of the nerve ends is carried out has a significant effect on the reaction of the nerve, and can determine the method of repair at the time of re-exploration.

For such a decisive choice there has been remarkably little discussion of the methods which would lead to the least epineurial and endoneurial fibrosis. There have been two principal aims. First, the nerve ends need to be placed in such a position that the natural elasticity of the nerve which causes retraction, and any tendency for further separation of the nerve ends through mobilization of the limb, will be eliminated. Second, the method of approximating the nerve ends should cause the least fibrosis between the nerve ends.

All types of suture material will produce local fibrosis (De Lee et al., 1977). If the nerve ends could be approximated without the use of suture material, a more advantageous situation would be obtained. Occasionally a complete division of the nerve substance has occurred but retraction of the nerve ends has been prevented by a persisting and intact strip of epineurium. In other cases the division has occurred just distal to a branch of the nerve, e.g. a division of the median nerve just distal to the palmar branch and this branch acts as a tie preventing significant separation. In most instances these natural ties have been removed.

The two nerve ends can be adapted or even slightly overlapped and stay sutures are inserted at a distance from the nerve division holding the stumps to the tissue bed and so preventing movement. Usually, the nerve ends are brought together and held with a few epineurial sutures at the line of division. If this method has to be chosen then the principle of using fine suture is still observed. It is preferable to use multiple 8/0 nylon sutures rather than 4/0 to 6/0 suture material. Prior to approximating the nerve ends a limited debridement of the damaged nerve tissue may be undertaken. Postoperatively the limb should be protected from excessive mobilization of the joints until definitive repair is performed 4—6 weeks later.

Secondary Nerve Repair
Timing
It is implied that re-exploration of the nerve is a planned procedure, decided upon at the initial exploration. This should occur when the skin wound has fully healed and the traumatic oedema has subsided, ideally between 4 and 6 weeks after injury. There are many factors which can produce a delay; failure of the wound to heal, failure of the surgeon at the time of primary closure to state whether he was satisfied with the formal suture, and difficulty in assessing the degree of regeneration (the advancing Tinel sign can only indicate that *some* fibres are regenerating into the distal stump). External factors such as multiple injuries, failure to diagnose the nerve injury at the time, closed injuries with a traction lesion in association with a fracture, may add to the delay.

There is general agreement that the damaged nerve should be explored within 6 months. It was considered that delay after 12 months had too poor a prognosis for secondary suture to be attempted. But as more nerve sutures are performed after 12 months this pessimistic view is being discarded. The possibility for return of sensation had always been more optimistic and it has been stated that some return of sensation could occur from 10 to 20 years after injury. The return of muscle function is obviously influenced by the degree of degeneration of the muscle fibres and the amount of interstitial fibrosis. It is now being accepted that the continued presence of fibrillation potentials on neurophysiological examination admits the potential for muscle innervation. Narakas (1977), from Lausanne, has noted recovery in muscles following surgical repair of brachial plexus palsies 5 years later. There are isolated examples of recovery occurring after even longer intervals.

Technique

The indications for either secondary epineurial repair or nerve graft will not be apparent until the neuroma has been exposed. It is preferable to anticipate the possibility of a nerve graft. The skin incision should allow the graft to lie beneath a healthy skin flap and the limits of the flap should cross proximal and distal to the suture lines of the graft. The lower limbs are prepared and towelled in case the sural nerves are required as the donor grafts. The initial exploration is performed under tourniquet control. The nerve is approached proximal and distal to the neuroma through healthy tissue. The neuroma is identified, isolated and freed from its bed. One of the following three situations might be encountered.

(1) The nerve ends are connected by an intervening neuroma.

(2) The proximal neuroma and the distal glioma are connected by a thin tube of epineurium (traction lesion).

(3) The nerve ends are completely separate.

In the first example the thick scar overlying the neuroma can be excised through a longitudinal incision and by dissecting circumferentially. A better assessment of the actual size of the gap is then obtained (*Fig. 6.4*).

However, it may not be possible to assess the extent of the peripheral nerve injury with accuracy even on microscopical examination. It can be difficult to distinguish between a complete lesion and a neuroma in continuity. In addition, even where the anatomical extent of the injury can be estimated with reasonable confidence, the proportion of the nerve that has preserved physiological function cannot be established simply by visual inspection. Terzis et al. (1976) has recommended the use of compound action potentials (CNAP) in the assessment of nerve injuries at operation, suggesting that recording of the CNAP could be useful not only to establish whether there was physiological continuity across the injury but also to establish whether particular fasciculi are capable of conducting nerve impulses. In 1965 Jacobson and Guth studied the regeneration of sciatic nerves following experimental injury in the rat and found that the amplitude of the CNAP was an indication of the number and size of the nerve fibres. Ballantyne and Campbell (1973) used the CNAP amplitude in the study of regeneration of injured peripheral nerves following epineurial repair. Kline and Nulsen (1968) have used the CNAP at operation and on the basis of the presence of a CNAP in the early postoperative period

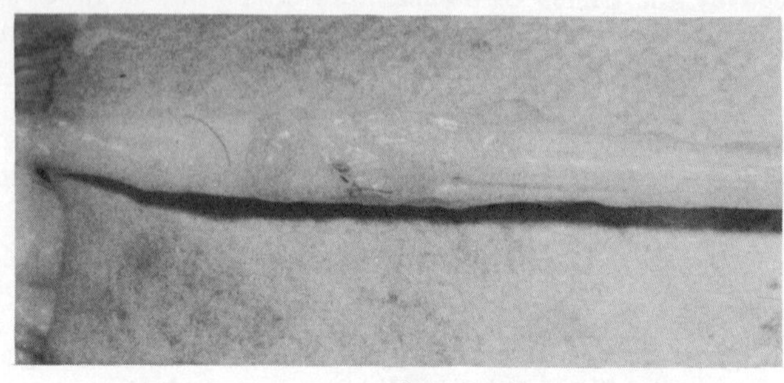

a

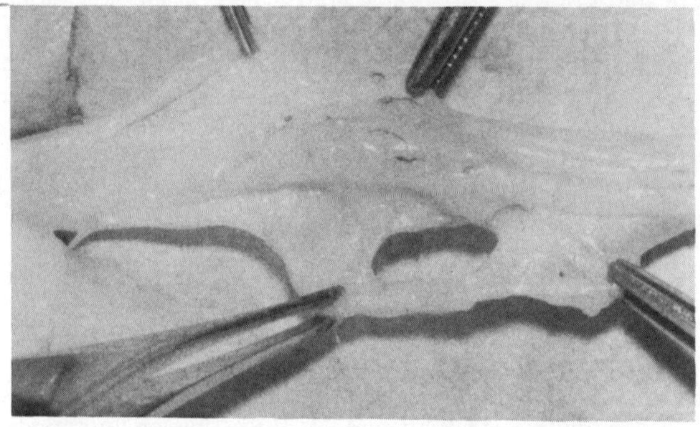

b

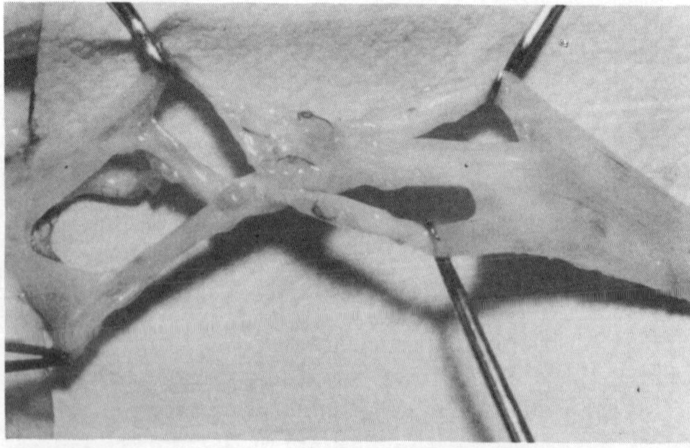

c

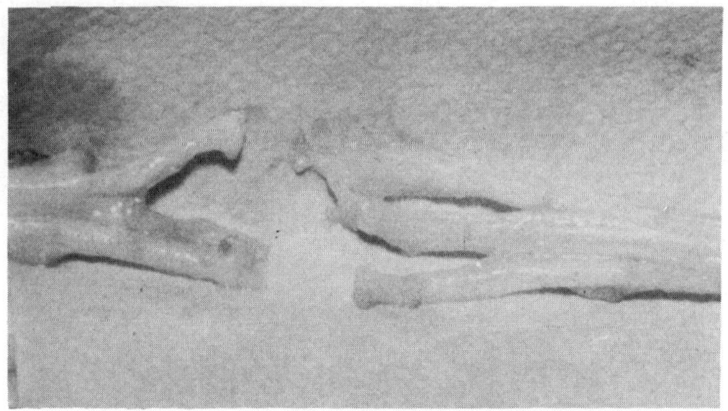

d

Fig. 6.4. a, Ulnar nerve neuroma. *b,* Longitudinal opening in thickened epineurium to expose fasciculi. *c,* Fasciculi separated to point of approximation. *d,* Excision of final scar; nerve prepared for a fascicular repair or nerve graft.

recommended leaving the neuroma alone, or performing a neurolysis, while the absence of a CNAP indicated surgical repair.

Our own limited experience has confirmed the practicality of obtaining CNAPs across lesions in continuity using portable electromyographic apparatus in theatre *(Fig. 6.5)* and also obtaining these from individual fasciculi across the neuroma with microtungsten electrodes placed proximal and distal to the neuroma. The amplitude of the CNAP could be compared with the CNAP of the normal nerve lying proximal to the neuroma. It has not as yet been possible to correlate the amplitude of the CNAP with the number of intact nerve fibres and so no quantitative conclusion has been drawn. There is the additional difficulty of preventing the stimulus spreading to adjacent fasciculi. However, further requirements of this technique could be of significant assistance in the management of lesions in continuity.

At present with neurophysiological techniques in their infancy, if there is doubt of the extent of the neuroma and the degree of endoneurial fibrosis this will be determined only by further surgical exploration. The neuroma can be approached either by (1) transverse incision into the neuroma; leading to the classical secondary epineurial suture (Seddon, 1975); or (2) longitudinal incision into the neuroma, leading to a possible secondary fascicular repair, but more probably to the insertion of inter-fascicular nerve grafts (Millesi et al., 1976).

Secondary Epineurial Suture (Fig. 6.6)
A sharp scalpel is used to cut in the mid-line between the retracted nerve ends and through the intervening scar tissue so as to separate them completely. Further sections are taken transversely from both the proximal and distal stumps until the normal axons pout into the wound proximally,

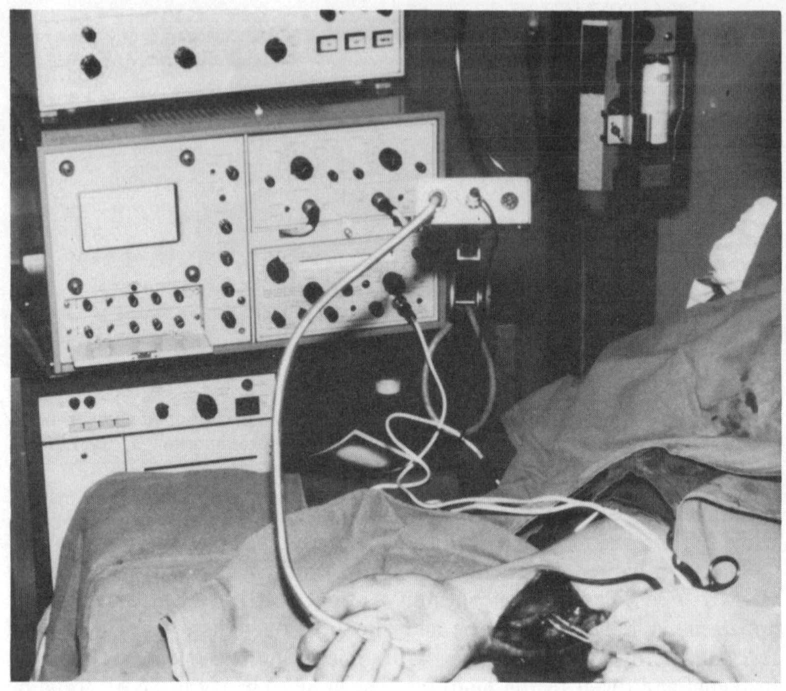

Fig. 6.5. Operative EMG with portable neurophysiological apparatus.

and in the distal stump, where Wallerian degeneration has emptied the
Schwann tubes of nerve fibres, removal of scarred tissue continues until a
discrete fascicular architecture is observed. Seddon (1975) used cut
sections for microscopy to determine the level of transection. The operating
microscope has allowed modification of this procedure as the intact
fasciculi can be identified clearly and observed directly with higher
magnification as exploration has proceeded.

The difficulty has remained in advising dogmatically whether a secondary epineurial repair should be performed. There is agreement that a nerve
suture should be accomplished with 'minimal tension' but there is no
agreement on the exact definition of this term. The experimental work of
Highet and Saunders (1943) on the adverse effect of tension on the nerve
suture line, the clinical report by Zachary (1954), who found that the
greater the gap the worse the prognosis, and the conclusion by Nicholson
and Seddon (1957) that the prognosis was affected adversely where there
had been extensive mobilization of the proximal nerve stump 'to close
even a moderate gap at the wrist' have each emphasized the unreliable
results of this type of secondary repair. Millesi (1975) has summarized the

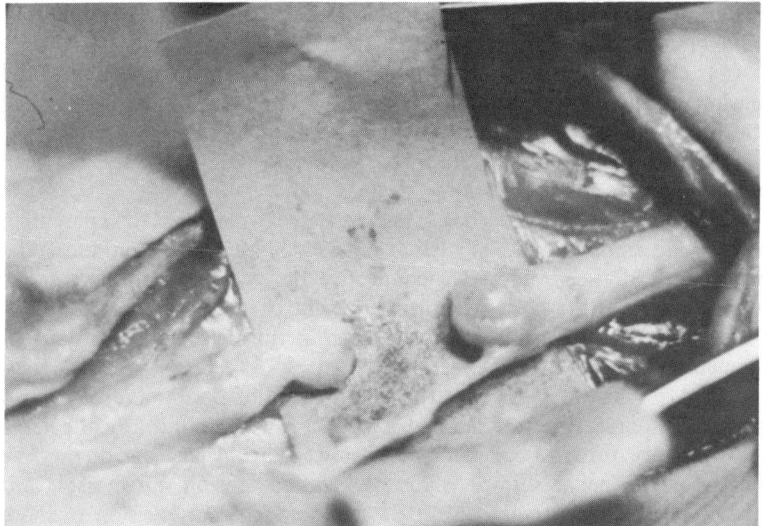

a

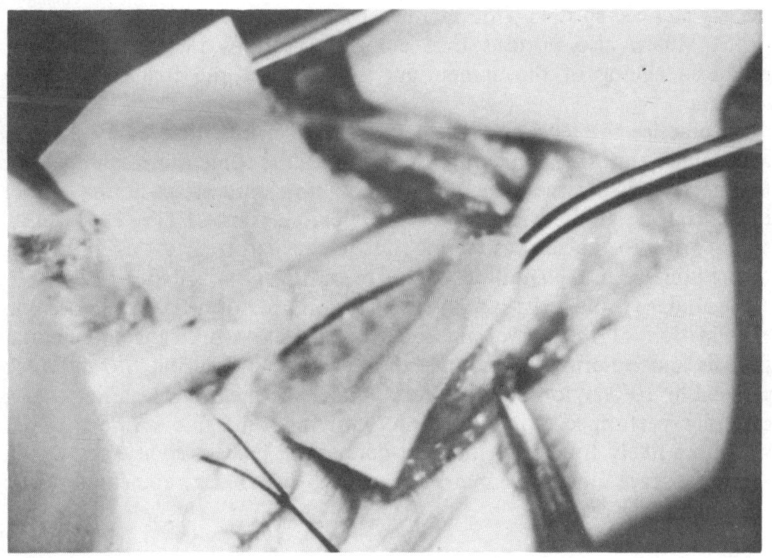

b

Fig. 6.6. a, Transverse incision through median nerve neuroma; separation of nerve ends limited by palmar branch of median nerve. *b*, Secondary epineurial repair with interrupted 8/0 nylon suture.

results of his extensive experimental studies on the effect of tension on nerve repair as follows.

(1) The extent of proliferation of the connective tissue is related to the tension at the site of suture. The greater the tension, the greater the scarring at the site of the sutures.

(2) There is a direct relationship between the length of the scar between both nerve ends and the tension.

(3) The proliferation of the connective tissue comes from the epineurial, perineurial and endoneurial tissue. The epineurial tissue produces the major part of the proliferative connective tissue. This connective tissue starts growing at the site of the suture, passing obstacles such as sutures on their outer side and displacing them inwards, thus causing loss of part of the neural diameter for regeneration.

(4) After simple division of the sciatic nerve of the rat a force of 5—6 grams is required to coapt the ends. When a gap is produced in the nerve the necessary force to coapt increases slowly until 4 per cent of the free length of the nerve stumps is lost, when the tension curve rises very steeply. Millesi noted that return of function after an excision of more than 4 per cent of the free nerve length was not as good as when less nerve had been excised, with correspondingly less tension. The best result was obtained when a precise length of nerve graft was inserted to exactly fill the gap and was sutured without any tension.

(5) Millesi also noticed that epineurial sutures tied under tension produced sliding of the epineurium distally over the free ends of the fasciculi.

In practice the tension of the nerve suture can be estimated by the ease with which an 8/0 nylon suture inserted into the epineurium can hold the two nerve ends together when the neighbouring joints are positioned either in neutral or, at the most, at $15°$ of flexion. Gaps of $1·5–2$ cm can be closed without the sutures tearing, but in gaps larger than this shortening of the bone, as in replantations, or nerve grafting is indicated.

Secondary epineurial repair is therefore performed if microscopic examination of the nerve ends has revealed no significant endoneurial fibrosis and a normal appearance of the fasciculi. Multiple 8/0 nylon or preferably 10/0 nylon sutures are used. It was mentioned earlier that a carefully performed 'approximation' with the same fine suture material was more likely to lead to the least connective tissue response and would therefore leave a neuroma more amenable to a secondary epineurial suture than to a nerve graft.

Interfascicular Nerve Graft
After the thickened outer layer surrounding the neuroma has been excised it may be apparent that the amount of scar around the nerve ends is still extensive, and that further excision would leave a gap of more than 2 cm

in the nerve. The neuroma can be transected through its equator to allow free mobilization of the ends.

The operating microscope is now used. An easier entry into the neuroma is obtained by excising a circumferential strip of epineurium at the junction of normal nerve and the neuroma itself. The normal fasciculi lying inside can be dissected into groups and followed into the neuroma until they become fibrous ends. The extent of the fibrosis running longitudinally within the endoneurium of each fasciculus will differ and so after cutting back to the normal tissue the fasciculi will be of varying lengths. The epineurium is resected for about 0·5–1 cm from nerve ends. It is thought that too great an excision of epineurium could lead to harmful endoneurial vascular changes. Unless a digital nerve, or a similar small nerve with only a few fasciculi, is being prepared for grafting, each individual fasciculus should not be separated. In the median nerve with twenty or more fasciculi an end-on examination of the nerve end helps put the fasciculi into groups ensuring that five or six of these will take an individual graft.

Excision of the epineurium has two advantages; it prevents or delays harmful scarring at the suture line while perineurial healing is taking place, and it allows a greater presentation of the fasciculi as they are free from the tight confines of the epineurial sheath. In cable grafting techniques the grafts were applied directly onto the flat interface of the cut nerve end. This interface is too small to take more than three sural nerve grafts while the diminutive distal stump might be large enough for only one or two. It also required an epineurial suture. The interfascicular nerve grafting technique allows a much greater Schwann tube volume to carry the regenerating nerve fibres. Although small the distal stump, like the proximal stump, can be separated into as many equal groups.

There has been much discussion on the possibility of joining fasciculi of the same modality together (i.e. motor—to—motor or sensory—to—sensory fasciculi) to enhance the quality of recovery. Millesi (1975) described his technique of drawing maps of the fascicular patterns of the two nerve ends and linking by grafts similar groupings. Sunderland (1978) had shown loose functional concentrations of motor and sensory fibres, particularly in the distal parts of the nerve, and it was felt important that this ana-tomical arrangement should be made use of. Hakistan (1968) attempted to define individual fasciculi by their sensory or motor character using the combination of an awake patient and a neurophysiological study of the distal muscles shortly after injury. Millesi's method has been criticized on the basis that the plexiform nature of the fasciculi within the nerve alters so much over a few millimetres that any attempt to join two apparently similar groups would not succeed. Sunderland's study (1968) showed that the fasciculi did not have an individual functional pattern.

Nevertheless, interfascicular nerve grafting can succeed in producing a good sensory and motor recovery (*Fig. 6.7*). The explanation probably lies in the diffuse spread of motor and sensory axons throughout the fasciculi

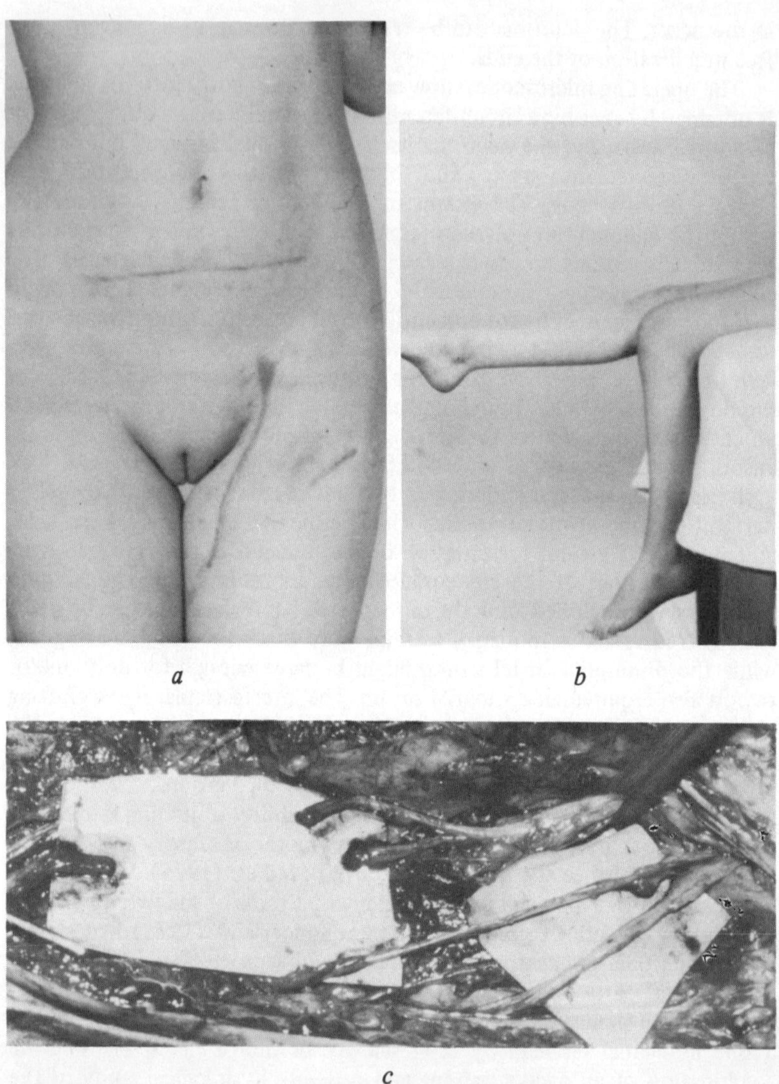

a

b

c

even at the most distal levels, and in the fact that an individual axon by collateral sprouting both at the site of the parent axon and at its terminal branching can overcome the loss due to misdirection of many of the other regenerating axons. For this reason, at the time of fascicular separation prior to grafting, the nerve ends are divided into quadrants or equal areas, and the nerve graft is placed between a similarly placed quadrant in the proximal and distal stumps.

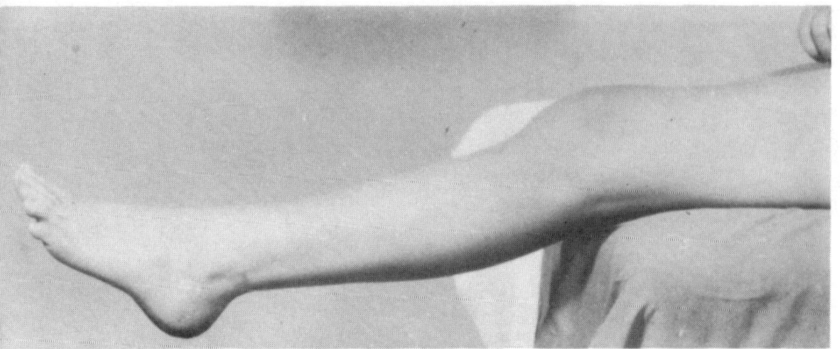

d

Fig. 6.7. a, Longitudinal scar in left groin associated with division of femoral artery, vein and femoral nerve (after revascularization of limb). *b,* Six months after injury. No active extension of left knee and no neurophysiological evidence of reinnervation. *c,* Operation: Femoral nerve neurolysis and sural nerve graft inserted into 5 cm nerve defect. *d,* 9 months after operation—active extension of left knee.

Each fascicular group is cut transversely to show a flat face to which the nerve graft is applied and held with a single 10/0 nylon suture (*Fig. 6.8*), the suture being taken through the perineurium of the fasciculus and the epineurium of the graft. In an awkward wound two sutures may be required to hold the function stable. The graft is laid in the best soft tissue bed even if this requires by-passing a local area of scarring, tendon or bone, and sutured in a similar manner to the prepared distal stump. The graft is slightly longer than the gap and is sutured without tension. The graft anastomoses lie interlocked, producing added stability, by reason of varying fascicular lengths. The tourniquet should be released before suturing and any significant epineurial bleeding controlled with a bipolar microcoagulator. A limited amount of blood is helpful as an adhesive factor between the nerve grafts and the nerve ends. The environment around the nerve grafts should have a good blood supply; this applies not only to the soft tissue bed but also to the overlying skin. If the skin is thin, scarred or adherent it is preferable to replace it with a full thickness skin flap; this can be done either prior to the grafting or as a combined procedure. As the graft has been inserted with the neighbouring joints in neutral or perhaps some extension, exercise of the digits can begin within 48 hours. This may be of importance if a tenolysis has been performed. Full movement of the neighbouring joints are allowed as soon as skin healing is complete. It is felt that the patient's own work and social activities are the best forms of physiotherapy and they are encouraged to return to work long before any signs of recovery have occurred.

Results of Interfascicular Nerve Graft
There have been few reports in the UK literature on interfascicular nerve grafts. Millesi et al. (1976) reported a series of grafted median, ulnar and

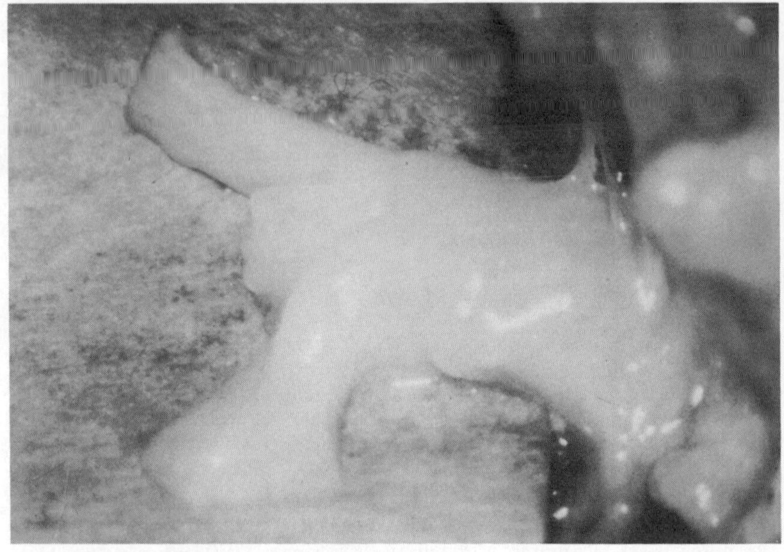

a

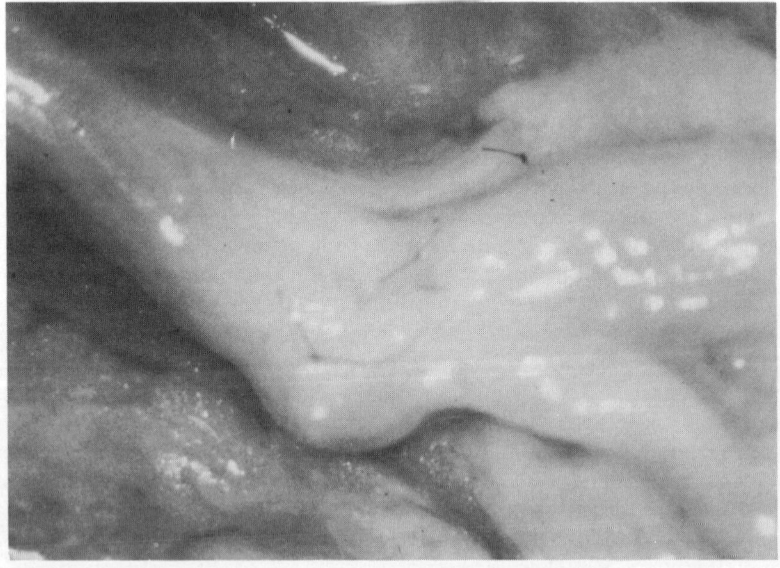

b

Fig. 6.8. a, Proximal nerve stump separated into three groups of multiple fasciculi. *b,* Sural nerve grafts inserted using single 10/0 nylon suture.

radial nerves with a minimum period of follow-up of two years. He assessed the results with the Medical Research Council system of grading for sensory and motor recovery. In 43 median nerve grafts he found 82 per cent had recovered M3 or more, all 39 ulnar nerve grafts had recovered at least M2, and 77 per cent of 13 radial nerve grafts had achieved M4 or M5. McFarlane and Mayer (1976) using Millesi's technique but taking the ante-brachial cutaneous nerve, rather than the sural nerve, as the donor graft performed a secondary repair of 13 digital nerves and found that 11 of the 13 patients had recovered two point discrimination between 7 and 20 mm. Tallis et al. (1978) studied neurophysiologically 16 sural nerve grafts used for the repair of median and ulnar nerve injuries up to two and a half years postoperatively. They found that there was a slow but sustained improvement during this period with motor conduction velocities across the graft reaching 40–80 per cent of normal. Sensory nerve action potentials were obtained in 44 per cent of the repaired nerves 18 months postoperatively, although in all cases the amplitude of the potentials, and their velocity were greatly reduced. The sensory nerve action potentials were not recordable before 18 months. In a few cases studied beyond the second year, it appeared that some improvement occurred even in the third year.

Millesi et al. (1976) has emphasized that the results of nerve grafting where the gap had been over 5 cm showed a worsening prognosis. Our own studies support this view, although in the radial nerve with its high proportion of motor fibres compared with sensory fibres and the good tissue bed often found in the upper arm, longer grafts can be used with success. Our longest sural nerve graft inserted into a radial nerve defect of 12 cm following a fracture of the shaft of the humerus has achieved M5 wrist extension and grade 4 finger extension, but as yet limited functional extension of the thumb (*Fig. 6.9*)

Donor Nerve Graft

The nerve chosen should have the following characteristics: (1) thin with sufficient available length, and limited branching; (2) easily accessible; (3) a large fibre content; and (4) cause minimal functional loss after its removal.

The two nerves that best meet these requirements are the sural nerve and the superficial radial nerve. For major nerve injuries a good length of donor nerve is required and this has favoured the use of the sural nerve. For small defects in digital nerves the superficial radial or the medial cutaneous nerve of the arm are preferred.

The excision of the sural nerve can provide between 30 and 40 cm in length. Its branches occur at the level of the lateral malleolus, except for the sural communicating nerve which has variable sites for branching from its parent trunk. On occasion it can branch as distal as the lateral malleolus, but more commonly in the mid-calf.

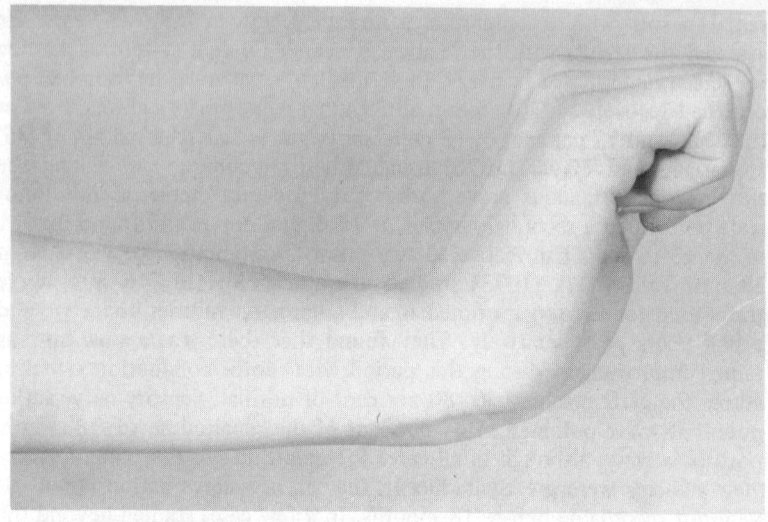

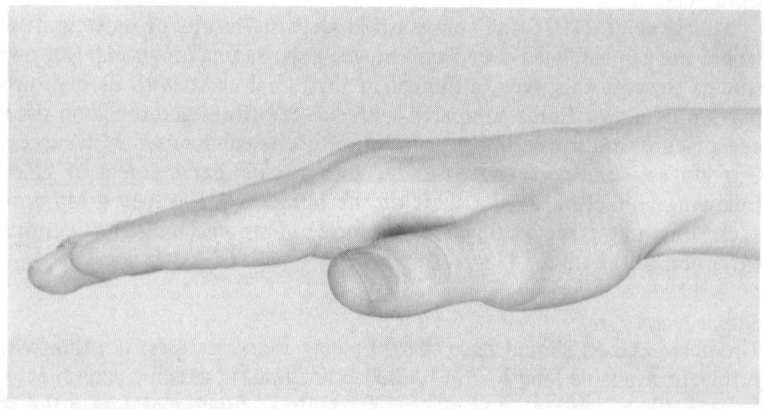

Fig. 6.9. *a*, 12 cm radial nerve defect repaired with 4 sural nerve grafts showing active wrist extension two years after surgery. *b*, Extension of digits two years after surgery.

When the need for grafting has been established the sural nerve is excised with the patient under a general anaesthetic. A sandbag is placed beneath the ipsilateral buttock. A small transverse incision is placed midway between the upper prominence of the lateral melleolus and the tendo Achillis. The sural nerve is isolated, divided and by gentle traction the proximal part of the nerve can be palpated in the posterior calf. Multiple transverse incisions are used to excise the nerve until the popliteal fossa is reached. In the upper third of the calf the sural nerve lying beneath the deep fascia may also lie deep between the muscle bellies of gastronemius, so that a longitudinal incision may be required to aid its removal. The proximal nerve stump should not be divided as proximal as the popliteal fossa in case of damage to the popliteal nerve trunk. It is cauterized and allowed to retract beneath the deep fascia.

Staniforth and Fisher (1978) examined 50 legs of 45 patients who had had removal of the sural nerve for grafting. No trophic ulcers had occurred. The loss of sensation was never complete and pain could still be felt on pin prick; the sensory disturbance varied from a small triangular area to an area that extended to include the fifth toe. Of the patients 8 out of 45 found the sensory change to be unpleasant and 5 found the scars to be an appreciable disability. Forty per cent of the patients were noted to have tenderness related to the proximal nerve stump but none of these warranted further surgery. One patient suffered a deep vein thrombosis.

It is essential that the sacrifice of one nerve to repair another should provide an overall advantage to the patient and that any disadvantages are weighed against the method of repair.

Taylor and Ham (1976) first described the use of a free vascularized nerve graft to bridge a 24 cm defect in a median nerve. The superficial radial nerve together with its arterial supply, the radial artery, were taken and a microsurgical anatomosis performed to re-establish blood flow at the time of nerve suture. Taylor and Watson (1978), reporting to the British Orthopaedic Association, showed from experimental studies the improved regeneration that occured in vascularized free nerve grafts compared with a non-vascularized nerve graft. They cited other instances in massive injuries where it was possible to take a free vascularized nerve graft from an irreparably damaged limb to salvage a major nerve defect in the opposite limb.

BRACHIAL PLEXUS INJURY

In recent years there has been a shift in opinion on the management policy of these brachial plexus injuries. Yeoman and Seddon (1961), after reviewing 36 patients with complete brachial plexus palsies, concluded that amputation of the arm combined with a shoulder arthrodesis and the provision of a prosthesis offered a better functional result than either repair of the brachial plexus or of no repair at all. Ransford and Hughes (1977) in a ten year follow-up of 20 patients with complete lesions noted that whether the patients had been left with a flail arm or had had amputation, both groups had come to terms with their disability and they felt there was little to choose between the two forms of treatment. More use was made of the fitted prosthesis if the dominant limb had been involved, but only 2 out of 13 were true prosthetic users, while in the non-dominant limb prosthetic use was much modified. They concluded that discussion of amputation should be delayed until 12 months after injury, and that management should be concentrated on intensive re-habilitation and retraining rather than cause delay by advising early amputation and prosthetic fitting.

Millesi (1977) reported on 56 patients who between 1964 and 1972 had an elective exploration of the brachial plexus for partial or complete palsies. By using a combination of interfascicular nerve grafts and neurolysis he achieved significant improvement in function in 68 per cent of the patients. As he noted, surgical explorations in the past had been adversely influenced by the extensive nerve defects that are encountered and the dangers of neurolysis which might have damaged intact fasciculi. The present use of the operating microscope and the improved results of nerve grafting have meant a re-appraisal of this pessimistic view. For example in 20 of his cases with complete lesions, 15 of 18 patients had obtained protective sensation, and some useful function in some part of the limb had been obtained in 10 of 18 patients.

There are now a number of surgeons re-evaluating the place of surgery in the treatment of brachial plexus palsy. Narakas (1977) reported his personal experience after reviewing 660 cases of brachial plexus palsy of which he had operated upon 176. His experience had shown that on exploration adequate proximal cervical root stumps were often available for nerve reconstruction, and that repair of C5, 6, 7 trunks gave the best chance of recovery whilst repair of C8—T1 trunks gave very poor results. The significant recovery in some cases had showed the need for a renewed evaluation of the surgical repair of these devastating injuries. For a patient with a flail arm, or with very limited use of this arm, any form of recovery can be of immense help.

REFERENCES

Ballantyne J. P. and Campbell M. J. (1973) Electrophysiological study after surgical repair of sectioned human peripheral nerves. *J. Neurol. Neurosurg. Psychiat.* **36**, 797.

Bora F. W. (1967) Peripheral nerve repair in cats: the fascicular stitch. *J. Bone Joint Surg.* **49A**, 659.

Bora F. W., Pleasure D. E. and Didizian N. A. (1976) A study of nerve regeneration and neuroma formation after nerve suture by various techniques. *J. Hand Surg.* **1**, 138.

Bunche H. J., Furnas D. W., Gordon L. et al. (1977) Free osteocutaneous flap from a rib to a tibia. *J. Plast. Reconstr. Surg.* **59**, 799.

Cabaud H. E., Rodkey W. G., McCarroll H. R. et al. (1976) Epineurial and peri-neurial fascicular nerve repairs: a critical comparison. *J. Hand Surg.* **1**, 131.

DeLee J. C., Smith M. T. and Green D. P. (1977) The reaction of nerve tissue to various suture materials: a study in rabbits. *J. Hand Surg.* **2**, 38.

Edshage S. (1964) Peripheral nerve suture. A technique for improved intraneural topography evaluation of some materials. *Acta Chir. Scand.* Suppl. **331**, 1.

Fujimaki A., O'Brien B. M., Kuxata T. et al. (1977) Experimental micro-anastomosis of 0·4—0·5 mm vessels. *Br. J. Plast. Surg.* **30**, 269.

Gordon L. and Bunche H. J. (1978) Universal operating table. *J. Hand Surg.* **3**, 101.

Goto Y. (1967) Experimental study of nerve autografting by fascicular suture. *Arch. Jpn. Chir.* **36**, 478.

Grabb W. C., Bement S. C., Koepke G. H. et al. (1970) Comparison of methods of
    peripheral nerve suturing in monkeys. *J. Plast. Reconstr. Surg.* **46**, 31.
Hakistan R. W. (1968) Fascicular orientation by direct stimulation: an aid to
    peripheral nerve repair. *J. Bone Joint Surg.* **50A,** 1178.
Hayhurst J. W. and O'Brien B. M. (1975) An experimental study of microvascular
    technique, patency rates, and related factors. *Br. J. Plast. Surg.* **28,** 128.
Highet W. B. and Sanders F. K. (1943) The effects of stretching nerves after suture.
    Br. J. Surg. **30,** 355.
Jabaley M. E., Burns J. E., Orcutt B. S. et al. (1976) Comparison of histological and
    functional recovery after peripheral nerve repair. *J. Hand Surg.* **1,** 119.
Jacobsen J. H. and Suarez E. L. (1960) Microsurgery in anastomosis of small vessels.
    Surg. Forum **11,** 243.
Jacobson S. and Guth L. (1965) An electrophysiological study of the early stages of
    peripheral nerve regeneration. *Exp. Neurol.* **11,** 48.
Kline D. G. and Nulsen F. E. (1972) The neuroma in continuity: its pre-operative and
    operative management. *Surg. Clin. North Am.* **52,** 1189.
McFarlane R. M. and Mayer J. R. (1976) Digital nerve grafts with the lateral ante-
    brachial cutaneous nerve. *J. Hand Surg.* **1,** 169.
Millesi H. (1975) Treatment of Nerve Lesions by Fascicular Free Nerve Grafts. In:
    Michon J. and Moburg F. (ed.). *Traumatic Nerve Lesions of the Upper Limb.*
    Edinburgh, Churchill Livingstone, p. 91.
Millesi H. (1977) Surgical management of brachial plexus injuries. *J. Hand Surg.* **2,**
    367.
Millesi H., Meissl G. and Berger A. (1976) Further experience with interfascicular
    grafting on the median, ulnar and radial nerves. *J. Bone Joint Surg.* **58A,** 209.
Morris J. H., Hudson A. R. and Weddell G. (1972) A study of degeneration and re-
    generation in the divided rat sciatic nerve based on electron microscopy. *Z.
    Zellforsch.* **124,** 76.
Narakas (1977) Personal communication.
Nicholson O. R. and Seddon H. J. (1957) Nerve repair in civil practice: the results of
    median and ulnar nerve lesions. *Br. Med. J.* **2,** 1065.
O'Brien B. M. (1977) *Microvascular Reconstructive Surgery.* Edinburgh, Churchill
    Livingstone.
Ohtsuka H., Torigai K. and Shioya N. (1977) Two toe-to-finger transplants in one
    hand. *J. Plast. Reconstr. Surg.* **60,** 561.
Orgel M. G. and Terzis J. K. (1977) Epineurial versus perineurial repair: an ultra-
    structural and electrophysiological study of nerve regeneration. *J. Plast.
    Reconstr. Surg.* **60,** 80.
Ostrup L. T. and Fredrickson J. M. (1976) Microvascular surgery. *Scand. J. Plast.
    Reconstr. Surg.* **10,** 18.
Paul R. L., Goodman H. and Merzenick M. (1972) Alterations in mechanoreceptor
    input in Brodmann's areas 1 and 3 of the postcentral hand area of macaca
    mulatta after nerve section and regeneration. *Brain. Res.* **39,** 1.
Ramon y Cajal (1928) In: May R. M. (ed.), *Degeneration and Regeneration of the
    Nervous System* (1959), vol. 1. New York, Hafner.
Ransford A. O. and Hughes S. P. F. (1977) Complete brachial plexus lesions. *J. Bone
    Joint Surg.* **59B,** 417.
Salvi V. (1973) Problems connected with the repair of nerve sections. *Hand* **5,** 25.
Schenk R. R. (1978) Rectus femoris muscle and composite skin transplantation by
    micro neuro-vascular anastomoses for avulsion of forearm muscles: a case
    report. *J. Hand Surg.* **3,** 60.
Seddon H. (1975) *Surgical Disorders of the Peripheral Nerves,* 2nd ed. Edinburgh,
    Churchill Livingstone.

Serafin D., Georgiade N. G. and Smith D. H. (1977) Comparison of free flaps with pedicle flaps for coverage of defects of the leg and foot. *J. Plast. Reconstr. Surg.* **59**, 492.

Smith J. W. (1964) Microsurgery of peripheral nerves. *J. Plast. Reconstr. Surg.* **33**, 317.

Staniforth P. and Fisher T. R. (1978) Effects of sural nerve excision. *Hand (in press)*.

Sunderland S. (1978) *Nerves and Nerve Injuries*, 2nd ed., Edinburgh, Churchill Livingstone, p. 31.

Tallis R., Staniforth P. and Fisher T. R. (1978) Neurophysiological studies of autogenous sural nerve grafts. *J. Neurol. Neurosurg. Psychiat.* **41**, 677.

Tamai S., Tatsumi Y., Shimuza T. et al. (1977) Traumatic amputation of digits: the fate of remaining blood. *J. Hand Surg.* **2**, 13.

Taylor G. I. and Ham F. J. (1976) The free vascularised nerve graft. *J. Plast. Reconstr. Surg.* **57**, 413.

Taylor G. I., Miller G. D. H. and Ham F. J. (1975) The free vascularised bone graft. *J. Plast. Reconstr. Surg.* **5**, 533.

Taylor G. I. and Watson N. (1978) One stage repair of compound leg defects with free, revascularised flaps of groin skin and iliac bone. *J. Plast. Reconstr. Surg.* **61**, 494.

Terzis J. K., Dykes R. W. and Hakistan R. W. (1976) Electrophysiological recordings in peripheral nerve surgery: a review. *J. Hand Surg.* **1**, 52.

Terzis J. K., Sweet R. C., Dykes R. N. et al. (1978) Recovery of function in free muscle transplants using microneurovascular anastomoses. *J. Hand Surg.* **3**, 37.

Urbaniak J. R. (1977) Digital replantation (Letter to the Editor). *J. Hand Surg.* **2**, 82.

Weilland A. J., Villarreal-Rios A., Kleinert H. E. et al. (1977) Replantation of digits and hands: analysis of surgical and functional results in 71 patients with 86 replantations. *J. Hand Surg.* **2**, 1.

Wise A. J., Topuzlu C., Davis P. et al. (1969) A comparative study analysis of macro and microsurgical neurorrhaphy technique. *Am. J. Surg.* **117**, 566.

Yamamoto K. (1974) A comparative analysis of the process of nerve regeneration following fascicular and epineurial suture for peripheral nerve repair. *Arch. Jpn. Chir.* **43**, 276.

Yeoman P. M. and Seddon H. J. (1961) Brachial plexus injuries: treatment of the flail arm. *J. Bone Joint Surg.* **43B**, 493.

Zachary R. B. (1954) *Peripheral Nerve Injuries.* Medical Research Council Report. No. 282. London, HMSO.

David Dandy

7 Arthroscopy of the Knee in Injury

INTRODUCTION

The arthroscope is no substitute for clinical judgement and does not supplant the clinical history as the most useful single investigation in the assessment of a knee injury. Carefully listening to the patient's account of the injury and subsequent events can provide at least as much information as the clinical examination, radiography, and arthroscopy combined, and will usually reveal which of the four main components of the knee — synovium, ligaments, bone or menisci — have been damaged. Although the characteristic clinical features of injury to each of these structures, which are set out below, will provide much information, the exact nature and extent of the injury is sometimes still obscure when all clinical means of examination have been exhausted. In these circumstances, arthroscopy may be indicated.

Synovium

The synovium is irritated to some extent in almost every knee injury, whether caused by direct or indirect violence. A simple traumatic synovitis may either follow a direct blow to the knee without disruption of other structures, or may be associated with damage to ligaments or menisci. An injured knee which has never had an effusion at any stage is uncommon, but not unknown. The effusion of fluid that follows synovial irritation alone takes several hours to appear and must be distinguished from a swelling that develops within a few minutes, which can only be due to haemorrhage into the joint and is an indication that a major injury has occurred.

Ligaments

Because the function of ligaments is to absorb energy, they will fail only under very great stress, such as the football tackle or a fall from a motorcycle. They do not rupture as the patient is getting out of the bath or changing the wheel on a car. Disruption of the vascular synovium that covers the cruciate ligaments may cause a haemarthrosis, but damage to the joint capsule or the medial or lateral ligaments alone cannot cause a haemarthrosis since the damage is outside the synovial cavity, although a simple synovial effusion may follow any ligament injury whether inside or outside the synovial cavity.

Bone and Articular Cartilage

Fractures are generally revealed by radiographs, but may easily be missed. This is particularly true of osteochondral fractures of the femoral condyle or the patella and avulsion of the tibial spine, which may be followed by a haemarthrosis and can give rise to a fat fluid level on the plain radiograph. Any patient who gives a history of sudden pain within the knee as he twists should be suspected of having an osteochondral fracture, particularly if there is an unexplained haemarthrosis.

Flakes of articular cartilage without underlying bone may also be sheared off without great violence. Because no vascular structure is damaged in such an injury there is no haemarthrosis, but an effusion, mechanical symptoms, and pain are usual. These lesions cannot be seen on a plain radiograph, but are easily demonstrated by arthrography or arthroscopy.

Menisci

One of the first things the surgeon finds on taking up arthroscopy is that meniscus injuries are rarer than he had been led to believe. The characteristic features of true meniscus symptoms are mechanical, e.g. true mechanical locking of the knee, or a definite sensation of something going out of place within the knee. These episodes generally occur without extreme violence; for example, when getting out of a car, rising from the kneeling position, or putting on a pair of socks.

Because the meniscus is avascular, damage to the meniscus alone cannot result in a haemarthrosis. A small effusion and a little joint-line tenderness, probably the result of trauma or traction of the menisco-synovial junction, is not uncommon.

TIMING OF ARTHROSCOPY

Patients with knee injuries fall into two categories. Some attend either the accident department or orthopaedic clinic as an emergency shortly after their knee has been injured, and others attend later with established symptoms long after the acute effects of injury have settled. These two groups present very different problems of assessment and management, and will be considered separately.

THE ROLE OF ARTHROSCOPY IN ACUTE INJURY

Arthroscopy makes three main contributions to the management and assessment of the acutely injured knee.

Haemarthrosis

Because haemorrhage can occur only if a vascular structure is damaged, a large haemarthrosis is almost invariably associated with a major knee injury and should not be allowed to pass undiagnosed or untreated. Arthroscopy is invaluable in the diagnosis of a haemarthrosis of unknown origin, and it is not uncommon to find at arthroscopy an undisplaced fracture line, for example in the tibial spine, which had escaped notice on the plain radiograph.

A tense haemarthrosis is painful and can result in prolonged, and sometimes permanent, restriction of movement. Simple needle aspiration of a haemarthrosis is usually unrewarding, and a formal arthrotomy to evacuate blood is unjustified, but the haematoma can easily be expressed through the arthroscope cannula and the joint irrigated thoroughly until the fluid leaving the joint is clear. Even if nothing else is done, the patient will be relieved of pain, and evacuation of the clot will allow the knee to recover more quickly.

Elimination of Delay

Before the advent of arthroscopy, it was not uncommon for the acutely injured knee to be wrapped in a bulky wool and crepe bandage, or even a plaster cylinder, for a period of two or more weeks until the synovitis had subsided so that the knee could be examined without the handicaps of swelling, joint effusion or pain. Apart from the muscle wasting and joint stiffness that follows such immobilization, few patients can afford to be away from their work or sport for several weeks until a diagnosis is made. The arthroscope makes such a delay unnecessary.

Exploratory Arthrotomy

Some surgeons advise that the knee should be opened and explored after certain injuries such as a fracture of the tibial plateau, when a meniscus may have been driven into the fracture site, or rupture of the anterior cruciate ligament, when there is often an associated meniscus injury. The necessary examination can now be done arthroscopically through a 5 mm incision without adding needless surgical trauma to the damage already present and with the extra benefit that the knee can be examined more thoroughly than at arthrotomy.

Operative Technique

The operative technique used is that described by Dr R. W. Jackson of Toronto (Jackson and Dandy, 1976b). The most suitable instrument is a standard diagnostic arthroscope approximately 5 mm in diameter. Small diameter instruments are of little value in examination of the acutely injured knee.

The examination is best done under general anaesthesia, and the surgeon should not miss the opportunity to examine the knee thoroughly under anaesthesia. More can be learned about the integrity of the ligaments from such an examination than from arthroscopy itself.

Although the synovium can be better assessed without the application of a tourniquet, it is prudent to elevate the leg and apply a tourniquet before examining an acutely injured knee. If this is not done, haemorrhage of the engorged and inflamed synovium is likely to make arthroscopy unnecessarily difficult.

Before inserting the telescope, the joint should be cleared of all clots and blood through the cannula by repeated filling and emptying with normal saline, assisted by occasional flexion of the knee to dislodge stubborn clots and bloody puddles from the popliteal fossa. This may take 10–15 minutes, and can consume two or more litres of saline.

It is important to watch for swelling of the calf and subcutaneous tissues during this procedure because irrigation fluid may escape from the joint through a defect in the joint capsule. To find a tense distended calf when the towels are removed is at best embarrassing, and at worst can cause ischaemia of the calf.

Anti-inflammatory Drugs

If the injured knee is not affected by synovitis before arthroscopy, it almost certainly will be afterwards. It is therefore sensible to support the knee in a firm wool and crepe bandage for at least 24–48 hours after injury, and to prescribe a non-steroidal anti-inflammatory drug such as ketoprofen, for 7–14 days. While not all surgeons are convinced of the efficacy of these drugs, they can do little harm and may well help the synovium to settle more rapidly.

LATE EFFECTS OF INJURY

It is unfortunate that few patients with knee injuries are seen by an orthopaedic surgeon within two weeks of injury. There are many reasons for this, among them the fact that most injuries settle spontaneously without specific treatment so that, until they are convinced that the symptoms are not going to go away on their own, most patients are understandably reluctant to visit a surgeon who might advise an operation. Some patients are referred to orthopaedic out-patient departments with an inevitable delay, while others remain under the care of sports medicine physicians, trainers, or misguided enthusiasts who believe their vocation is to save their patients from the ministrations of a knife-happy surgeon. While these factors can result in an avoidable delay before treatment is instituted, it is not practicable for all acutely injured knees to be seen immediately by a surgeon with an interest in the knee and some compromise is inevitable, depending on local circumstances.

The role of the arthroscope in the management of the late effects of injury can be considered according to the structures involved.

Synovium

Although the synovitis that follows acute injury (*Fig. 7.1*) usually settles within a few weeks of injury, it may persist for many months if the patient continues with sport or other vigorous activity in the mistaken belief that anything which hurts must be doing good. If a large synovial effusion persists without a history of recurring locking or collapsing of the knee or other clinical evidence of a major undiagnosed knee injury, the effusion may settle with rest, if necessary enforced by the application of a plaster cylinder and with the help of a non-steroidal anti-inflammatory drug. If the synovium does not subside with these measures, arthroscopy is indicated to exclude a surgically treatable lesion.

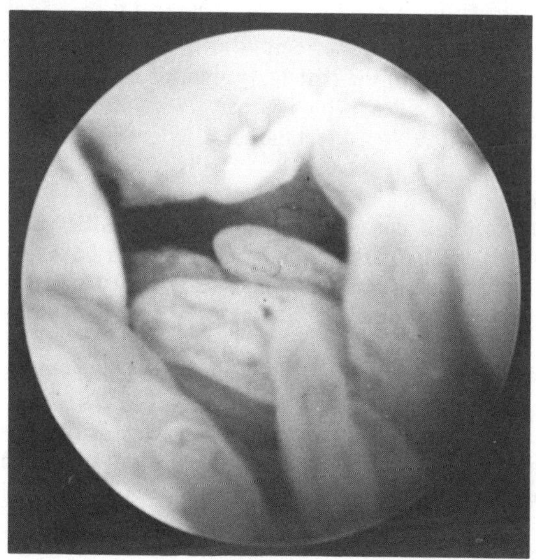

Fig. 7.1. Acute synovitis. The synovial fronds are thickened, hyperaemic and rounded.

The same problem of a persistent synovitis may follow arthrotomy, particularly meniscectomy, if the patient has returned to full activity before the synovium has had time to recover completely after the operation. Once again, rest and anti-inflammatory drugs should be advised, reserving arthroscopy, which itself irritates the synovium to some extent, for those patients whose effusion persists despite rest and drugs.

Synovial adhesions are sometimes found in the knee after arthrotomy or other injury, and may be ruptured by distension of the joint with irrigation fluid, or divided, preferably by the closed technique. Although division of adhesions is a simple non-destructive procedure that occasionally produces dramatic relief, the results are more often disappointing.

Synovial Fold Syndrome

The synovial fold syndrome is attracting much attention. In the normal knee there is a fold or shelf of synovium extending from the antero-medial edge of the patella into the medial gutter, which is easily felt and sometimes mistaken for a loose body or meniscal fragment. This fold, which becomes thickened and inflamed when the rest of the synovium is inflamed and is a useful clinical guide to the state of the synovium, also appears to be particularly vulnerable to trauma and may remain tender, thickened and swollen long after the rest of the joint has recovered.

The synovial fold syndrome should be considered whenever a patient presents with a tender synovial fold and persistent pain around the patella or the inner side of the flexed knee, especially if there is a history of direct trauma. The fold can easily be seen at arthroscopy when it appears as a shelf below and medial to the patella, running at right-angles to the medial suprapatellar fold, or plica, which it may cross. The fold, or shelf, can easily be divided by the closed technique.

Synovial Disease

When patients with a chronic inflammatory synovitis such as gout or crystal synovitis sustain a knee injury they may attribute the onset of the symptoms to the injury, however minor that may be. Arthroscopy will reveal the synovial pathology, and a biopsy can be taken by the closed technique.

Special attention should be paid to younger patients who have effusions in both knees. Investigation of such patients should include a blood sedimentation rate and an agglutination test, such as the Rose-Waaler. It should also be remembered that Reiter's disease is not unknown in vigorous athletic males.

Ligaments

Arthroscopy should not be necessary to determine whether the ligaments of the knee are intact. Ligament injuries are characteristically associated with a clear history of direct trauma to the knee and subsequent collapsing under stress, notably when changing direction while running at speed or landing after jumping for a ball. If the diagnosis is not obvious from the clinical history, the ligamentous laxity will probably be apparent on clinical examination, and any residual doubt should be dispelled by examination under anaesthetic.

Every knee undergoing arthroscopy should be examined carefully under general anaesthetic with the patient fully relaxed (*Fig. 7.2*). A swift grapple with the patient's leg in the anaesthetic room immediately after induction of anaesthesia is of no more help than examination with the patient awake, and the examination is best deferred until full relaxation has been achieved. Special attention should be paid to the integrity of the anterior cruciate ligament, and to the pivot shift test of Macintosh or jerk test of Hughston.

Despite the precedence of the history and examination, the arthroscope does have a part to play in the assessment of patients with ligament injuries. For example, a meniscus lesion may be associated with a torn ligament and these two elements of the injury can be difficult to separate on the basis of the history and clinical examination alone. The arthroscope will also reveal whether the articular cartilage has been damaged by the abnormal movement that can follow a ligament injury, and permits a dynamic assessment of the joint to be made. In particular, the meniscus

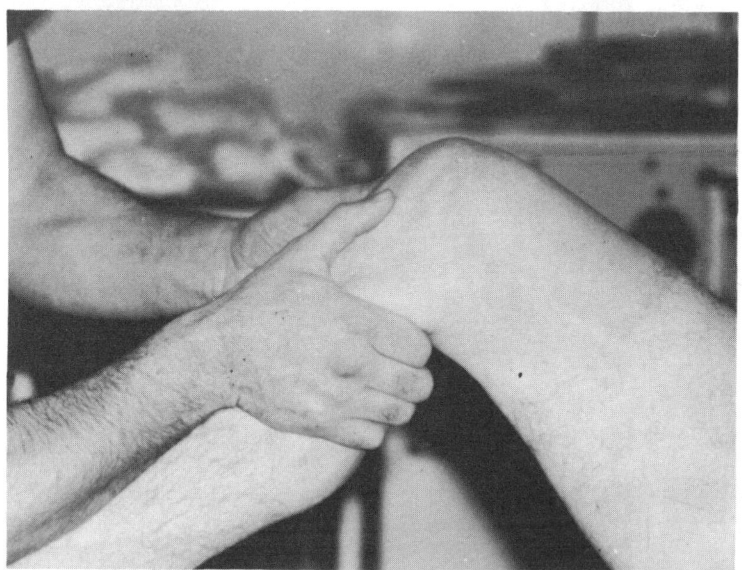

Fig. 7.2. Examination under anaesthetic. The opportunity to assess the anterior cruciate ligament with the patient fully relaxed should not be overlooked.

can be watched as the joint is manipulated, and the full extent of its abnormal movement determined. The meniscus can be distorted in the absence of an anterior cruciate ligament (*Fig. 7.3*).

The anterior cruciate ligament, if ruptured at its proximal attachment, may remain as a tag which is sometimes long enough to be caught between the joint surfaces and cause mechanical symptoms. Such a tag may be removed very simply by the closed technique or at arthrotomy.

Posterior Cruciate

Deficiency of the posterior cruciate ligament can cause the knee to collapse when the patient descends stairs or places weight upon the flexed knee. If the arthroscope is inserted from the antero-lateral route the ligament cannot usually be seen unless the anterior cruciate is absent, when it may be seen throughout its length, but the fat pad which obscures the femoral

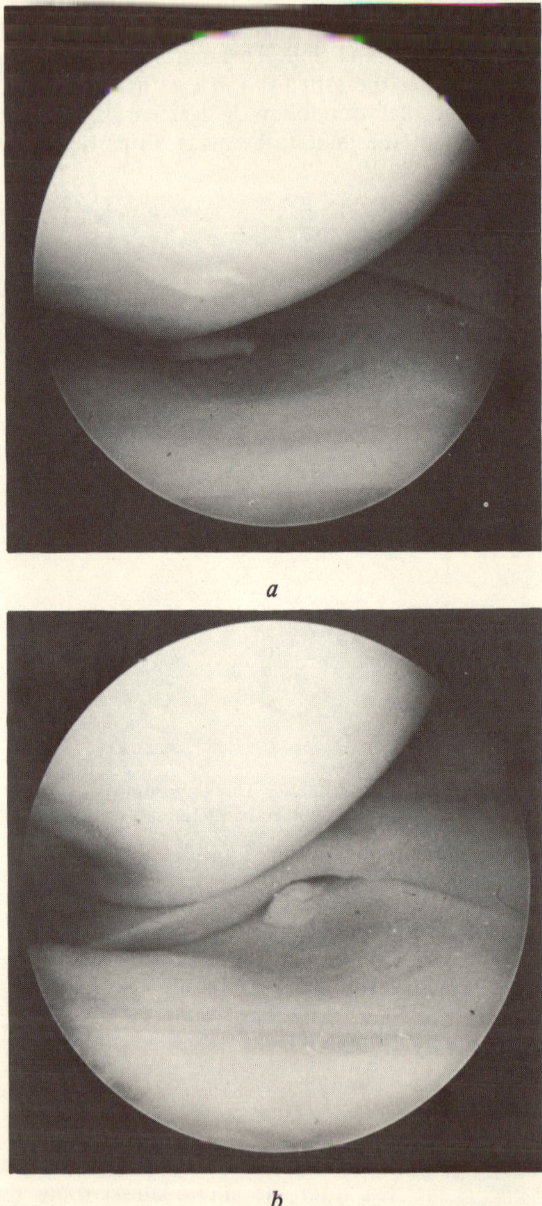

a

b

Fig. 7.3. Abnormal movement of medial meniscus in the presence of a ruptured anterior cruciate pigament. *a,* The femoral condyle is well forward of the meniscus when the tibia is held back. A small loose body can be seen. *b,* When the tibia is pulled forwards, the meniscus is drawn beneath the femoral condyle.

attachment of the ligament is sometimes inflamed and haemorrhagic after an acute injury. The posterior cruciate ligament is best seen arthroscopically from the postero-medial route.

Bones and Articular Cartilage
Early Osteoarthritis
Irregularity of the joint surfaces whether due to trauma or degenerative change is often associated with a catching sensation, which the patient may describe as 'locking'. These episodes usually follow a sharp twist with the knee straight or almost straight, and may be followed by an effusion. Unless the degenerative changes are gross or there is a fracture, the plain radiograph will be normal and the patient is then in danger of undergoing an unnecessary meniscectomy. If the symptoms are due to early osteo-arthrosis, the removal of one of the few remaining normal structures within the joint, viz. the meniscus, is unlikely to relieve the symptoms and will almost certainly make them worse.

Patients affected by early osteoarthrosis are at least as likely to sustain a meniscus injury as those who are not, and arthroscopy enables the surgeon to warn his patient that some residual symptoms may persist after the offending meniscal fragment has been removed. Neither the patient nor the surgeon should expect perfection from a knee affected by osteo-arthrosis.

Osteochondral Fractures and Chondral Flaps
Occasionally, the arthroscope will demonstrate an unexpected osteo-chondral fracture, or detachment of a chondral flap (*Fig. 7.4*). These lesions, though uncommon, often give rise to the symptoms of pain, catching and locking of the knee that are typical of a torn meniscus. Apart from demonstrating the cause of the patient's symptoms, arthroscopy has little to offer these patients, and does not make the clinician's task any easier. Most patients would much prefer to hear that a damaged meniscus has been removed than to learn that the weight-bearing surface of the joint has been damaged beyond repair (*Fig. 7.5*). Perhaps the only advantage of arthroscopy in such cases, apart from avoiding a needless arthrotomy, is the opportunity to observe the lesion as the knee is flexed and extended so that its relationship to the weight-bearing arc of movement of the knee can be determined.

Popliteus Tendon
The popliteus tendon can be avulsed from the femur with a bony fragment which may be seen on the plain radiograph. Although this lesion is rare, the surgeon should consider it in patients with pain and tenderness over the lateral femoral condyle. The popliteus tendon should be inspected whenever there is tenderness around the lateral side of the knee without obvious ligamentous laxity, and is best seen with the knee flexed to 20°

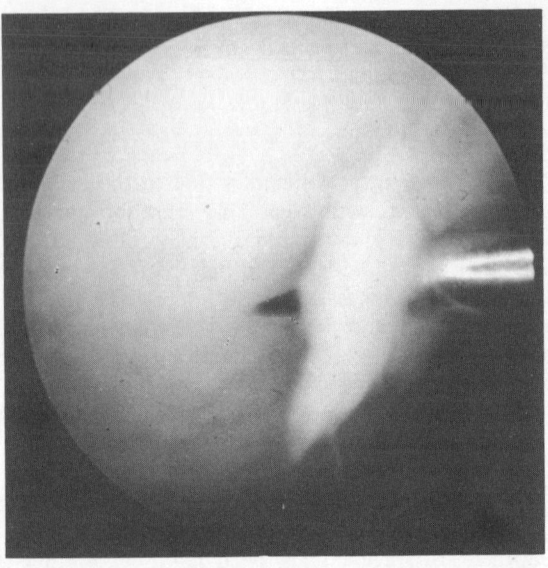

Fig. 7.4. Chondral flap. A small flap of articular cartilage is examined with a percutaneous needle.

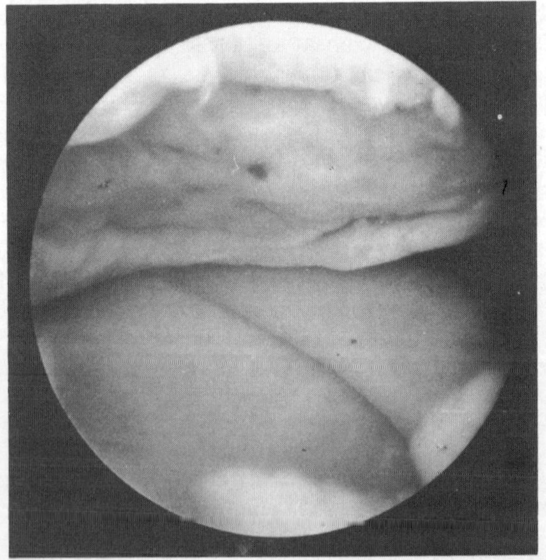

Fig. 7.5. Osteochondral fracture. A large segment of the weight-bearing surface of the medial femoral condyle has been sheared off to form a loose body.

Meniscus

The value of arthroscopy in the management of meniscus injuries depends very much on the surgeon's philosophy of meniscal function. If the surgeon believes that the meniscus serves no useful purpose and can be totally extirpated with impunity, as in the case of an appendix or tonsil, he will find little use for the arthroscope. If, on the other hand, he believes that the meniscus is there for a reason and should not be wantonly excised, the arthroscope will be of enormous value in determining which menisci are damaged and which can be preserved.

There is now a convincing body of evidence to show that knees which have undergone meniscectomy have a poor outlook (Gear, 1967), with a 30–35 per cent chance of giving rise to troublesome symptoms of one kind or another within 10 years (Huckell, 1965) and a 25 per cent chance of exhibiting radiographic changes of early osteoarthritis within 5 years (Jackson, 1967). Whether this poor prognosis results from the injury that caused the meniscus lesion, the presence of a damaged meniscal fragment, the trauma of operation, or the fact that the meniscus has been removed is uncertain, but the first two possibilities are made unlikely by the report of Zaman and Leonard (1978), who reviewed the late results of meniscectomy in children between the ages of 3 and 16 years and found that the prognosis was particularly bad if a normal meniscus had been removed.

For these and other reasons, it is unwise to remove a meniscus unless there is a good reason to suppose it is the cause of the patient's symptoms. The arthroscope is perhaps at its most useful in preventing the surgical error of removing a normal meniscus.

Partial Meniscectomy

To remove only the damaged part of the meniscus is easier technically than a total meniscectomy, and has the added advantages that the patient recovers more quickly and with better long-term results (Aarstrand, 1954; Tapper and Hoover, 1969; Jackson and Dandy, 1976a; McGinty et al., 1977; Editorial, 1978).

The most common type of partial meniscectomy is the removal of a 'bucket handle' fragment from the medial compartment, but it is also possible to remove isolated flaps or tags of damaged meniscal material. Sometimes these tags are over 2 cm long (*Fig. 7.6*); which result from a bucket handle fragment becoming detached, usually posteriorly, to behave as a loose body in the medial gutter of the knee. In other cases, meniscal flaps may be raised from either the upper or lower surface of the meniscus as the result of a horizontal split. When 'bucket-handles' are removed, the rim should be examined with a blunt hook in case there is a second split parallel with the first and likely to generate a second fragment, an established disadvantage of partial meniscectomy of any type (Cargill and Jackson, 1976; Fowler, 1976).

When flaps or tags are excised, care should be taken to ensure that the

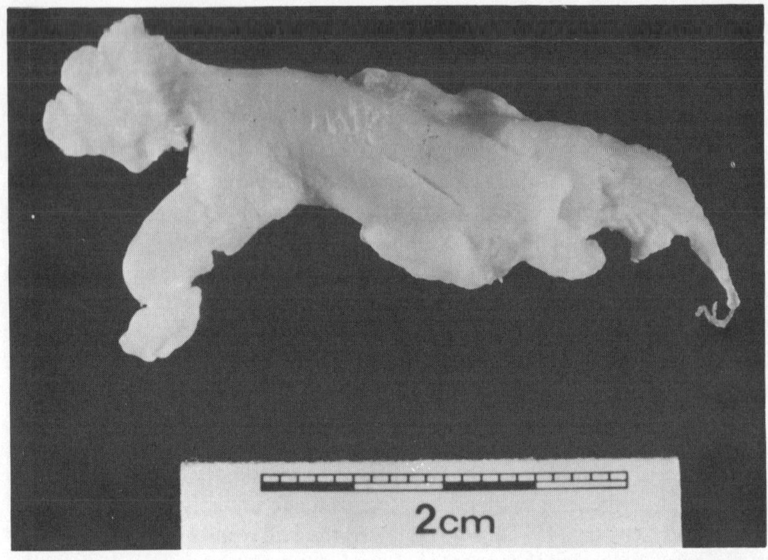

Fig. 7.6. A meniscal tag. This tag is over 3 cm long, and was attached at one end only. The edges of the meniscus had become rounded and smooth.

peripheral rim is intact, and that all loose meniscal tissue is removed until a firm and even rim remains.

Small horizontal splits without an associated flap or tag may often be demonstrated in an otherwise normal meniscus. Most surgeons are embarrassed by the removal of a normal meniscus, and there is a great temptation to attribute the patient's symptoms to a tiny fissure. It is not easy, however, for the critics of total meniscectomy to understand how a minute crevice in an avascular and insensitive structure such as the meniscus can be responsible for any important symptoms. Many other structures in the knee may, on careful examination, be found to bear crevices or fissures. The anterior cruciate ligament, for example, may be bifid, and longitudinal splits are not uncommon. We do not hear of the anterior cruciate ligament being excised in these circumstances, yet it is just as logical as a total meniscectomy for a small horizontal tear in an otherwise intact meniscus. Routine total colectomy for trivial bowel disorders was abandoned long ago, and wholesale total meniscectomy deserves the same fate.

Partial meniscectomy must not be taken as an excuse for excision of the anterior or posterior half of the meniscus alone, which can lead to the remaining half of the meniscus becoming degenerate, swollen and painful, and acting as a block to movement. If the meniscal rim is completely ruptured, as in a severe radial ('parrot-beak') tear, the whole meniscus must be removed (*Fig.* 7.7).

The degenerate meniscus presents a difficult problem. Total meniscectomy cannot be avoided if the entire meniscus is affected by cystic degeneration, but more commonly a slightly degenerate meniscus is found in a knee affected by early osteoarthrosis, with articular cartilage

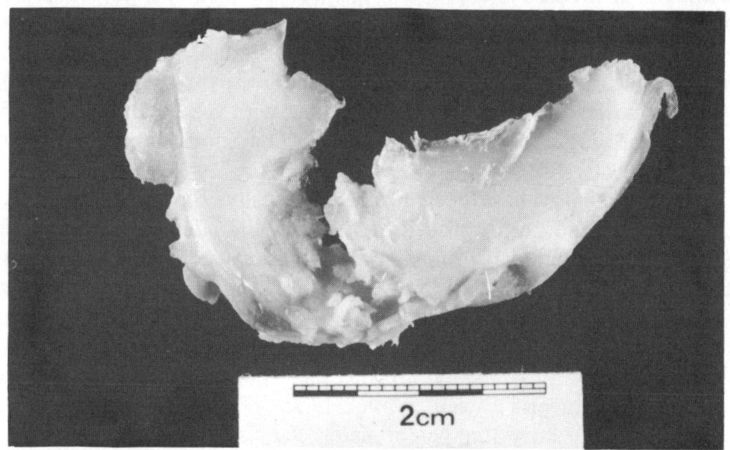

Fig. 7.7. Radial tear of the lateral meniscus. The tear extends completely through the meniscal rim of the under surface of this lateral meniscus.

degeneration and long synovial fronds. It would be surprising indeed if the meniscus did not share in the degenerative change affecting the rest of such a knee. While it is hard to see how the diseased articular cartilage can be made more healthy by removal of the meniscus, it is probably justifiable to trim any small degenerative flaps or tags from the meniscal margin by the closed technique to reduce further trauma to the articular cartilage.

Technique

The thorough examination of the meniscus at arthroscopy begins with visual inspection. As the arthroscope is brought from the suprapatellar pouch into the medial compartment, the medial menisco-synovial junction is seen and should be inspected carefully. It is easy to miss a peripheral split in this area if the loose segment of meniscus has fallen back into its normal position, particularly if there is localized synovitis at the menisco-synovial junction.

The meniscal edge should be inspected next while a valgus strain is applied to the knee, and the tibia rotated internally and externally. It is easy to see the meniscal edge throughout its length, but the back of the posterior third is a blind-spot for the arthroscope, although a lesion of the posterior horn can be inferred if the edge of the posterior third is unduly prominent. Having passed this difficult area the arthroscope may be passed lateral to the medial femoral condyle and the posterior horn inspected in far greater detail than is possible with the naked eye at arthrotomy.

The arthroscope should then be withdrawn slightly into the inter-condylar notch, and the anterior cruciate ligament examined. The femoral attachment of the posterior cruciate ligament, covered by a fat pad, can be examined conveniently at this point before the arthroscope is passed into the lateral compartment of the knee. If a varus strain is then applied to the joint, the edge of the lateral meniscus can be seen throughout its length. Any irregularities of its edge should be noted, with special attention to the intercondylar notch to be certain that it does not conceal a 'bucket handle' fragment.

When the menisci have been inspected visually, they may be probed with a hypodermic needle placed at the joint-line and passed below the meniscus. The accurate placement of this needle is difficult at first, but with practice it becomes possible to place it just under the meniscus so that the meniscus may be turned up and its under-surface exposed. The needle may also be used as a sweeper to bring out any flaps lurking beneath the posterior horn. By inserting the needle a little higher, into the substance of the meniscus itself, a 'bucket handle' fragment can sometimes be demonstrated but random percutaneous stabbing should be avoided.

If the 'needle trick' fails to reveal a meniscal lesion, a blunt hook may be inserted from the antero-medial route and passed beneath the femoral condyle to examine the posterior third of the meniscus, just as it can be examined with a blunt hook at arthrotomy. Unless this is done, peripheral tears of the posterior third in the blind area are easily missed.

Much of the posterior third of the meniscus is a blind area and it is therefore fortunate that most meniscal lesions likely to cause symptoms can be demonstrated by inspection, sweeping with the needle or probing with the blunt hook. To say that any lesion which cannot be so demon-strated cannot be causing symptoms is comforting but probably untrue. If no lesion of the posterior horn can be demonstrated, but is still suspected on the basis of the clinical findings, a double contrast arthrogram may be indicated. Arthrography is sometimes considered an alternative to arthroscopy but it should be borne in mind that the technique of arthrography is no easier to learn than arthroscopy and that a radiologist with considerable experience of the technique is required if reliable results are to be obtained.

Discoid Menisci

The lateral meniscus is of variable width and it may be hard to decide whether the meniscus is truly discoid, or just within the range of normal. A truly discoid meniscus can be quite difficult to demonstrate, probably because the arthroscopist looks first for the meniscal margin to align himself in the lateral compartment, and becomes confused and disoriented if such an obvious landmark is missing. The appearance of 'wall to wall meniscus' is remarkable but may be an incidental finding and not a cause of symptoms. The usual complaint associated with a discoid lateral meniscus is a block to full extension of the knee without pain or effusion. Unless the arthroscope demonstrates that the discoid meniscus is damaged, it need not be removed. The long-term results of total lateral meniscectomy, particularly in children, are demonstrably bad and an otherwise asymptomatic loss of full extension is probably the lesser of two evils.

Retained Fragments

The retained fragment of meniscus is grossly overrated as a cause of symptoms after meniscectomy (Dandy and Jackson, 1975). If the patient's symptoms are unchanged by meniscectomy the most likely explanation is that the meniscus was not responsible for the original symptoms. Occasionally, a long fragment of meniscus is seen and can easily be removed with the closed technique or at arthrotomy, but it is often very difficult to attribute the patient's continued symptoms to the presence of this fragment and the clinical results of excision are unrewarding.

ARTHROSCOPIC SURGERY OF THE KNEE

The technique of performing surgical procedures inside the knee under arthroscopic control and without the need for a wide arthrotomy is known variously as closed surgery, arthroscopic surgery, or endoscopic surgery. The technique has now become standard practice in a few centres.

The principal advantage of the technique is the minimal disturbance of the skin, subcutaneous tissues, joint capsule and synovium. The preservation of these tissues hastens the patient's recovery and makes rehabilitation less arduous so that, using the closed technique, it is now usual for patients to walk out of hospital without crutches or sticks the day after their meniscus operation and to return to work within a few days if they are engaged in a sedentary occupation, or within 10–14 days if their work is heavy (Dandy, 1978). Such a reduction in the period of disability, hospital admission, and rehabilitation has obvious economic and social advantages both to the patient and to those who provide health care.

A second benefit of the technique is that it becomes possible to determine the effects of intra-articular elements of an operation now that they are not overshadowed by the effects of arthrotomy. It is an interesting observation that mechanical symptoms such as clicking or catching within the joint can be relieved by removal of a comparatively small detached fragment of meniscus while the aching and swelling that follows heavy use of knees with early osteoarthritis remains unchanged. 'Inhibition' of the quadriceps and severe pain on attempted straight leg raising do not occur after arthroscopic surgery and are clearly the result of the incision necessary to open the joint.

Arthroscopic surgery also has its disadvantages. The arthroscopic novice always encounters great difficulty in knowing exactly what it is that he sees down his instrument, and few surgeons feel really confident with their arthroscopic technique until they have done 50 or more arthroscopies. Before embarking on a closed operation the surgeon must have complete confidence in his arthroscopic findings, or considerable damage may be done. Probably the main disadvantage of this technique is that it could lead to widespread intra-articular devastation in the hands of the inexperienced enthusiast.

The second disadvantage is the length of the operation itself. At first, a closed partial meniscectomy may take almost two hours to perform, but with practice, and with the development of the appropriate instruments, it is now exceptional for a closed partial meniscectomy by the double puncture technique to take longer than 45 minutes from insertion of the irrigation needle to the last stitch, 30 minutes being more usual. When the technique is developed further, it may well be possible to remove a 'bucket handle' fragment of the meniscus in 10–15 minutes without admitting the patient to hospital.

The obvious criticism of the sceptic is that the view obtained through the arthroscope is not as good as that obtained at arthrotomy. While it is certainly true that the anterior part of the joint cannot be seen as clearly through an arthroscope as at arthrotomy, the posterior attachments of the menisci and other structures tucked away in obscure recesses can be seen in much more detail and with the advantage of magnification. Synovial biopsy, division of synovial folds, and trimming of the irregular meniscus can be all done under magnification, and in these circumstances the arthroscope offers the same advantages as an operating microscope elsewhere. If the surgeon can see more at arthrotomy than at arthroscopy, he is either using the wrong arthroscope, or the right arthroscope wrongly.

Technique

Either single or double puncture techniques may be used, and both are best done after elevation of the leg and inflation of a tourniquet. For the single puncture technique an operating arthroscope is used incorporating irrigation, a telescope, fibre-light guide and a channel for operating instruments. The addition of a channel to carry operating instruments inevitably increases the diameter of the instrument, and thus the size of the wound necessary for insertion. The instruments that can be passed down such an arthroscope must be small and delicate, and may not be strong enough to deal with a tough meniscus. The telescope may also be reduced in diameter to minimize the bulk of the instrument but to do so involves a reduction in the field of vision. The instrument itself is more complex in design than a simple diagnostic arthroscope and thus more difficult to manipulate within the knee. The fact that the operating instruments run in a cannula parallel with the telescope brings the advantage that there is no difficulty in identifying the tip of the instrument within the knee, but also the disadvantage that the instrument cannot be manoeuvred without moving the telescope itself.

The need to use a complicated and rather bulky instrument with a thicker barrel, a narrow angle of vision and delicate instruments which can move only in one plane weigh heavily against the advantages of making only one incision. It may also be that the larger incision necessary to insert such an instrument is more disruptive of the joint capsule than the two smaller incisions used for the double puncture technique.

The double puncture technique requires two separate incisions, one for the arthroscope and one for the instruments. Experience so far suggests that for procedures within the suprapatellar pouch, the most suitable place for insertion of the operating instruments is the lateral side of the joint, at the usual point of insertion of the irrigation needle. It is advisable to identify the tip of the irrigation needle with the telescope and to manipulate the structures to be cut or divided with its tip to ensure that instruments can reach their target if inserted from this approach.

For operation on the menisci, the instruments may be inserted through a short cannula immediately medial to the patellar tendon, and approximately 5 mm above the wound used for insertion of the arthroscope. Positioning the instruments at this point makes it possible, rather surprisingly, to operate on either the medial or the lateral meniscus and the need for a medial insertion of the telescope is rare.

The instruments are inserted through a short cannula of the same diameter as that of the arthroscope. At present, the cannula does not have a tight seal or effective valve, and an assistant able to place a finger over the end of the cannula after the instrument has been withdrawn prevents a gush of irrigation fluid striking the observer or surgeon unexpectedly.

When inserting the operating instruments from the antero-medial route, the knee should be flexed to approximately 60° and the arthroscope held in the intercondylar notch by an assistant. Care must be taken that the trocar does not strike the arthroscope during insertion. This can be prevented by ensuring that the tip of the arthroscope is pointing downwards and that the trocar is aimed upwards from its point of insertion, which should itself be above the insertion of the telescope. The surgeon will quickly find that he has insufficient hands with which to manipulate two instruments and the patient's leg, but this problem may be overcome if the surgeon sits, resting the patient's foot between his own knees. With practice, the knee may be manipulated surprisingly well in this way.

It is advisable to use the straight ahead 0° telescope, because it is much easier to bring the tip of the operating instrument in front of the lens. If an oblique or side-viewing lens is used, the telescope can be directed laterally so that the instruments pass in the same plane as the direction of vision, making orientation easier, and these manoeuvres can be practised outside the operating theatre. The basic operating instruments include a blunt hook with which to probe the meniscus and apply traction to it, a

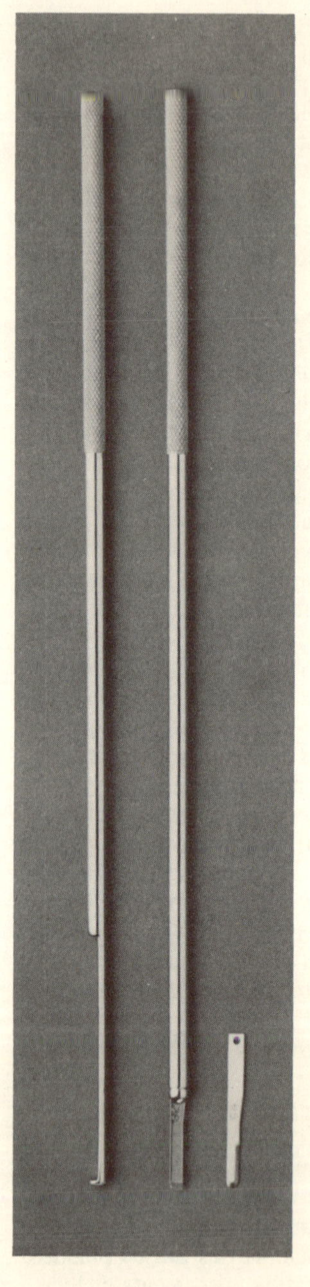

a

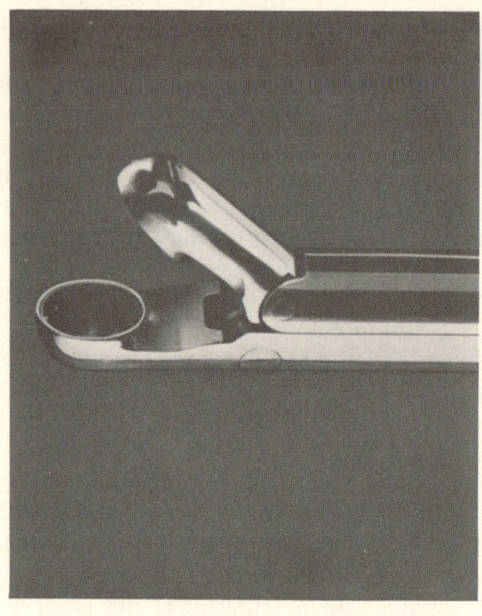

b

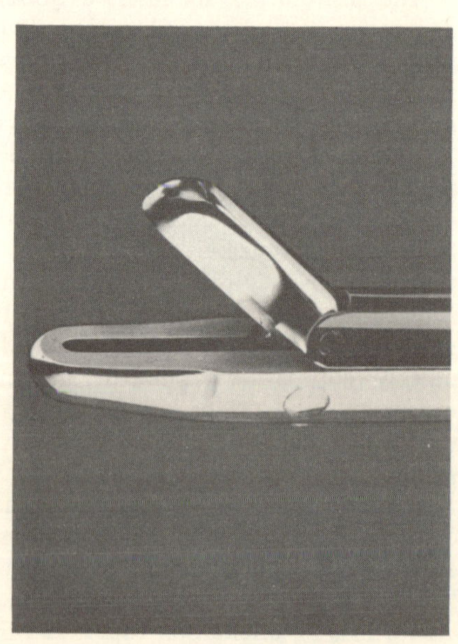

c

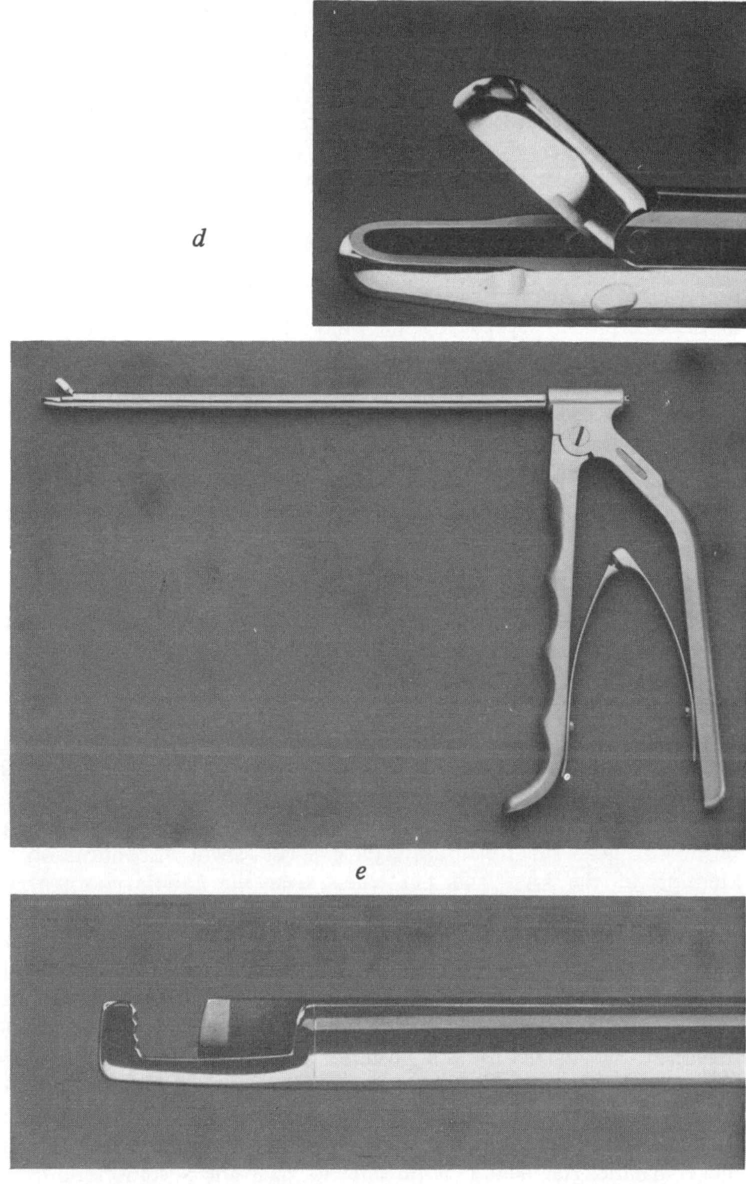

Fig. 7.8. Operating instruments for closed meniscectomy: *a*, blunt hook and long-handled knife. *b*, cup forceps. *c*, punch scissors. *d*, meniscal punch, *e*. meniscal punch. *f*, guillotine. (*Reproduced by kind permission of Chas. F. Thackray Ltd., Leeds.*)

pair of punch scissors with which to cut meniscus, a punch to trim the meniscus, cup forceps, a long-handled knife, and a guillotine consisting of a knife-blade fitted with a hook (*Fig. 7.8*). Identification of the tip of the operating instruments may be difficult, and it is essential that the operating instruments are moved with great care. The temptation to make blind stabs, chops or cuts when the tip of the instrument is out of sight must be resisted at all costs. Until the cerebellum develops the necessary circuits and neural pathways for manipulation of the instruments, there are two other ways in which the tip of the instruments can be found. If the instruments have been inserted from the antero-medial route, the inter-condylar notch, which is easy to identify, can be used as a 'reporting base' for the instruments by passing them into the notch for recognition. The alternative method is to feel the barrel of the arthroscope with the operating instrument, which is then slid along the arthroscope to its tip. This technique is less satisfactory and should be avoided in tight areas of the knee such as the medial or lateral gutter, but is useful if the target, e.g. a loose body, is elusive.

Closed Partial Meniscectomy

It is essential to delineate the exact anatomy of the meniscus lesion before inserting the operating instruments so that a surgical strategy can be formulated. To this end, the lesion may be placed in one of the following categories and treated accordingly.

Circumferential Tears

Circumferential or 'bucket handle' tears fall easily into four types.

The first is a complete 'bucket handle' tear which extends to the anterior meniscal attachment, with the meniscal fragment locked in the intercondylar notch. Such lesions may cause surprisingly little disability, but may cause a small effusion after exercise, slight discomfort on full extension of the knee and tenderness over the anterior horn of the meniscus, presumably due to stretching or irritation of the synovium at the anterior attachment of the meniscus.

For this, as for all meniscal lesions, the operating instruments should be inserted initially from the antero-medial route. The posterior attachment of the meniscus is best divided first for two reasons. Firstly, if the anterior attachment is cut before the posterior attachment the fragment may disappear into the posterior fossa, and prove extremely difficult to retrieve. Secondly, if the tear extends as far as the anterior horn and the operating instruments are inserted immediately above the anterior attachment of the 'bucket handle' fragment it is possible to grasp the posterior end of the fragment with forceps and pull it out through the wound before it is divided at its anterior attachment, simplifying the operation enormously (*Fig. 7.9*).

The posterior attachment can be divided with the straight knife, the

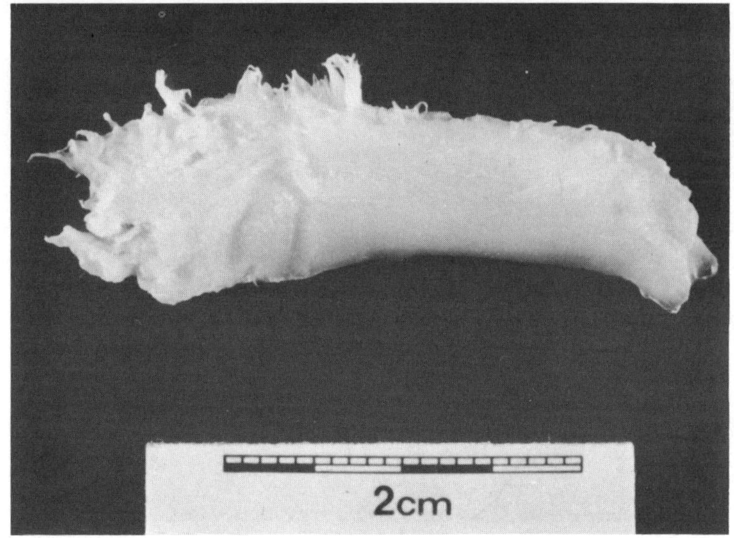

Fig. 7.9. 'Bucket handle' fragment of medial meniscus removed by the closed technique.

punch scissors or the guillotine. To pass the guillotine around the posterior attachment is difficult but when this can be done, repeated cutting with the guillotine will either divide the meniscal attachment completely or weaken it so that it can easily be avulsed or cut with the scissors. Once the posterior attachment is divided, the posterior horn can be trimmed with cup forceps until none remains.

Attention can then be turned to the anterior attachment which, if the fragment cannot be withdrawn through the skin, can usually be divided with the guillotine, supplemented if necessary by the scissors (*Fig. 7.10*). Great care should be taken at this stage in case the meniscal fragment escapes and floats around the knee as a loose body. Identification and retrieval of such a fragment can be tedious and protracted, but this difficulty can be avoided if the irrigation is turned off and the knee held still as soon as it is clear that the fragment is free. The meniscal fragment should then be seized at its end with grasping forceps and withdrawn.

A large 'bucket handle' fragment is usually too big to bring through the cannula, in which case the cannula can be withdrawn together with the meniscus. If the fragment is particularly large or has been grasped at its middle instead of its end, a small No. 15 blade may be passed along the side of the cannula while applying gentle traction to the meniscal fragment to enlarge the capsular incision until the fragment is delivered. Once the fragment has been removed, attention should be directed to the anterior

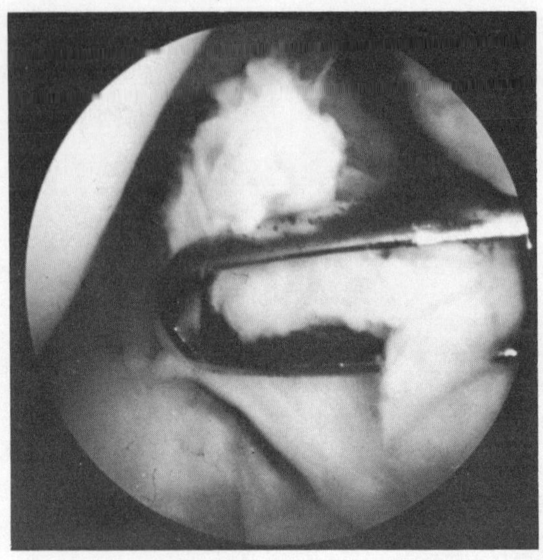

Fig. 7.10. Division of the anterior attachment of the 'bucket handle' tear by the closed technique, using punch scissors.

attachment which may once again be trimmed with the operating instruments until a clean and healthy rim remains.

The second type of circumferential tear is that in which there is true locking of the knee, i.e. a mechanical block to extension. Such a patient will almost certainly have a 'bucket handle' tear with the tear starting at the posterior meniscal insertion extending into the anterior half of the meniscus, but stopping short of the anterior meniscal insertion. The smaller the block to extension, the further forward is the tear likely to extend.

This pattern of tear is comparatively simple to deal with, the principal difficulty being that of bringing the cutting instruments to the anterior attachment of the fragment. When this has been achieved the fragment may be withdrawn and the rim trimmed in the usual way (*Fig. 7.11*).

The third type of circumferential tear is that which involves the posterior horn only and is manifest by locking of the knee in full flexion. The patient may become wary of flexing the knee fully and will thus avoid it subconsciously so that the history of locking, though definite, may be very infrequent. If such a history is present the knee should be fully flexed under anaesthetic and particular attention paid to the posterior horn with the blunt hook and probing needle at arthroscopy. These fragments can be difficult to remove neatly and may need to be taken out piecemeal with the cup forceps and punch (*Fig. 7.12*).

The fourth type of lesion resulting from a circumferential tear is the

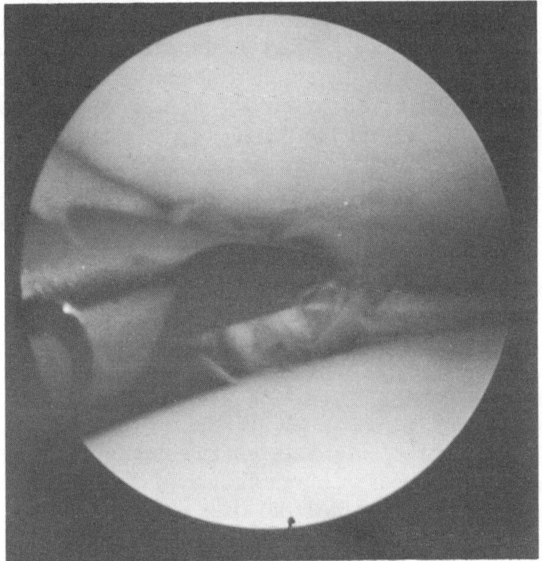

Fig. 7.11. Trimming the meniscal rim by the closed technique after removing a meniscal flap.

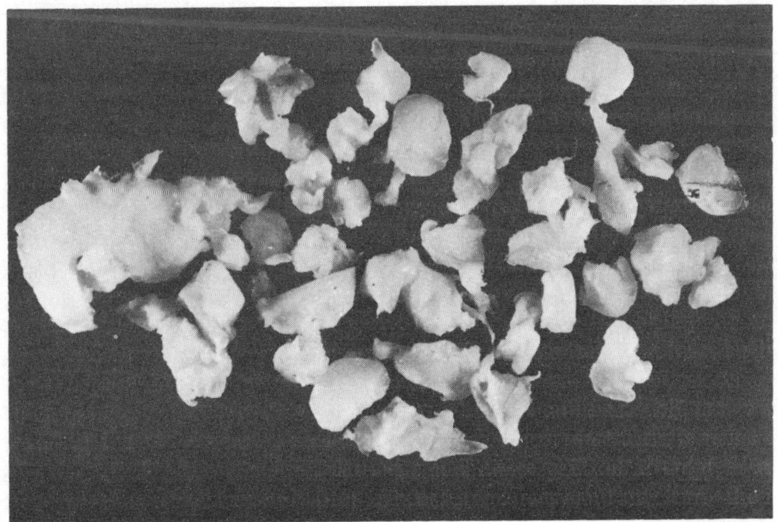

Fig. 7.12. Meniscal fragments. These fragments constituted a 'bucket handle' fragment of the medial meniscus which had dislocated to the centre of the joint.

detached bucket handle which presents as a long tag of meniscal tissue (*see Fig. 7.6*). These tags almost always become detached posteriorly, the symptoms being caused by the anteriorly based remnant. It is noticeable that if the fragment has been present for months or years it will become smooth and rounded as will the margin of the meniscus from which it arose. This observation offers great encouragement to those who advocate partial meniscectomy for it demonstrates that a torn edge of meniscus will eventually become smooth. They may be dealt with exactly like the first two types of circumferential tear, except the first part of the procedure, detachment of the posterior horn, has already been done.

Flaps

Flaps of meniscal tissue give rise to a transient sensation of catching or clicking when the leg is twisted, and do not cause true locking. They may conveniently be classified into superior and inferior types according to their origin from the upper or lower surfaces of the meniscus, and further subdivided into anterior and posterior flaps according to their attachment to make a total of four fypes. A fifth type is the anterior horn tag which gives rise to pain on hyperextension, and when viewed through the arthroscope seems much larger than its true size.

The classification of meniscal flaps in this way is of value when operation is planned. Inferiorly based flaps can be seized and avulsed with the cup forceps, but the upper surface is usually intact in such lesions and need not be touched. Superiorly based flaps are easier to remove, but the meniscus usually needs to be trimmed back to healthy tissue (*Fig. 7.13*). Anteriorly based flaps can be removed with the guillotine.

The rare anterior flaps are difficult to examine arthroscopically because they lie so close to the lens of the instrument. Care should be taken that the lesion seen is indeed the meniscal flap and not a piece of synovium lying close to the lens, appearing unnaturally white because of its proximity to the light source. They may be removed with cup forceps.

The 'parrot beak' tear affecting the lateral meniscus is a radial tear affecting the mid-portion of the lateral meniscus. Particular attention should be paid to both upper and lower surfaces of such a lesion to determine whether or not the tear extends right through the peripheral margin. There is no alternative to total meniscectomy if the rim is completely divided (*see Fig. 7.7*) but if it is intact, the damaged part of the meniscus alone may be trimmed away until a healthy rim is seen.

Degenerate menisci have already been mentioned. Slight irregularity of the inner edge of the meniscus, horizontal fissuring and irregularity of the posterior horn are normal findings in the elderly patient. These irregularities may be trimmed by the closed technique, but such a procedure would not warrant arthrotomy. The posterior horn is the usual site of such irregularity, and can be inaccessible unless the knee is manipulated care-

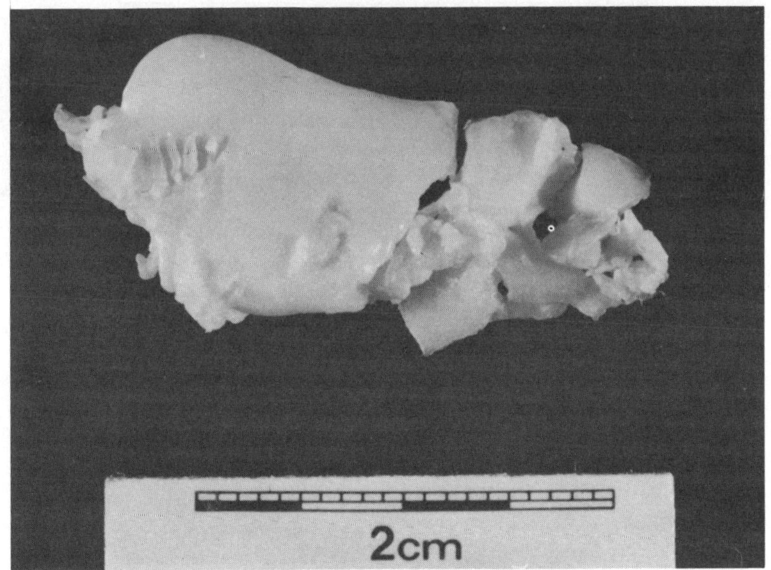

Fig. 7.13. A large meniscal flap removed by the closed technique.

fully. It is easy to damage the articular cartilage while trimming the posterior horn, and great caution should be exercised.

Loose Bodies
Identification of a loose body with the arthroscope is considerably easier than grasping and removing it. Once identified, any attempt to seize the loose body with operating instruments may result in its skating away into some remote fastness of the joint such as the popliteal fossa, when an arthrotomy may be needed for its removal. If the fragment can be identified and directed to the suprapatellar pouch or to the medial or lateral gutter, it may sometimes be secured with a percutaneous needle (*Fig. 7.14*) and held there until it is either grasped with forceps, or a small incision made over it. If the loose body is successfully grasped, and it is obviously too large to be withdrawn through the stab incision used for insertion of the cannula, a Number 15 blade may be passed beside the cannula to enlarge the capsular incision and allow the loose body to be delivered, as described for large meniscal fragments.

Postoperative Management
Although the wounds necessary for a closed operation are small they are nevertheless stab wounds and take as long to heal as any other wound. The synovium, too, responds unfavourably to arthroscopy, and to the slight trauma of the operating instruments.

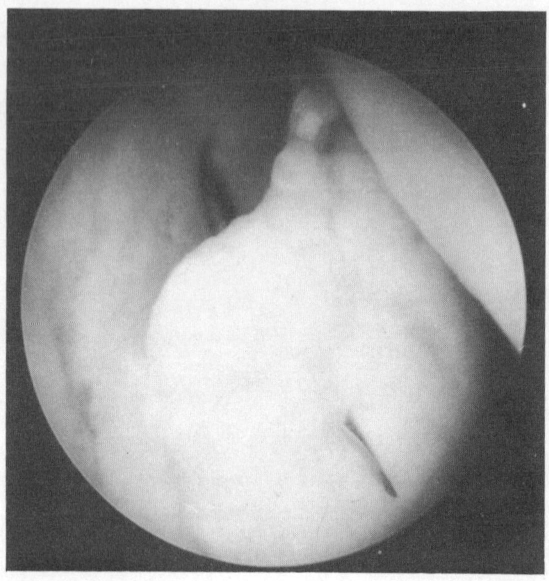

Fig. 7.14. A loose body, which had arisen from osteochondral fracture of the patella, is transfixed by a percutaneous needle.

To reduce the inevitable synovitis that follows injury of any kind, the knee should be dressed with orthopaedic wool and a crepe bandage and the bandage retained for at least seven days. Failure to do this may result in a persistent effusion. A non-steroidal anti-inflammatory drug, e.g. ketoprofen, 50 mg three times a day, may also help the joint to settle and can do little harm.

Physiotherapy is hardly necessary. Proper instruction in quadriceps exercises is useful, and ultrasound to the wounds, especially the medial wound, may speed the resolution of postoperative inflammation.

Learning Arthroscopic Surgery

Like all endoscopic procedures, arthroscopy and arthroscopic surgery are difficult techniques to learn. Once the surgeon is confident with the arthroscope, there are a number of 'exercises' which can be undertaken before a major closed procedure is attempted. The simplest such exercise is to identify the tip of the irrigation needle in the suprapatellar pouch. When confidence in identifying the needle has been acquired, and the effect of rotating the oblique or side viewing telescope observed, the surgeon may progress to the examination of the under-surface of the meniscus with a probing needle. Accurate placement of the needle is easier if the area of meniscus beneath which the needle is to be inserted is examined closely with the arthroscope so that the skin is transilluminated.

With practice, the needle may be passed immediately beneath the meniscus at the first attempt.

The next step is to take a biopsy of the synovium either from the lateral patellar or the antero-medial approach. When fully confident with the manipulation of the biopsy forceps and the arthroscope together, the surgeon may proceed either to trimming a degenerate meniscus, excising a flap or tag in the anterior half of the joint, or probing a doubtful meniscus with the blunt hook. When all these manoeuvres can be accomplished with confidence and ease, the surgeon may proceed to what is at present the tour de force of arthroscopic surgery — the removal of a 'bucket handle' fragment.

Acknowledgement

Figs. 7.1–7.7 and 7.9–7.14 *reproduced by courtesy of Addenbrooke's Hospital, Cambridge.*

REFERENCES

Aarstrand T. (1954) Treatment of meniscal rupture of the knee-joint: a follow-up examination of material where only the ruptured part of the meniscus has been removed. *Acta Chir. Scand.* **107**, 146.

Cargill A. O'R. and Jackson J. P. (1976) Bucket handle tear of the medial meniscus. *J. Bone Joint Surg.* **58A**, 248.

Dandy D. J. (1978) *Br. Med. J.* **1**, 1099.

Dandy D. J. and Jackson R. W. (1975) The diagnosis of problems after meniscectomy. *J. Bone Joint Surg.* **57B**, 349.

Editorial (1978) Partial meniscectomy preferred. *Br. Med. J.* **1**, 1091.

Fowler A. W. (1976) Partial meniscectomies for bucket handle tears of the medial meniscus. *J. Bone Joint Surg.* **58B**, 136.

Gear M. W. L. (1967) The late results of meniscectomy. *Br. J. Surg.* **54**, 270.

Huckell J. R. (1965) Is meniscectomy a benign procedure?: a long term follow-up study. *Can. J. Surg.* **8**, 254.

Jackson J. P. (1967) Degenerative changes in the knee after meniscectomy. *J. Bone Joint Surg.* **49B**, 584.

Jackson R. W. and Dandy D. J. (1976a) Partial meniscectomy. *J. Bone Joint Surg.* **58B**, 142.

Jackson R. W. and Dandy D. J. (1976b) *Arthroscopy of the Knee.* New York, Grune & Stratton.

McGinty J. B., Guess L. F. and Marvin R. A. (1977) Partial or total meniscectomy. *J. Bone Joint Surg.* **59A**, 763.

Tapper E. M. and Hoover N. W. (1969) Late results after meniscectomy. *J. Bone Joint Surg.* **51A**, 517.

Zaman M. and Leonard M. A. (1978) British Orthopaedic Association Meeting, 6.4.78.

W. M. Steel

8 External Skeletal Fixation in Fracture Treatment

INTRODUCTION

In the UK surgeons have a background of sound conservative management of fractures. Our fracture clinics allow close surveillance of patients treated in plaster and our training of nurses, technicians and surgeons has led to the wide dissemination of skills in the manipulation, immobilization and rehabilitation of limb injuries. The fears of inadequacy and dangers of plaster and the dire consequences to the joint of weeks in a cast that are expressed by some European surgeons are based on ignorance of sound conservative techniques.

Nevertheless, we are beginning to add the best of the European techniques of internal fixation onto a foundation of well tried conservatism. Controversy in certain areas is bound to continue and this is healthy, but few would dispute the place of internal fixation for certain injuries, particularly in the treatment of joints. If we are to employ such techniques it is only prudent to seek the most successful of European methods. The gradual introduction of AO techniques into British orthopaedics is therefore a sound progression in fracture surgery.

It is now time to consider a further significant development in fracture treatment: the use of external skeletal fixation. Just as internal fixation was practised for many years so external fixation has been available for at least four decades. However, the progress in these areas has been the introduction of improved engineering design, detailed research of biomechanical aspects and careful clinical appraisal of the methods. As a consequence we can now add to our armamentarium, not a Heath Robinson contraption, but a system which has been well tried and tested by European surgeons of high repute.

The previous indiscriminate use of external apparatus did not give the principle the credit that it deserved but there is now increasing support for external skeletal fixation. The most generally popular apparatus is that devised by Hoffmann and modified by Vidal which is used occasionally for pelvic fractures but mainly for open, comminuted fractures, and infected pseudarthrosis, especially of the tibia.

In the simpler fractures, simpler devices have been used, differing mainly in the strength of the side bars and the means whereby the transfixing pins are attached to them and compression or distraction are applied.

In the USSR, compression—distraction apparatus has been used for many years in the treatment not only of fresh, old, malunited, ununited and infected fractures but also of congenital and other deformities, in the correction of contractures and the performance of arthrodesis. The apparatus used in the USSR varies in detail but is based upon taut Kirschner's wires that are attached to circular or semicircular frames (*Fig. 8.1*) but it is almost unknown in the UK.

In the circumstances, it seems best at this stage to indicate current practice in the UK rather than to try to analyse critically the different methods, which are for the most part unfamiliar.

HISTORICAL DEVELOPMENT

Systems of external skeletal fixation date back to the mid-nineteenth century when Malgaigne (1853) described percutaneous fixation for fractures of the patella. Further early developments followed in France with the design by Lambotte (1907) of an external anchorage which became the prototype of subsequent models. Cuendet (1936) introduced the concept of percutaneous pins transfixing the bone on both sides of the fracture with a tie bar on each side. The method which is widely used in Europe and which is at last finding favour in the UK derives from the equipment designed by Hoffmann (1938). Improvements on the original model have been made by Vidal (1968) as a result of his extensive experience with the system and following the bio-mechanical survey conducted by Adrey (1970). Connes (1973) analyses the Hoffmann system in great detail and describes the indications and results of this technique of fracture fixation. This work, which is in English, is the 'guidebook' for those contemplating an introduction to this method.

Reports from Scandinavia have confirmed the value of the Hoffmann system, particularly in the highly selected group of patients with open tibial fractures unsuitable for other forms of fixation. Felländer (1963), Olerud (1973) and Karlström and Olerud (1975) have each reported favourably on their experience with the Hoffmann device.

It will be no surprise to learn that external skeletal fixation was introduced in the USA during the same period. Roger Anderson (1934) is credited with the earliest work, followed by the Stader (1937) method and the Haynes (1939) device. Reports of large series of fractures treated by these techniques appeared in the 1940s and several military establishments used external fixation extensively during World War II. Lewis et al. (1942) and Shaar et al. (1944) described their experience with the Stader apparatus, whilst Naden (1949) reported 237 fractures treated by the Roger Anderson method. In all these series, however, external fixation was used extensively for closed fractures, and was not limited in any way to the open, comminuted fracture. Needless to say there were complications, notably pin-track sepsis, and the American devices did not provide the rigidity or versatility of the Hoffmann system. Enthusiasm was dampened and virtually extinguished by a report of a survey conducted by the

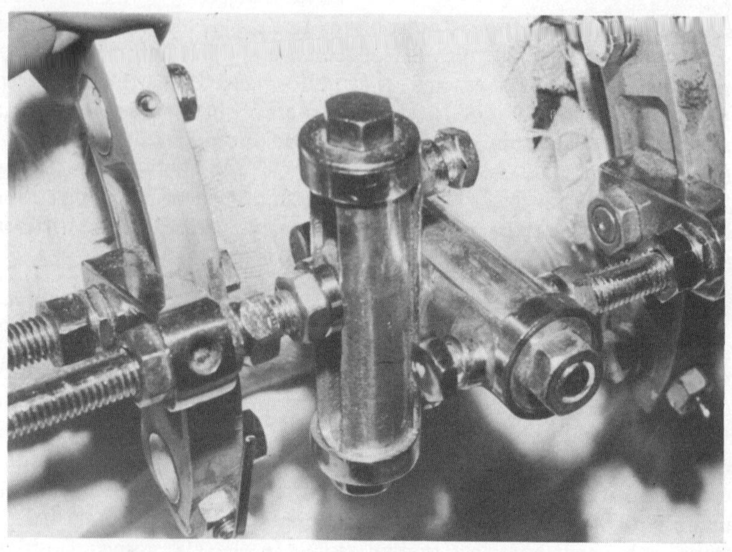

a

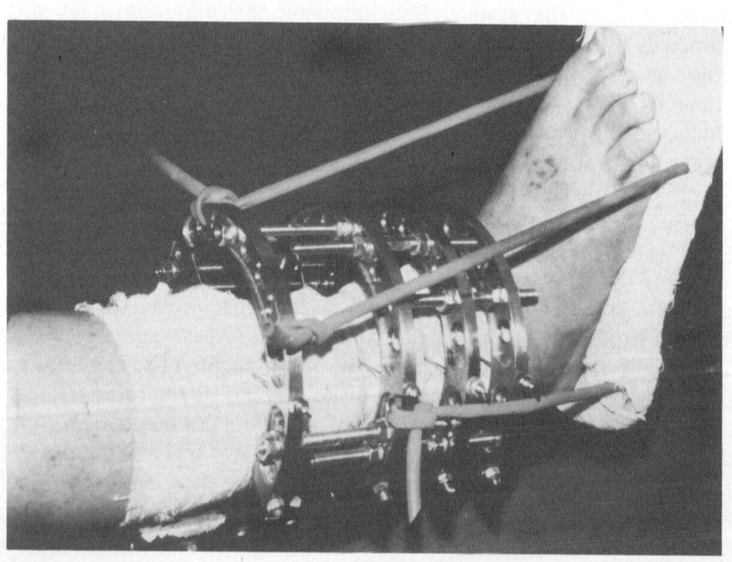

b

Fig. 8.1. a, The Volkov apparatus showing in detail how some of the adjustments are carried out. *b*, Kalnberz's apparatus.

Committee on Fractures and Traumatic Surgery of the American Academy of Orthopaedic Surgeons summarized by Johnson and Stovall (1950) from which it was concluded that the use of external fixation should be restricted to specialized centres with experience of the method. Thereafter reports in the American literature relating to external fixation are largely confined to the use of pins above and below the fracture incorporated in a cast, which is not strictly external skeletal fixation. Indeed, in a recent analysis of the reasons for failure of treatment in open tibial fractures by Rosenthal et al. (1977) no mention is made of the use of external skeletal fixation although the paper surveys the recent American experience in Vietnam and in civilian practice.

Developments in the UK have followed an even more conservative pattern. Apart from the occasional use of pins incorporated in plaster, leg-lengthening machines or the Roger Anderson device, British surgeons have eschewed external skeletal fixation. Papers by Dwyer (1973), Ronen et al. (1974), Rezaian (1977) and Wynn-Jones (1978) have drawn attention to the possibilities of external fixation, particularly in the difficult open tibial fractures, but the series are small and the devices have not been widely used by others. The use of percutaneous pins has of course been used widely in facio-maxillary surgery and in areas of orthopaedic surgery other than fracture surgery. Maxillary fractures are frequently treated by external skeletal fixation attached to the skull cap or halo device. The halo has been widely used in conjunction with pelvic or femoral fixation in the management of scoliosis. Leg-lengthening by percutaneous pins attached to a frame has been practised safely for many years by Anderson (1952) and the Edinburgh school with few complications. Care of the pin-track, prevention of movement, and precise skin puncture should prevent sepsis and osteomyelitis. It is therefore surprising that treatment of fractures by percutaneous pin fixation attached by bars should have been viewed with such disfavour by British and American surgeons.

Perhaps the increasing contact which has been made with European surgeons in connection with internal fixation techniques has made British orthopaedic surgeons more aware of other developments in fracture surgery in Continental Europe. Certainly there is an awakening of interest in external skeletal fixation and it is hoped that we shall benefit from the experience of French, German and Scandinavian authors and add this technique to our armamentarium.

INDICATIONS FOR USE

The principal indications for the use of external fixation are as follows.

1. In the management of open fractures with marked comminution or loss of bone.
2. In the treatment of infected pseudoarthroses.
3. In severe pelvic fractures.

Open Fractures

Conservative Treatment

The combination of a shattered long bone and extensive soft tissue damage poses an almost insurmountable problem to the conservative surgeon. Adequate immobilization, maintenance of length and correction of deformity by means of plaster fixation or traction is virtually impossible. Add to this the necessity for regular dressing, grafting and possible flap cover of the wound and the condition taxes surgical skill to the limit.

The incidence of infection in Nicoll's (1964) series of conservatively treated tibial fractures was 15 per cent, and of non-union 55 per cent. Even if union is achieved and healing of soft tissue obtained it is often at the expense of bone shortening and deformity.

Plating

The use of plates and screws in the management of long bone fractures, especially the forearm and tibia, has become extensive. It may be an admirable technique where soft tissue damage is minimal and bone destruction does not preclude stability. However, where the wound cannot be closed over the plate and fracture, or where there is gross shattering of the bone, the method is unsuitable. Burwell (1971), otherwise an enthusiast of plating, stated that 'the large wound with severe damage to soft tissue is often not well suited to plating' and goes on to suggest the use of an intramedullary device. Five of his twelve septic cases had severe open fractures.

Intramedullary Fixation

When the soft tissue defect is large intramedullary fixation is a much more attractive method of fixation than plating, provided that stability can be obtained. However, it is not suited to grossly comminuted fractures. Harvey et al. (1975) in an enthusiastic review of this technique for open fractures of the tibia quote gross comminution as one of their contra-indications.

Advantages of External Fixation

There is undoubtedly a need for a technique which will permit coincidental stabilization of a severely comminuted fracture and management of a large soft tissue wound. This type of injury is not rare. In our unit during the last eighteen months 7 patients have fulfilled the criteria for external fixation by presenting with such injuries. All have been the result of high velocity trauma on the roads: 2 were pedestrians, 4 were motorcyclists and 1 was involved in a lorry collision. The protection of the motorcyclist's skull may have resulted in less loss of life but we are now faced with the dreadful limb injuries in these hitherto fatally injured young people. The completely unprotected lower limbs are most vulnerable to severe trauma in high-speed road traffic accidents. The pedestrian is also exposed to this type of injury, and the tibia, by reason of its subcutaneous position, is most frequently involved.

The aim of external fixation in open, comminuted fractures is to achieve sufficient skeletal stability so that plaster, traction or internal fixation is unnecessary. Free access to the soft tissue wound is permitted enabling the use of free grafts, distal flaps or continuous irrigation and secondary healing by granulation. There is no doubt that the Hoffmann system achieves these aims.

Even in the most unstable fracture stability can be obtained by the double frame method. Such is the versatility of the system that not only can local dressings and grafts be applied to the wound but primary cross-leg flaps were used in two patients and a secondary cross-leg flap in one other. No additional plaster or fixation was required and stability of the cross-leg flap was obtained by management of the second leg in the Hoffmann apparatus.

The use of external fixation in the primary treatment of patients will be largely confined to fractures of the tibia because the combination of extensive bone comminution and soft tissue wounding is almost exclusively a tibial problem. Connes (1973) noted that the system was rarely used for primary treatment other than in the tibia but it is being applied to other bones as well (Kamhin et al., 1978).

Infected Pseudo-arthrosis

The infection rate in open fractures is closely related to the extent of soft tissue wounding and to the degree of vascular insufficiency of bone and soft tissue. In a series reported by Nicoll (1964) 22 (15 per cent) of 144 open fractures treated conservatively became infected. In Burwell's (1971) series of plated tibial fractures, the infection ratio was very similar: 14 per cent. Almost identical figures were quoted by Olerud and Karlström (1972) in a series treated by AO osteosynthesis and by Hamza et al. (1971) using intramedullary nailing. However, lower figures have been claimed by Harvey et al. (1975) using intramedullary nails without reaming.

Therefore it appears that approximately one in seven open tibial fractures become infected. Infection is not unknown in femoral fractures and occasionally it occurs in upper limb injuries. Some of these infected fractures can be adequately managed by external plaster fixation and local treatment through a window. There is, however, an appreciable risk that loss of stability will result and this seems to be a potent factor in prolonging infection. Even if the infection settles, non-union almost inevitably persists.

The proponents of internal fixation maintain that rigid fixation should be continued even in the presence of sepsis and that this assists healing and avoids non-union (Hicks, 1970). Problems arise in cases where there is no rigid fixation either because it has not been used initially or where the primary fixation has been inadequate and has broken or become loose as sepsis developed. In these circumstances there is a need for a method which will provide stability of the fracture, permit debridement of the wound and allow continuing treatment of the sepsis. External skeletal fixation fulfills these requirements. It has been used extensively in France in the treatment of infected non-union. Judet and Letournel (1968) have a special unit in Paris for the treatment of such cases. With the use of external skeletal fixation, thorough debridement, decortication of bone and prolonged irrigation and drainage, they have achieved remarkable success.

The more conservative approach to fractures in the UK is slowly changing. Internal fixation is being widely practised in closed fractures as well as open injuries and there will inevitably follow a spate of infected pseudarthroses. To deal with this problem we must be familiar with the techniques perfected by our European colleagues, and in particular we should be acquainted with external skeletal fixation devices.

METHODS OF EXTERNAL SKELETAL FIXATION

Recent Systems

The earlier devices of Stader (1937), Roger Anderson (1934) and Haynes (1939) have not been the subject of any recent reports. Ad hoc arrangements such as those described by Wynn-Jones (1978) are the product of individual ingenuity. The incorporation of pins into plaster is widely practised in the USA as noted by Anderson et al. (1974) and offers a compromise between simple plaster fixation and external skeletal fixation although it lacks many of the advantages of external skeletal fixation. The use of methylmethacrylate to connect transfixion pins has been reported by Inove et al. (1975) and Aron (1976). It is a convenient technique in fractures of the finger bones but lacks the strength, rigidity and versatility of more sophisticated apparatus. Of more interest are commercially available systems which have sufficient versatility to be adapted to various types of fracture.

A relatively new system (*Fig. 8.2*) devised at the East Birmingham Hospital by Dwyer (1973) involves two-plane fixation with pins fitting into circumferential rings above and below the fracture. Loaded springs allow compression. His indications are similar to those discussed and further reports on this technique are awaited.

This system is very similar to that used in the USSR by Gudushaury, Volkov, Ilyzarov and by Kalnberz of Riga, where it is usually described as compression—distraction apparatus (Personal Communications, 1978). By using wires with bent ends as hooks, separate fragments can be drawn into place. There are many ingenious uses for the apparatus, which is apparently used more for the management of malunion than for the

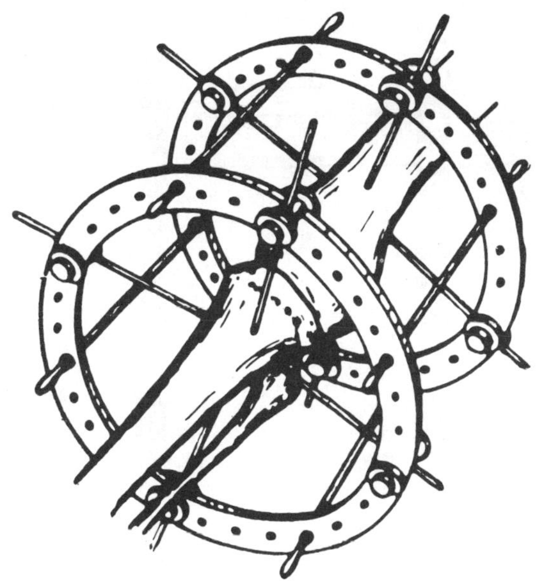

Fig. 8.2. East Birmingham external compression device. (*Reproduced from Dwyer (1973) by kind permission of 'Injury'.*)

treatment of fresh and complicated fractures. Unfamiliarity with the language leads to ignorance of their methods. However, there is currently a scheme of collaboration between British and Soviet surgeons on the subject of external skeletal fixation. It is anticipated that as a result of this effort we will be able to compare their techniques with other established methods.

Another system recently introduced (*Fig. 8.3*) was described by Rezaian (1977). Initially developed for leg-lengthening he employed it in ten complicated tibial fractures. The apparatus has similarities to older methods of leg-lengthening which in their turn were occasionally used for external fixation of fractures. Further reports by other authors will help to assess the value of this technique as compared with the more widely used systems.

In the German-speaking world an external fixation system has been developed by the AO school. They too have recognized that internal fixation has its limitations and that for open, comminuted tibial fractures and for infected pseudarthrosis, there is a need for external fixation. Their 'fixateur externe' differs only in detail from the Hoffmann apparatus but in principle there is the same emphasis on rigidity, adaptability and the ability to compress or distract the bony fragments.

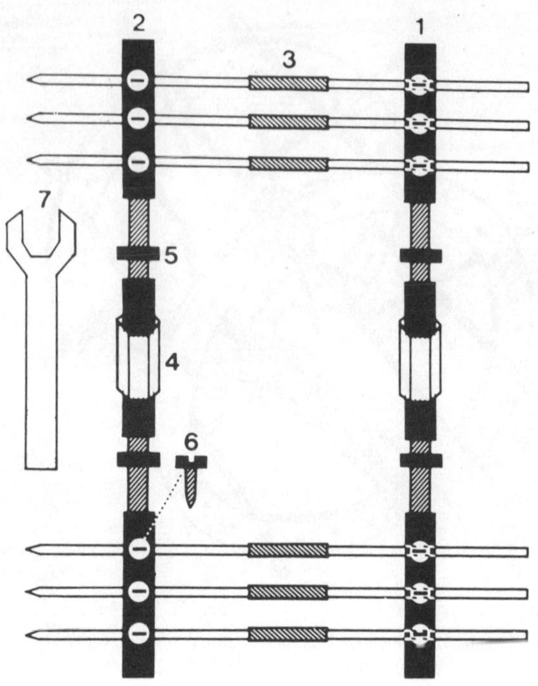

Fig. 8.3. The Rezaian apparatus. 1, Lateral bar, 2, Medial bar. 3, Thread pin. 4, Turn-buckle. 5, Nut. 6, Grab screw. 7. Spanner. (*Reproduced from Rezaian (1977) by kind permission of 'Injury'.*)

Hoffmann Technique

At the present time the most widely used system of external skeletal fixation is undoubtedly the Hoffmann (*Fig. 8.4*).

The basic principles of the technique are as follows.

1. *a.* Two groups of three pins are placed — one on each side of the fracture.

   b. The pins are parallel. This is achieved by using a special guide.

   c. Ideally the pins should be as near as possible to the fracture.

   d. The pins are introduced manually using a drill brace to avoid thermal necrosis.

   e. An incision of 1 cm is made at the site of introduction to avoid skin necrosis or infection.

2. *a.* Ball joints are applied to each group of three pins about 15–20 mm from the skin.

   b. The ball joints are held together by vertical bars, thus forming a double frame — anterior and posterior.

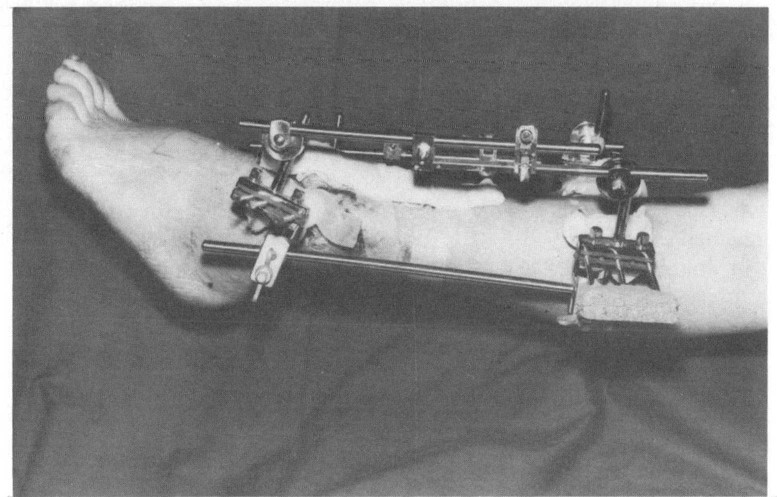

a

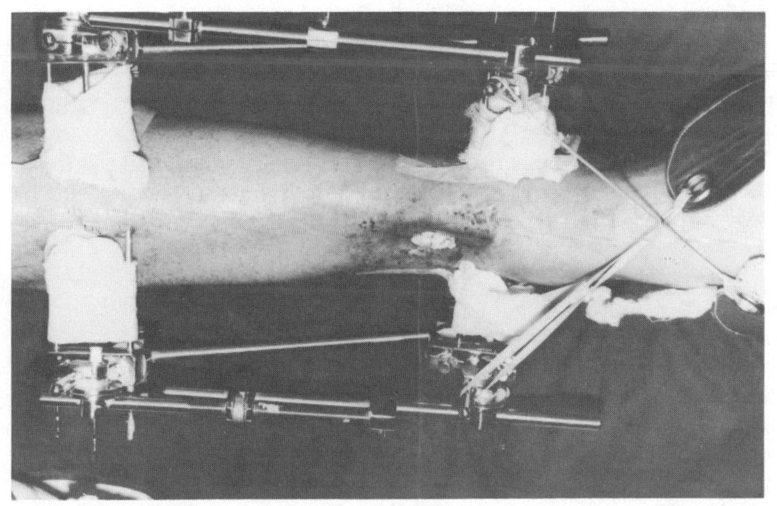

b

Fig. 8.4. The Hoffmann external fixation system in situ.

3. Four long bars then connect each corner of the frame; these can be used:

    a. In compression when a slider bar with an adjustable knurled nut is used.

    b. In distraction using the above system in reverse.

    c. In neutralization when the mounting is locked without any adjustment.

4. This basic double-frame anchorage can then be modified to suit the individual case.

In double fractures of the tibia, groups of three pins are placed above the upper fracture and below the lower fracture. Two or three central pins are introduced between the fractures. Two separate systems can then be employed with compression of one fracture and neutralization of the other if necessary.

Stable fractures can be compressed by the apparatus. This would apply in cases of transverse or short oblique fractures without severe loss of bone substance. Short oblique fractures may be made more stable by the use of an inter-fragmentary screw and then compressed by the external fixation.

When the fracture is unstable due to comminution or loss of bone the frame is used without compression. Additional internal fixation by wires, pins or screws may be used to aid reduction or stability.

External skeletal fixation is rarely indicated in the treatment of recent fractures except in the tibia. When used in the femur special precautions are necessary to avoid damaging the femoral vessels. Whilst a lower group of pins can safely be introduced in the frontal plane, pins in the middle or upper part of the femur should not transfix the bone. Threaded pins which do not traverse are used in groups in planes at right-angles to each other. Because of the versatility of the system adequate stability can still be obtained.

Similarly, in the humerus and forearm bones, where again external skeletal fixation is very rarely used in fresh fractures, transfixion is dangerous and a less rigid fixation on the outer side of the humerus is used.

Pelvis

External skeletal fixation has a special part to play in serious fractures of the pelvis, especially where there is disruption of the symphysis and sacro-iliac joints. Three threaded pins are inserted into each iliac crest just posterior to the anterior iliac spine. An 'A' frame mounting is constructed in such a way as to permit free access to the skin of the lower abdomen and thus allows freedom of movement for the patient (*Fig. 8.5*). The technique is described by Connes (1973) and by Slätis and Karaharju (1975).

In associated fractures of the acetabulum a third group of threaded pins may be inserted into the outer surface of the upper femur and tied onto the anchorage.

This system can be used with an orthopaedic table in distraction to disengage the posterior pelvic arch, traction is then employed to reduce the upward displacement of the hemi-pelvis, and finally compression is applied to stabilize the reduction.

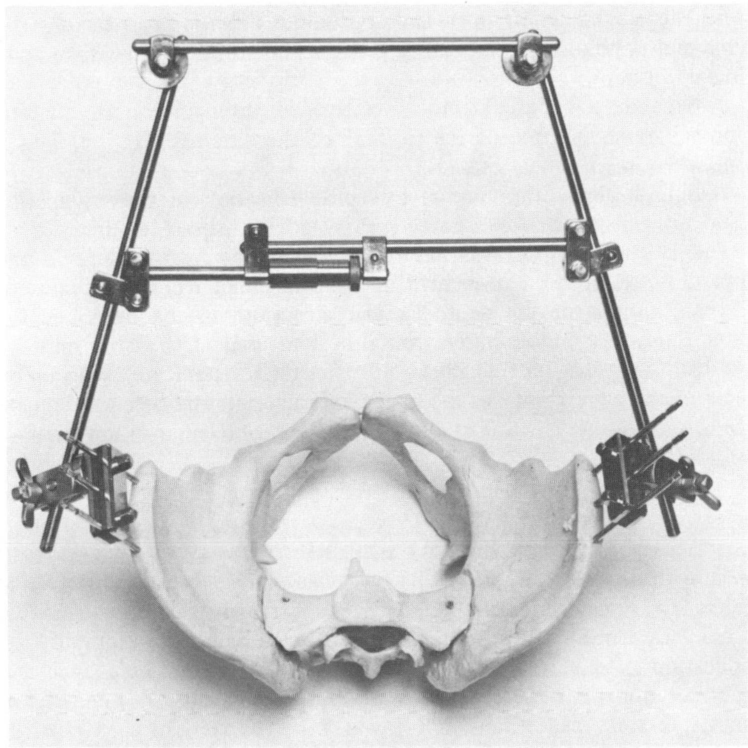

Fig. 8.5. Trapezoid compression frame mounting for the pelvic fractures. (*Reproduced from Slätis and Karaharju (1975) by kind permission of 'Injury'.*)

Infected Pseudarthrosis

The other major group of patients in which external skeletal fixation is indicated in those with infected non-union of a long bone.

The technique employed in the introduction of the Hoffmann system differs little from the methods used in the fresh fractures. If possible, compression is used or bone resected to allow compression, which is then maintained. Where there is bone loss, this is not possible and in rare cases the system may be used in distraction to maintain limb length.

Details of management of infected non-union using the Hoffmann frame are given by Connes (1973) as follows.

1. Internal fixation devices are removed.

2. Radical excision of necrotic or infected bone and soft tissue is performed.

3. The bone ends are freshened by osteo-periosteal decortication and if necessary trimmed to aid stability.

4. The fixation is maintained in compression if possible.

5. The wound is left open and continuous irrigation carried out with saline and antibiotics until healthy granulations form; this may take up to three months.

6. Secondary bone grafting is performed through a postero-lateral approach removing one of the tie bars of the external fixation. This is done when irrigation has ceased.

7. Skin healing often occurs by epithelialization of the granulation tissue but split-skin grafts or, rarely, cross-leg flaps may be required.

The Hoffmann apparatus has been used in the femur, humerus and forearm bones in the management of infected pseudarthroses. Because of the vulnerability of the neuro-vascular structures in the thigh and the upper limb, the double-frame frontal system used in the tibia must be modified. Threaded pins which do not transfix the bone are used and, by virtue of the adaptability of the system of ball joints and tie bar, adequate stability can be obtained. Details of the anchorage techniques are given by Connes (1973).

CLINICAL EXPERIENCE

Because few surgeons in the UK have yet had much experience of external skeletal fixation and because details are important it is perhaps justifiable to use 7 cases dealt with during the last eighteen months to exemplify the application of the Hoffmann apparatus. All 7 fractures were open and occurred in patients involved in road traffic accidents: 4 were motor-cyclists, 2 were pedestrians and 1 was a lorry driver. In each case the patient suffered multiple injuries, three of the patients having ipsilateral femoral fractures. These were leg injuries of the most severe type and in one instance the leg was cold and pulseless on admission.

The Hoffmann double frame was applied as a primary procedure in 5 patients, while in the other 2, treated before external skeletal fixation was obtainable, primary treatment with plates had been employed (Table 8.1).

The indication for external skeletal fixation in the primary and one of the secondary cases was a grossly unstable fracture with comminution or segmentation plus a major soft tissue injury. Treatment of the skin defect involved split-skin grafting in 4 patients and the use of cross-leg flaps in 3. In 2 of the cross-leg flap cases the procedure was carried out as a primary measure, as well as external skeletal fixation of the fracture. The

Table 8.1. Summary of Cases

Case (age)	Tibial injury	Other injuries	Primary bone treatment	Primary soft tissue treatment	Secondary bone treatment	Secondary soft tissue treatment	Time to clinical union (months)
1 (38)	Open comminuted	Fractured lumbar vertebra	ESF	Cross-leg flap	Plaster cast		6
2 (26)	Open segmental	Open fracture of patella Fracture of malleoli	Plates and screws	Split-skin graft	ESF bone graft, plaster cast		18
3 (62)	Open comminuted	Open fracture of other tibia open fracture of patella	ESF	Wound closure	Plaster cast	Transposition flap	13
4 (57)F	Open comminuted	Fractured clavicle Fractured ribs	ESF	Split-skin graft	Plaster cast, blade-plate, bone graft		12
5 (44)	Open segmental	Fractured femur, pelvis and ribs	ESF	Split-skin graft			Not united
6 (19)	Open comminuted	Fractured femur	ESF	Cross-leg flap	Plaster cast secondary ESF and bone graft		13
7 (17)	Open segmental	Fractured femur	Plates and screw	Split-skin graft	ESF and bone graft	Cross-leg flap	Not known

ESF = External skeletal fixation

Hoffmann apparatus is sufficiently versatile to permit fixation of the fracture and allow a cross-leg flap at the same time.

Treatment of the Fracture

Two of the cases were admitted before the Hoffmann apparatus became available and were treated initially by plates and screws. These proved ineffective in stabilizing the extremely comminuted or segmental fractures and after external skeletal fixation became available the plates were removed and the Hoffmann device used.

In the remaining 5 cases external skeletal fixation was used as the initial management of the fracture.

No matter how effective the Hoffmann apparatus may be in achieving stabilization of the bony injury, the gross loss of skeletal material and the violence of the injury will prejudice bony union. One must therefore be prepared to carry out secondary cancellous bone grafting in many cases before union is established. Whether this is done when the external skeletal fixation is still in place or whether some other form of skeletal fixation is used will depend on individual circumstances. In this series two tibias have gone on to union without secondary intervention; one at thirteen months and the other at six months. Four patients have been grafted and one awaits grafting. Grafting has been carried out with external skeletal fixation in three and with internal fixation in one patient. Union has been achieved in three of these four patients within eighteen months of injury.

The Hoffmann apparatus was kept in place for periods of three to four months, being followed by plaster in most cases until union was achieved or by bone grafting and other forms of fixation, but external skeletal fixation can be maintained for much longer periods if required.

Treatment of the Soft Tissues

Primary cross-leg flaps were combined with external skeletal fixation in two cases. In a third patient, cross-leg flap and external skeletal fixation were applied at two months after injury. In each case excellent soft tissue healing was obtained without disturbing the progress of fracture immobilization.

In remaining cases split-skin grafts were used to heal the skin wounds.

Complications

Pin-track Sepsis

Pin-track sepsis was a significant problem in only one case and necessitated removal of the frame at four months and before union was established. Three months later it was possible to graft the tibia, again using external fixation.

Delayed Union

All of these fractures healed slowly, the earliest at seven months. Bone grafting has been or is likely to be, needed in four cases. The progress of union is related more to the severity of injury, the damage to soft tissue and the insult to the vascularity of the bone than to the method of treatment. Indeed, with conventional treatment union might be slower still because of the lack of rigid fixation to protect tenuous bony union.

Infection
One of the cases developed wound sepsis of serious extent but this settled and bony union was achieved.

Necrosis
The one case in which primary closure of the wound was attempted developed necrosis and secondary grafting had to be carried out. One of the advantages of external skeletal fixation is that the wound remains easily accessible for the appropriate method of skin cover.

CASE HISTORIES

1. *R.T:* a 38-year-old male involved in a motorcycle accident. In addition to an open fracture of the tibia he had a crush fracture of the lumbar vertebra.

The tibial fracture was extensively comminuted (*Fig. 8.6*) with a large soft tissue defect over it (*Fig. 8.7*). Primary treatment consisted of the application of the Hoffmann double frame apparatus (*Fig. 8.8*) and a cross-leg flap (*Fig. 8.9*). The flap was divided at 5 weeks (*Fig. 8.10*) and the patient was discharged home on crutches at 2 months with the frame in situ. Full weight-bearing in the frame was permitted at 10 weeks. On removing the frame at 16 weeks, the fracture felt firm (*Fig. 8.11*). A patellar tendon-bearing plaster was applied and at 6 months clinical union was established.

2. *D.R:* a 26-year-old male involved in a motorcycle accident. His injuries consisted of a penetrating wound of the knee, fractured patella, fractured malleoli and open segmental fracture of the tibia, all in the same leg (*Fig. 8.12*). The primary operative treatment comprised repair of the knee wound, plating of the two tibial fractures (*Fig. 8.13*), primary cancellous bone grafting. When Hoffmann apparatus became available 6 months later it was used to stabilize the un-united tibia (*Fig. 8.14*). Further cancellous grafting was performed. Wound sepsis occurred but settled without the need to remove the external fixation. The frame was removed after 5 months and a plaster cast applied. This was removed after 6 weeks (*Fig. 8.15*) and 18 months after the injury he was back at work with full movement of the knee and a united tibia.

3. *T.B:* a 62-year-old male involved in a collision between two lorries and trapped in his cab. He had bilateral open tibial fractures (*Fig. 8.16*) and an open fracture of the right patella. The initial management comprised excision of the patella, excision and suture of wounds and the application of heel traction of both legs. He recovered from a mild fat embolism and definitive surgery carried out on the 12th day consisted of plaster fixation of the right tibia, insertion of one intra-fragmentary screw and the Hoffmann double frame on the left tibia (*see Fig. 8.4 and Fig. 8.17*). The wounds over the left tibia were split-skin grafted. Three weeks later a cross-leg flap was considered to cover the exposed tibia but scarring of the opposite leg precluded this.

The frame was removed at 4 months and a local transposition flap used to cover the defect in the soft tissues. By 7 months skin healing was complete and after 13 months the tibiae were both clinically united (*Fig. 8.18*).

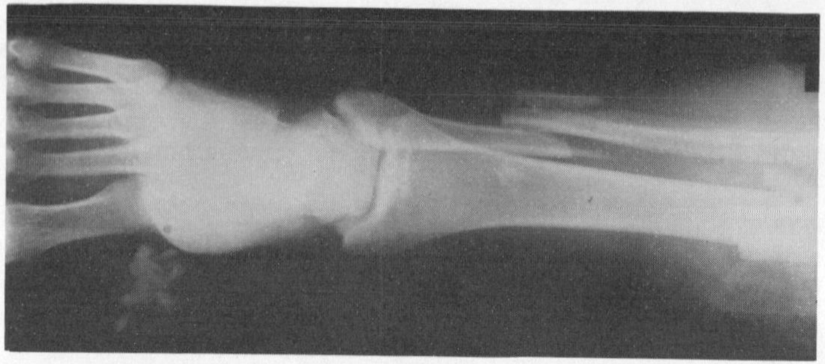

a

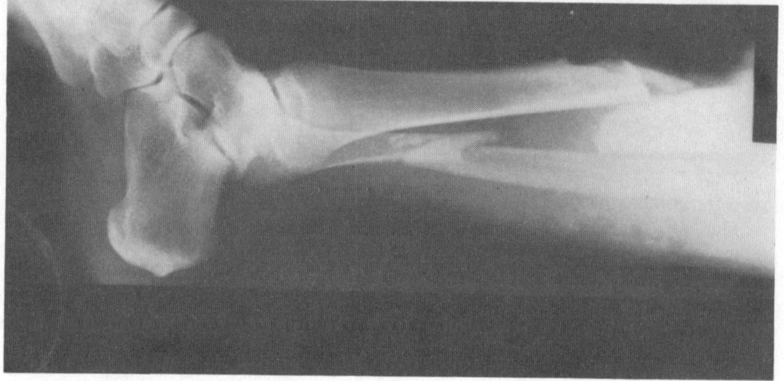

b

Fig. 8.6. Case 1. Comminuted tibial fracture.

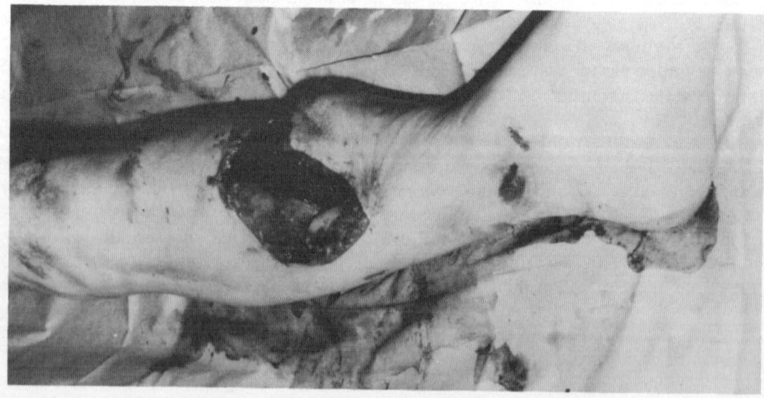

Fig. 8.7. Case 1. Associated soft tissue injury.

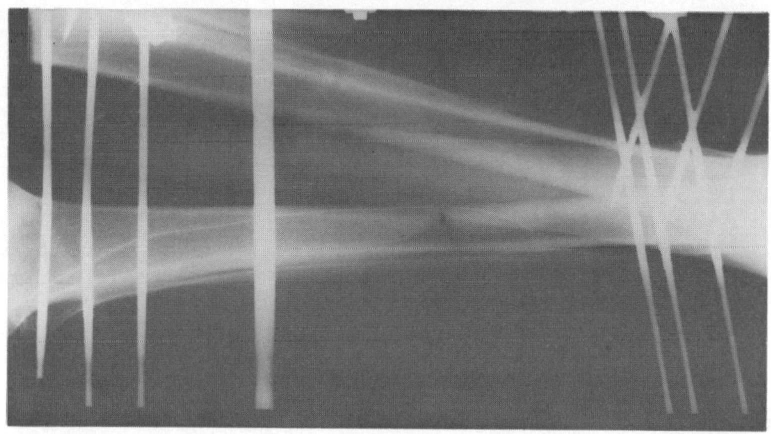

a

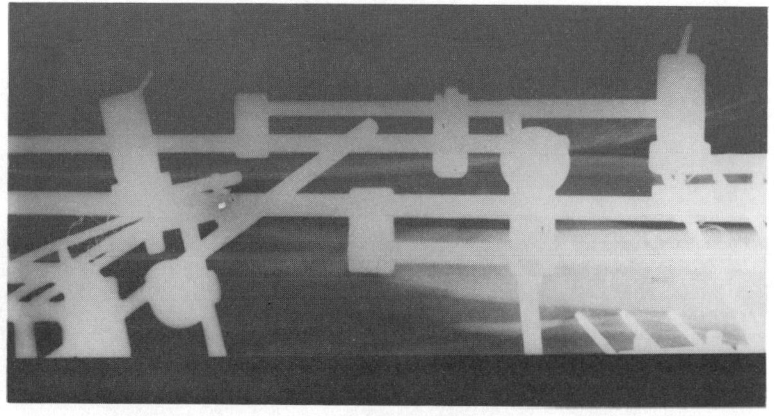

b

Fig. 8.8. Case 1. The fracture stabilized by a Hoffmann frame, also controlling a cross-leg flap.

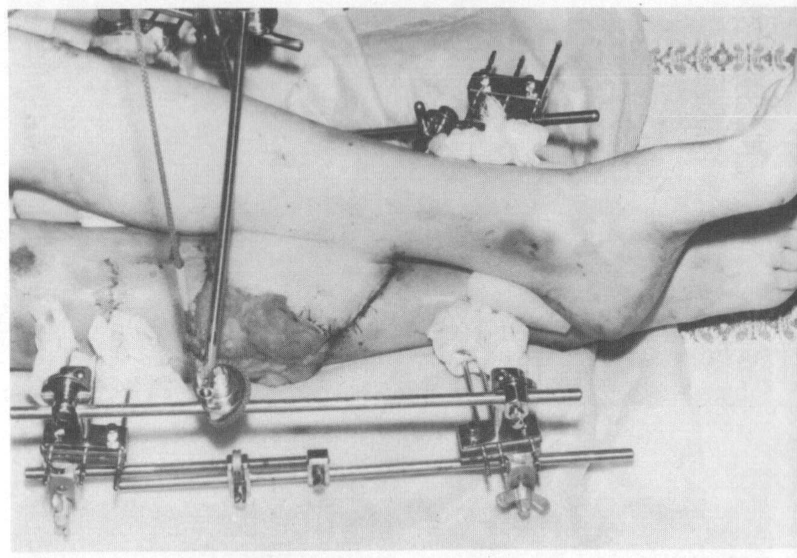

Fig. 8.9. Case 1. Primary cross-leg flap controlled by Hoffmann frame.

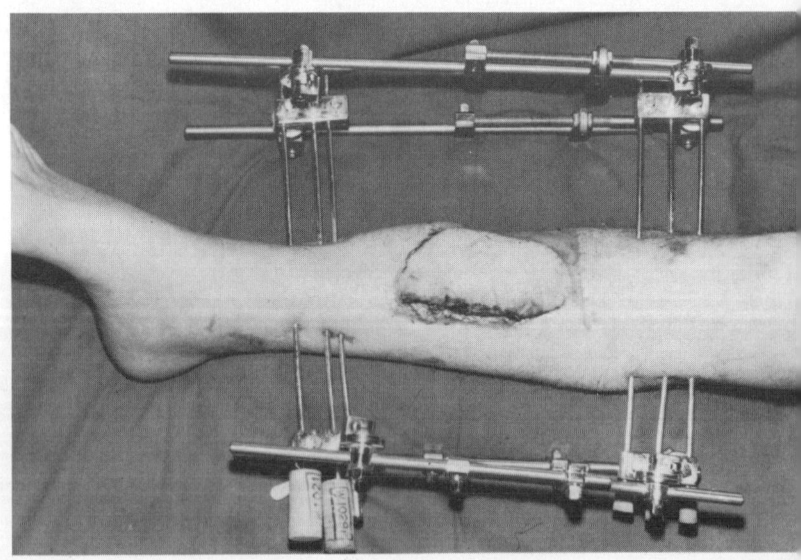

Fig. 8.10. Case 1. After flap separation.

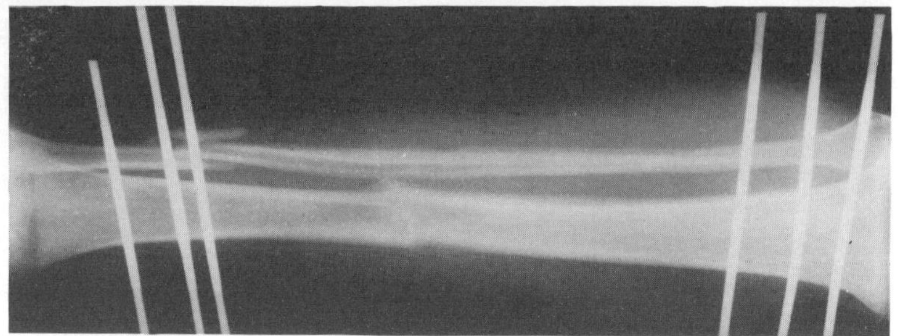

a

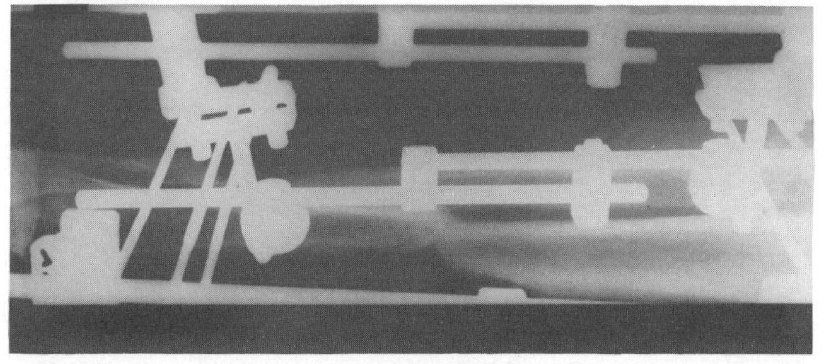

b

Fig. 8.11. Case 1. Position at sixteen weeks.

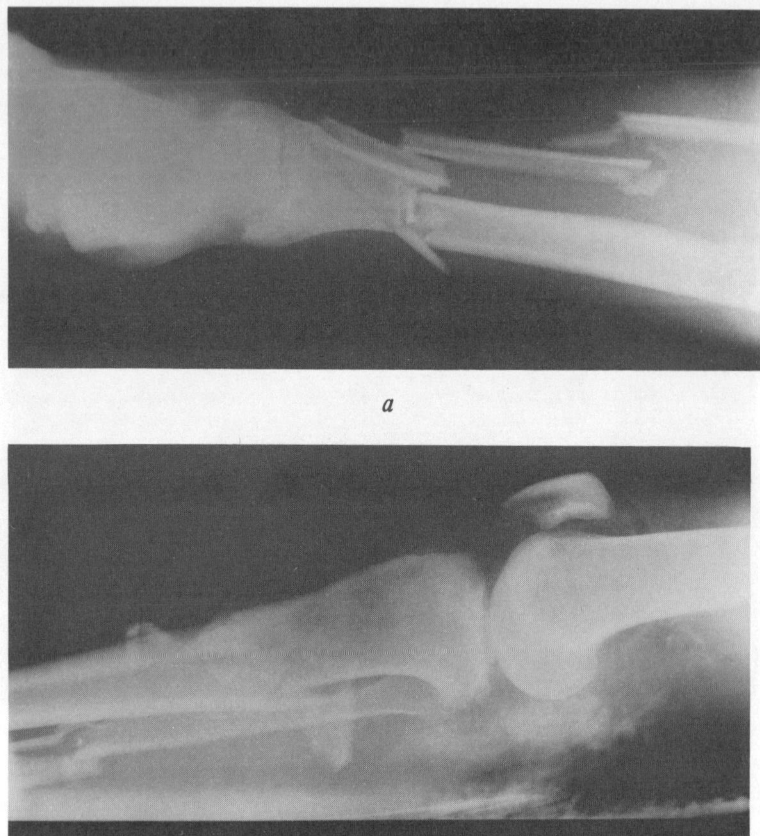

a

b

Fig. 8.12. Case 2. Comminuted segmental fracture of the tibia.

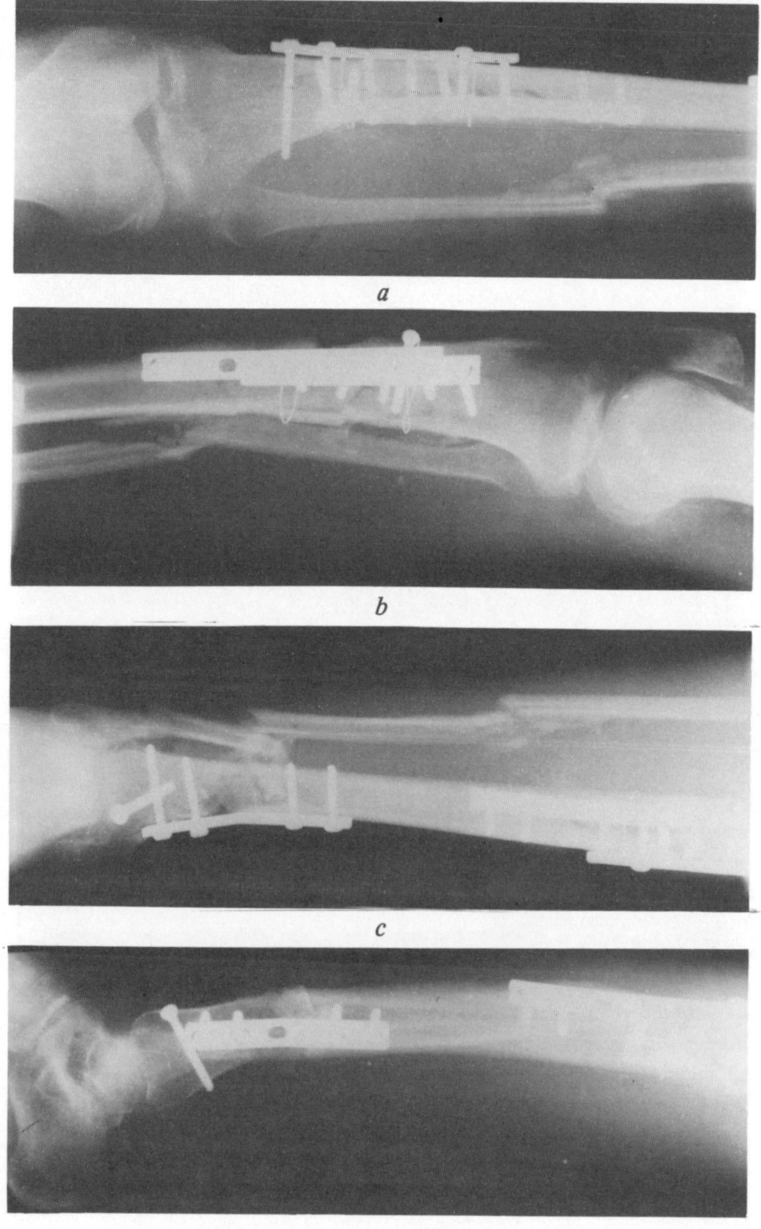

Fig. 8.13. Case 2. Primary fracture treatment by internal fixation.

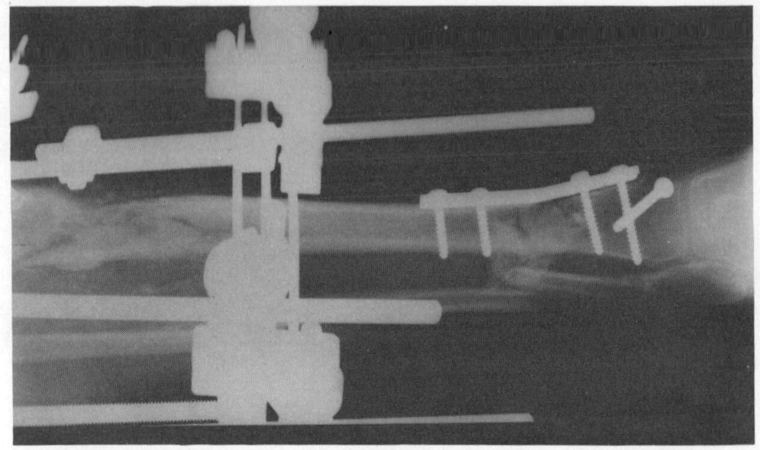

a

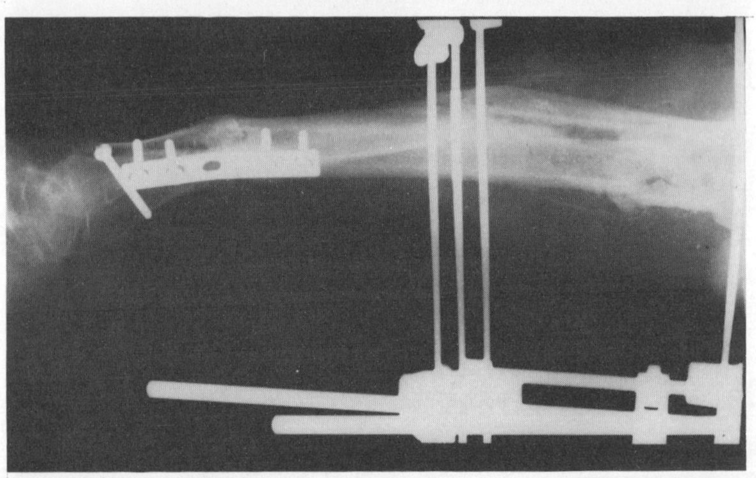

b

Fig. 8.14. Case 2. Hoffmann frame applied secondarily to fix the unstable upper tibial fracture.

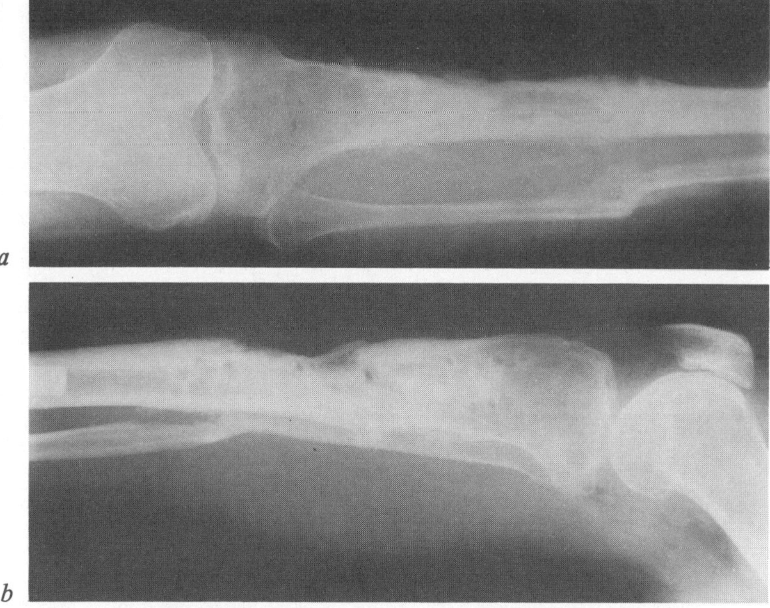

Fig. 8.15. Case 2. Five months after removal of external fixation.

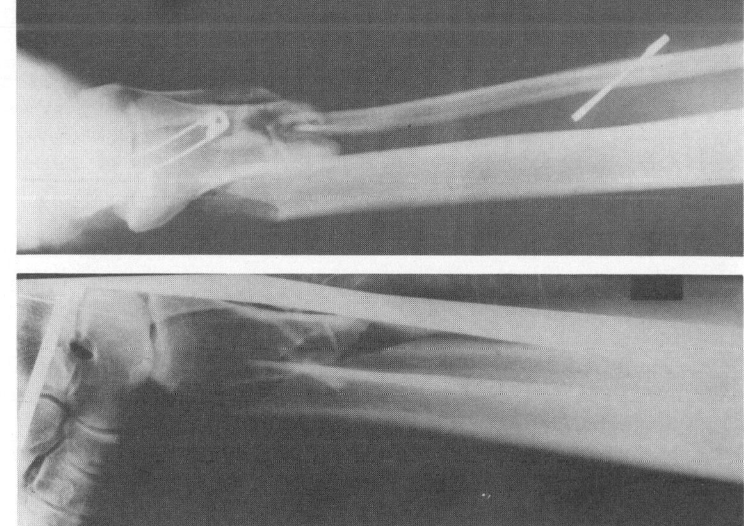

Fig. 8.16. Case 3. The right tibial fracture.

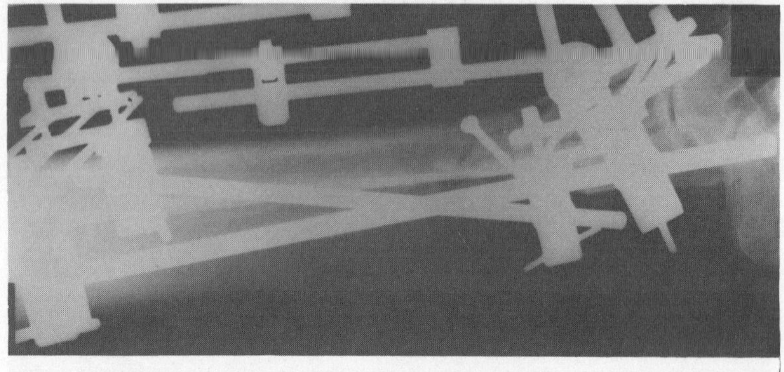

a

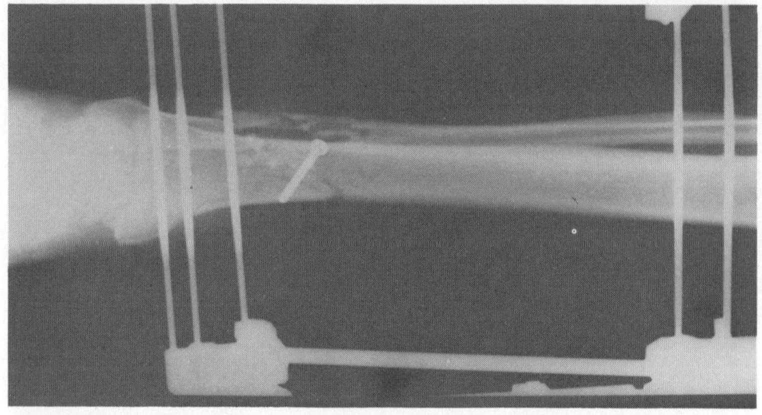

b

Fig. 8.17. Case 3. Radiographs following application of external skeletal fixation and one inter-fragmentary screw.

Whilst it is possible in many cases to achieve union and soft tissue healing in the open shattered tibia by conservative treatment, this is often at the expense of mal-union, shortening and joint stiffness. The advantage of external skeletal fixation are rigidity of fixation, adaptability to any bony situation, stability, allowing early movement of joints and accessibility in the management of the soft tissues. These are considerable advantages and should be weighed against the low incidence of complications.

These same advantages are available in the treatment of infected non-

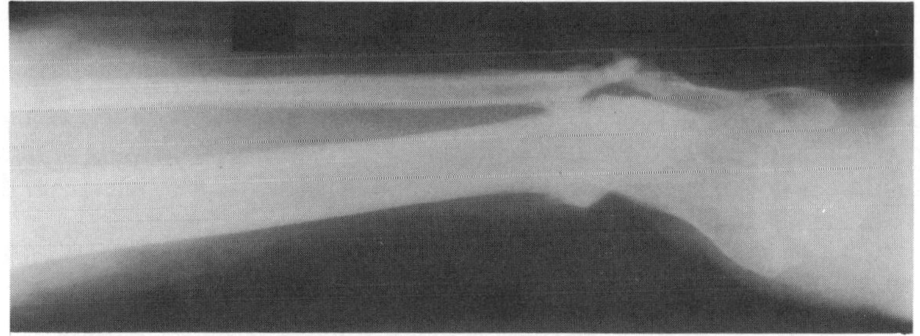

a

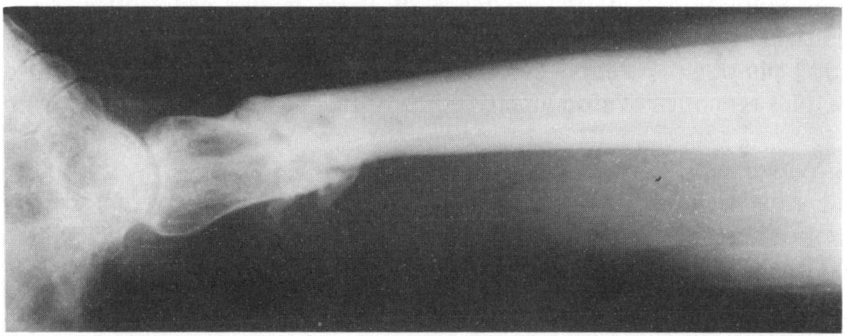

b

Fig. 8.18. Case 3. The tibial fracture at thirteen months.

unions. Perhaps our conservatism has had its blessing in the low incidence of this problem and hence the necessity for special methods of treatment has not been felt. Inevitably we will face the same problem of infected plated fracture as our friends in Europe and will need a reliable method of dealing with them. The experience in France, Germany, Austria, Switzerland and Scandinavia all points to external skeletal fixation as the method to choose in these circumstances.

It is likely that we will shortly be subjected to a barrage of external fixation systems just as we have in internal fixation of fractures and joint replacement surgery. Some of them may be an improvement but others will be merely advocating change for its own sake. It seems prudent to choose that technique which has been widely practised, carefully reported and critically analysed. The Hoffmann and AO methods fulfill these criteria and are already being tried on a small scale in the UK. Our experience with the Hoffmann frame in seven patients during the last eighteen months encourages us to persist with this technique in cases where the indications are clear.

DISADVANTAGES OF EXTERNAL SKELETAL FIXATION

Osseous Complications

1. *Loosening of Pins*

Loosening of pins may well be the result of thermal necrosis with secondary infection and occurs when power tools are used to insert the pins. Where stability is not secure, as in the humerus and pelvis, loosening may occur if the frame has to be maintained for long.

2. *Infection*

Pin-track sepsis was the major anxiety in the minds of earlier authors who condemned external skeletal fixation. Inadequate skin incisions, the use of power tools, poor stability and movement of the pins contributed to this poor reputation. Careful avoidance of these factors can reduce serious pin-track sepsis to a minimum. In Connes' (1973) series only 3 out of 1 000 pin-tracks required curettage for sepsis. Usually simple removal of the pins is enough to stop infection proceeding.

3. *Subsequent Internal Fixation*

Subsequent internal fixation is hazardous following external skeletal fixation and has rarely been successfully performed. The use of external fixation does therefore compromise future treatment.

4. *Osseous Sclerosis*

The appearance of sclerosis is a frequent factor in pseudarthroses healed by external apparatus and is the price paid for the stability and rigidity of the apparatus. The stresses are taken at the points of entry of the pins.

Articular Complications

1. *Stiffness of the Ankle*

An equino-varus deformity may develop due to the pins compressing the anterior tibial muscles. Care in pin placement and the use of a foot support are important details but some loss of ankle movement at the end of treatment is almost inevitable.

2. *Stiffness of the Knee*

Stiffness of the knee usually follows external fixation of the femur and is difficult to avoid.

ADVANTAGES OF EXTERNAL SKELETAL FIXATION

1. *Rigidity*

The essence of the system is rigidity of fixation even in the most unstable fracture.

2. *Versatility*

By means of the compression and distraction facilities, fractures may be reduced as well as fixed and can be compressed over a period as well as at the initial operation.

3. *Adaptability*
The ingenious use of ball joints and tie bars allows adaptations in the treatment of double fractures, in the use of the system in the upper limb and pelvis, in cross-leg flaps and in arthrodesis.

4. *Stability*
Complete skeletal stability allows mobilization of proximal joints (*Fig. 8.19*) and early ambulation of patients (*Fig. 8.20*).

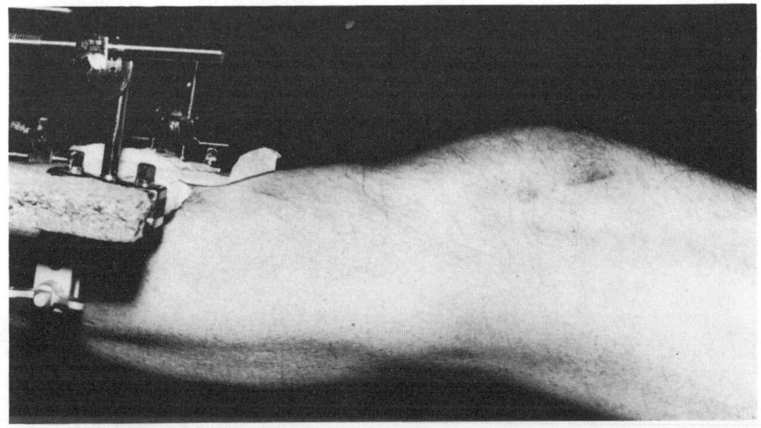

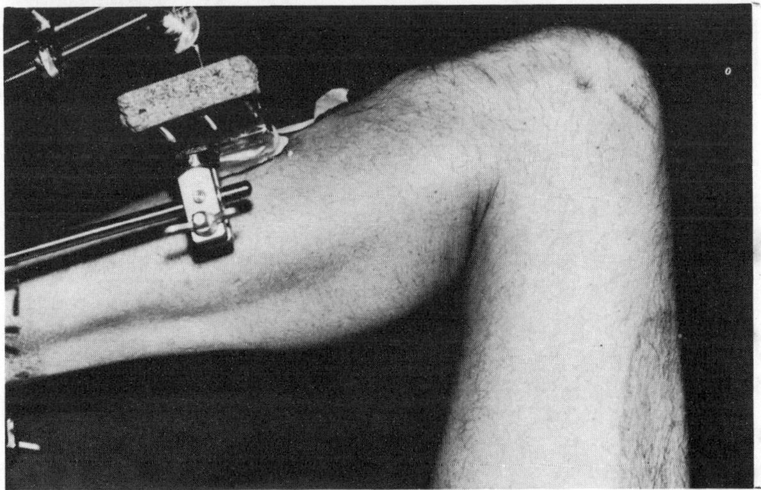

Fig. 8.19. Mobilization of the knee joint with Hoffmann apparatus in place.

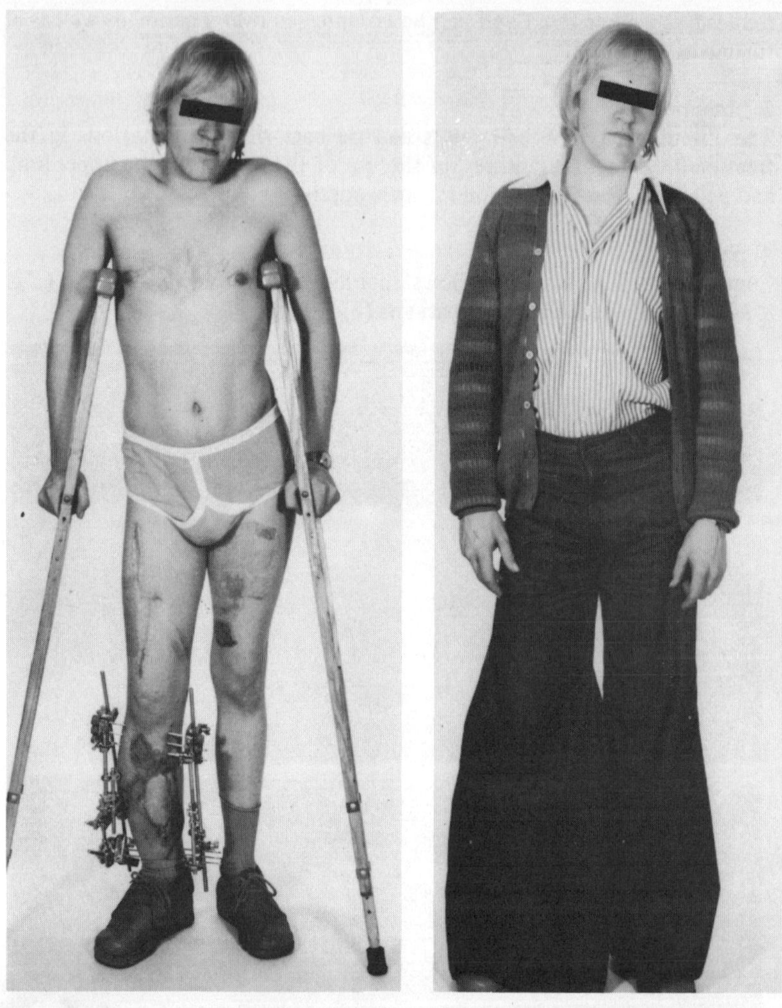

Fig. 8.20. The ambulant patient with Hoffmann frame.

5. *Accessibility*

Free access to the limb or wound permits associated treatment of bone or soft tissues. It is therefore possible to carry out removal of dead bone, bone grafting, local flaps and even cross-leg flaps without disturbing the stability of the fracture.

6. *Suspendability*

The apparatus may be suspended from conventional bed frames to facilitate dressings or irrigation (*Fig. 8.21*).

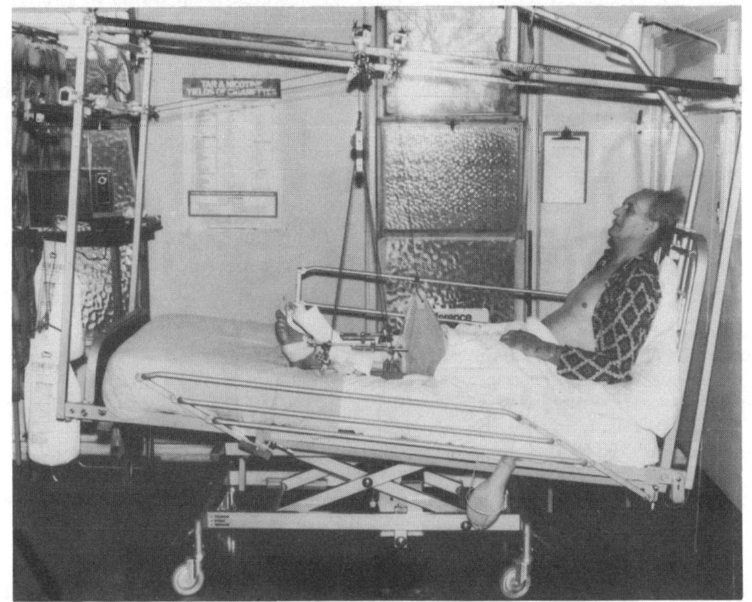

Fig. 8.21. The Hoffmann apparatus suspended from a bed frame.

7. *Anaesthesia*

The mounting can be applied under local anaesthesia.

With any new technique there is a danger of enthusiasm leading to incautious application of the method. Poor techniques and the flouting of strict indications will inevitably lead to complications and poor results. The ultra-conservatives will blame them on the new system rather than on its misapplication and progress will be halted. It is essential that new practitioners in this field seek advice from the experienced and adhere firmly to established techniques and case selection. In an area where the USA is tending to even more conservatism we cannot turn there as we have so often for consultation. Instead there should be a far greater emphasis on the European outlook in British fracture surgery. Language and the strangeness of the Continental hierarchical system are barriers which should be overcome. Senior trainees and established surgeons with the maturity to gain from their visits are beginning to seek links with western Europe, and there is collaboration between British surgeons and those in the USSR.

Although daunting at first sight, the application of external skeletal fixation is not demanding once the objective has been decided. Practice beforehand on a cadaver bone, careful attention to detail and meticulous care of pin-tracks will obviate complications. The apparatus is initially costly and a stock of four or six tibial anchorages is desirable in any large centre. However, for an outlay of about £2 000 the basic instrumentation and stock can be assembled. Thereafter, there will be a circulation of frames as they are used and removed. A relatively small outlay will be needed for additional items.

Acknowledgements

I am indebted to my colleagues in Stoke-on-Trent — A. K. Mitting, T. R. Fisher, Peter Hill and D. H. Edwards — who have been most helpful in allowing their cases to be included in the series reported.

REFERENCES

Adrey J. (1970) Le fixateur externe d'Hoffmann couplé en cadre. Étude bio-mécanique dans les fractures de jambe. Thèse, Montpellier University.

Anderson L. D., Hutchins W. C., Wright P. E. et al. (1974) Fractures of the tibia and fibula treated by cast and transfixing pin. *Clin. Orthop.* **105**, 79.

Anderson R. (1934) An automatic method of treatment for fractures of the tibia and fibula. *Surg. Gynecol. Obstet.* **58**, 639.

Anderson W. V. (1952) Leg-lengthening. In: Proceedings of the British Orthopaedic Association. *J. Bone Joint Surg.* **34B**, 150.

Aron J. D. (1976) Using methylmethacrylate to make external fixation splints. *J. Bone Joint Surg.* **58A**, 151.

Burwell H. N. (1971) Plate fixation of tibial shaft fractures. *J. Bone Joint Surg.* **53B**, 258.

Connos H. (1973) *Hoffmann's Double Frame External Anchorage.* Paris, Gead.

Cuendet S. (1936) Procède de réduction des fractures de la diaphyse des deux os de l'avant-bras à l'aide de l'appareil à broches jumelées. In: Vromant (ed.), *Livre Jubilaire Albin Lambotte.* Bruxelles, 129–136.

Dwyer N. St J. P. (1973) Preliminary report upon a new fixation device for fractures of long bones. *Injury* **5**, 141.

Felländer M. (1963) Treatment of fractures and pseudarthroses of the long bones by Hoffmann's transfixion method (osteotaxis) *Acta Orthop. Scand.* **33**, 132.

Hamza K. N., Dunkerley G. E. and Murray C. M. M. (1971) Fractures of the tibia. A report on fifty patients treated by intra-medullary nailing. *J. Bone and Joint Surg.* **53B**, 696.

Harvey F. J., Hodgkinson A. H. T. and Harvey P. M. (1975) Intra-medullary nailing in the treatment of open fractures of the tibia and fibula. *J. Bone Joint Surg.* **57A**, 909.

Haynes H. H. (1939) Treating fractures by skeletal fixation of the individual bone. *South. Med. J.* **32**, 720.

Hicks J. H. (1970) Sepsis in fractures. In: London P. S. (ed.), *Modern Trends in Accident Surgery and Medicine.* London, Butterworths, pp. 220–249.

Hoffmann R. (1938) Rotules à os pour la réduction dirigée, non sanglante, des fractures (osteotaxis). *Congrès Français de Chirurgie*, Paris, 601–610.

Inove S., Oheshi T. and Ichida M. (1975) Our external skeletal fixation for sup-purative pseudarthrosis of the tibia. *J. Jpn. Orthop. Assoc.* **50**, 21.

Johnson H. F. and Stovall S. L. (1950) External fixation of fractures. *J. Bone Joint Surg.* **32A**, 466.

Judet R. and Letournel E. (1968) Pseudarthroses suppurées de jambe. *Rev. Chir. Orthop.* **54**, 119.

Kamhin M., Michaelson M., and Waisbrod H. (1978) The use of external skeletal fixation in the treatment of fractures of the humeral shaft. *Injury* **9**, 245.

Karlström G. and Olerud S. (1975) Percutaneous pin-fixation of open tibial fractures. Double-frame anchorage using Vidal–Adrey method. *J. Bone Joint Surg.* **57A**, 915.

Lambotte A. (1907) *L'Intervention Opératoire dans les Fractures.* Bruxelles, Lamertin.

Lewis K. M., Breidenbach L. and Stader O. (1942) The Stader reduction splint for treating fractures of the shafts of the long bones. *Ann. Surg.* **116**, 623.

Malgaigne (1853) Considérations cliniques sur les fractures de la rotule et leur traitement par les griffes. *J. Connaissances Méd. pratiques,* **16**, 9.

Naden J. R. (1949) External skeletal fixation in the treatment of fractures of the tibia. *J. Bone Joint Surg.* **31A**, 586.

Nicoll E. A. (1964) Fractures of the tibial shaft. A survey of 705 cases. *J. Bone Joint Surg.* **46B**, 373.

Olerud S. (1973) Treatment of fractures by the Vidal–Adrey method. *Acta Orthrop. Scand.* **44**, 516.

Olerud S. and Karlström G. (1972) Tibial fractures treated by A.O. compression osteosynthesis: experience from 5-year material. *Acta Orthop. Scand.* Suppl. 140.

Rezaian S. M. (1977) A new external fixation device for treatment of complicated fractures of the leg. *Injury* **9**, 17.

Ronen G. M., Michaelson M. and Waisbrod H. (1974) External fixation in war injuries. *Injury* **6**, 94.

Rosenthal R. E., McPhail J. A. and Ortiz J. E. (1977) Non-union in open tibial fractures. *J. Bone Joint Surg.* **59A**, 244.

Shaar C. M., Kreuz F. P. jun. and Jones D. T. (1944) End results of treatment of fresh fractures by the use of Stader apparatus. *J. Bone Joint Surg.* **26**, 471.

Slätis P. and Karaharju E. O. (1975) External fixation of the pelvic girdle with a trapezoid compression frame. *Injury* **7**, 53.

Stader O. (1937) A preliminary announcement of a new method of treating fractures. *North Am. Vet.* **18**, 37.

Vidal J. (1968) Notre expérience du fixateur extérne d'Hoffmann à propos de 46 observations: les indications de son emploi. *Montpellier Chir.* **14**, 451.

Wynn-Jones C. H. (1978) A simple fixation method using wire and cement. *Injury* **9**, 329.

E. M. Eagling

9 Injuries to the Eye and Adjacent Structures

BLUNT INJURIES TO THE EYE AND ORBIT

Blunt injuries to the eye and orbit are common and may give rise to damage either directly to the eye or to the surrounding structures. A review (Eagling, 1974) of patients with this type of injury demonstrated a close relationship between the nature of the impact and the ensuing damage. Maximal damage to the eye itself is caused by small hard objects such as stones or lead pellets, or objects with a hard edge such as racquets, that strike the eye with considerable force. If the impact is on the cornea, complications such as lens damage and macular oedema can be expected, while a scleral impact has a high incidence of peripheral retinal damage. With large smooth objects such as footballs much of the force is arrested by the orbital margin, and intraocular damage is minimal; if the object is small enough to fit partly within the orbital margin, such as a fist, the whole orbital contents will be compressed, with maximal damage to the periocular structures.

Intraocular Damage following a Blunt Injury

A hyphaema (*Plate 1*) or bleeding into the anterior chamber of the eye, is the most common manifestation of a blunt injury. All significant blunt injuries will show this sign, with the exception of the rare injuries where the impact is confined to the sclera; these will show *commotio retinae*, or a white appearance of the affected retina, often accompanied by retinal and vitreous haemorrhage.

Other studies (Tönjum, 1966; Eagling, 1974) have confirmed that every patient with a visible hyphaema has a tear into the anterior face of the ciliary body, which gives rise to the haemorrhage into the anterior chamber. Other sources of bleeding may be splits of the pupil margin, or detachment of the peripheral iris root. The tears into the face of the ciliary body are known as 'angle recession', because they result in deepening of the drainage angle of the anterior chamber.

The importance of these tears is two-fold: firstly, there is a considerable risk of further bleeding for the first few days after injury, especially if the patient remains ambulant; they require admission to hospital for bed-rest during the period of risk. Secondary bleeding is often very severe and may fill the anterior chamber with bloodclot; this obstructs the outflow of aqueous humour, leading to an acute rise of intraocular pressure and severe pain. This complication will require surgical treatment.

Secondly, the damage in the region of the drainage angle may give rise to late glaucoma, a condition where a chronic rise of intraocular pressure leads to permanent loss of vision from optic nerve damage. After a severe blunt injury, the full circumference of the drainage angle may be damaged, and these patients are particularly at risk in developing this complication. They require long-term follow-up to detect and treat this complication before visual damage occurs.

The full extent of ocular damage cannot be assessed until the hyphaema has cleared. In a review of a large series of patients Eagling (1974) showed that in over 50 per cent of the patients, the hyphaema with minor angle recession was the only damage incurred, and recovery was complete. In the more severe injuries, other intraocular structures may be damaged: the lens may be dislocated or ruptured, and progressive changes lead to a cataract. The management of this complication will be discussed later. A contre-coup type of injury may affect the macular region; the force may be sufficient to rupture the choroid and outer layers of the retina, resulting in a large subretinal haematoma and permanent damage to central vision (*Plate 2*).

An important cause of preventable blindness following a blunt injury is the development of a retinal detachment. A prospective study (Eagling, 1974) demonstrated that the retinal breaks leading to a detached retina are produced at the time of impact, and careful examination of the peripheral retina with the indirect ophthalmoscope prior to discharge from hospital should allow early detection and treatment of this potentially blinding complication (*Plate 3*). Patients particularly at risk are those in whom the impact has been over the sclera, where the other signs of injury, e.g. hyphaema, may be slight.

Extraocular Damage following a Blunt Injury

A diffuse blunt injury will cause compression of the orbital contents; the force may be dissipated by causing a fracture of the infraorbital margin or orbital floor, but if this does not occur, the sudden compression and decompression of the orbital contents may result in massive retrobulbar haemorrhage and contusion of the oculomotor nerves. Blindness may occur from avulsion of the optic nerve.

With regard to fractures, it is common for zygomatic and infraorbital margin fractures to coexist with a fracture involving the orbital floor. The apparent alignment of the fractures may be good, but what is frequently missed is the downward displacement of the whole orbital floor, which may even be completely disrupted behind the infraorbital margin. This allows subluxation of the globe, with enophthalmos and intractable double vision in all positions of gaze.

A pure blow-out fracture of the infraorbital floor is less dramatic; it is very common and symptoms may be minimal. Damage to the infraorbital nerve results in an area of anaesthesia on the cheek, while communication with an air sinus produces crepitation of the eyelids, especially if the nose is blown forcefully. Problems arise only if the orbital tissues are trapped in the fracture line; this may tether the eyeball and restrict ocular movement. In mild cases, the restriction is limited to upward gaze, and recovery usually occurs within a few days. If there is marked entrapment, double vision may be present when looking straight ahead or on downward gaze, and this is extremely disabling. A duction test is performed under local anaesthesia to establish whether the restricted gaze is due to entrapment or muscle paresis, as either may occur after this type of injury. The patient is instructed to look in the direction of restricted gaze, and the movement is assisted by forceps. Mechanical restriction can be demonstrated in this way, and sometimes this test is curative.

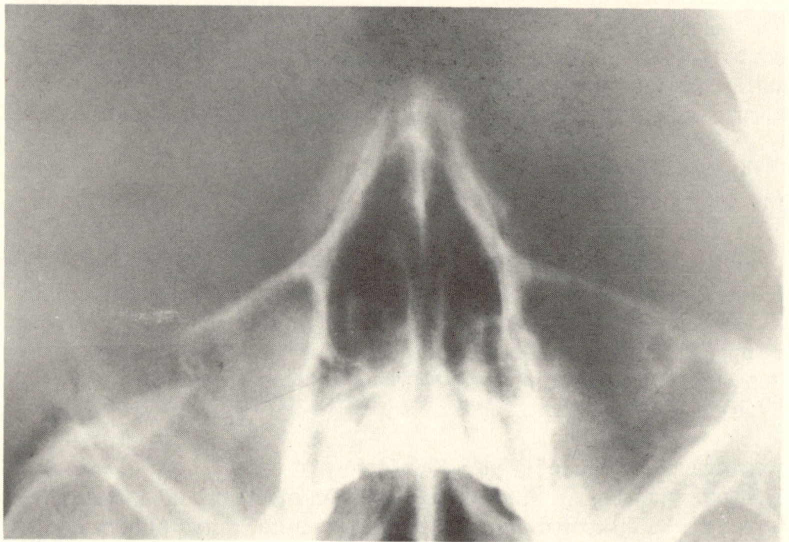

Fig. 9.1. Right orbital floor fracture demonstrated by occipito-mental view, with 30° down-tilt on X-ray tube.

Orbital radiographs should include a view of the orbital floor, obtained by an occipito-mental view with a 30° uptilt. This may show displacement along the fracture line, and protrusion of the orbital contents into the maxillary antrum, known as the 'hanging drop' sign. Gas shadows around the orbit confirm communication with an air sinus (*Fig. 9.1*).

The primary concern here is with function: a decision as to whether surgical intervention is required must be based not only on the alignment of the fracture, but also on the presence or absence of double vision. Exploration is best performed between five and ten days after injury; if there is simple entrapment, the orbital floor is explored from above, via a subperiosteal approach along the infraorbital margin, and the trapped tissues are freed. With a compound injury this approach is combined with an antrostomy so that the displaced orbital floor can be elevated from below. If there is a large defect in the orbital floor, a silicone implant may be used for support (Emery et al., 1972).

A report by Putterman et al. (1974) has tempered the earlier enthusiasm for surgical exploration of all patients with double vision, particularly where the problem has not been diagnosed early. A conservative approach is now adopted for patients with double vision on upward gaze only, as there is some risk that surgical intervention will damage further the trapped inferior rectus muscle, and provoke double vision on looking down, which is much more disabling.

Severe retrobulbar haemorrhage is usually found in the absence of orbital fractures. The eye is proptosed with limitation of movement in all directions. This is partly mechanical, but damage to the innervation of the extraocular muscles is common, and this can only be assessed when the haematoma has subsided. Rarely this type of injury results in total and irreversible blindness from avulsion of the optic nerve, when compression of the globe results in the optic nerve being squeezed out of the back of the eye. The pupil will show no direct light reaction and fundus examination will show massive retinal infarction which often becomes obscured by vitreous haemorrhage. The proptosis results in danger from exposure, and patients require treatment in hospital, with liberal applications of antibiotic ointment and a carbonet dressing to prevent dryness and infection. Recovery from oculomotor nerve damage is frequently slow and incomplete; surgical treatment for double vision is deferred for nine months to allow maximal natural recovery to occur. A new optical device, known as a Fresnel prism, can be temporarily affixed to the patient's glasses to relieve double vision. Basically, this is a series of prisms constructed in a thin sheet of plastic, which adheres to the spectacles by surface tension; these can be easily changed as the patient improves.

INJURIES TO THE EYELIDS
AND LACRIMAL DRAINAGE APPARATUS

In injuries resulting in multiple facial lacerations, or full thickness lid lacerations, there is a strong probability of an underlying ocular perforation, so careful examination of the eye should be performed before undertaking repair of the facial lacerations (*Plate 4*).

Full-thickness lid lacerations involving the lid margin should be referred to an ophthalmologist for repair. Thorough cleansing of the wound is important, followed by closure in layers, using an absorbable suture for the tarsal plate and for the muscle layers and fine nylon or silk for the skin. It is important to align the lash margin very accurately, and to leave this suture in place for two weeks, otherwise notching may occur.

Failure to cleanse the wound adequately and repair in layers results in keloid formation; the subsequent contracture deforms the eyelid, resulting in a cosmetic defect and exposure of the cornea. Secondary repair should be delayed for at least six months when possible, so as to avoid stimulating further fibroblastic activity. If exposure problems make early reconstruction necessary, an application of beta irradiation may help reduce further fibrosis.

Lid lacerations close to the medial canthus may involve the lacrimal drainage apparatus; the cut ends of the tear canaliculi will require identification and splinting with a soft silicone tube during healing.

A serious injury may occur in young children when they have fallen onto a pointed object. The external evidence of injury may be minimal — a tiny skin laceration or a small subconjunctival haemorrhage. A pointed object such as an umbrella or knitting needle can penetrate deeply, causing blindness from direct optic nerve damage, or intracranial infection from penetration of the orbital roof. If the child is too young to assess vision, the pupil reflex may provide evidence of optic nerve damage; skull X-rays should always be taken, and if there is any doubt about the child's general condition, the safest policy is to admit for observation.

PERFORATING EYE INJURIES

The last two decades have seen a marked change in the pattern of injuries causing ocular perforation. A comparison of two series reported from the Birmingham and Midland Eye Hospital in 1959 and 1976 (Roper-Hall, 1959; Eagling, 1976) shows that there has been a marked fall in the incidence of perforating injuries from industrial accidents (Table 9.1).

Table 9.1. Birmingham and Midland Eye Hospital: causes of perforating eye injuries, compared over 27 years.

Cause	1959 per cent	1976 per cent
Road accident	2	31
Child play	27	26
Industrial	41	15
Domestic	20	14
Assault, bombs	1	8
Outdoor	6	4
Sport	3	2

Accidents to children and in the home remain common causes of perforating eye injuries, and the incidence from assault and terrorism has significantly increased. However, the most dramatic change has been in the incidence of injury due to road traffic accidents; this has risen from 2 per cent in 1959 to 31 per cent in 1976. Since the injuries arise from recoil onto the edge of a shattered windscreen, bilateral perforation is not uncommon. The use of laminated instead of toughened glass for windscreens and compulsory wearing of seatbelts would dramatically reduce the incidence of serious eye injuries (Soni, 1973; Mackay, 1976).

Recognition of a perforating eye injury is extremely important. After a major injury, blood and intraocular contents, such as vitreous gel, may be seen oozing from under closed eyelids; if this is seen the eye should not be disturbed further, and expert assistance should be sought (*Plate 5*). A sterile dressing should be lightly applied over both eyes, and the patient kept lying down. If X-ray examination is required for other injuries, the radiographer must be warned of the presence of an eye injury.

Small ocular perforations may be more difficult to see, but any distortion of the pupil or shallowness of the anterior chamber with hyphaema indicate a full thickness corneal laceration (*Plate 6*).

Major advances in the repair of perforating eye injuries have been made in the last twenty years. With microsurgical techniques, an accurate watertight wound closure can be achieved, and the anterior chamber reconstituted with physiological saline (*Fig. 9.2*). Corneal wounds are repaired with fine 10/0 monofilament nylon, which reduces fibrovascular scarring of the wound, with an improved visual result. Prolapsed iris may be replaced with safety providing that it is viable and the wound uninfected. In major perforating injuries, radical surgery at the time of repair to remove blood, damaged lens and prolapsing vitreous may prevent subsequent intraocular fibrosis, progressing to loss of vision from retinal detachment (Coles and Haik, 1972; Eagling, 1975). With these techniques the percentage of patients achieving good vision (6/12 corrected or better) after a perforating injury has risen from 45 per cent in 1959 to 68 per cent in 1975 (Eagling, 1976).

The prognosis is related to the extent of the injury; 25 per cent of perforating injuries are extensive, involving both anterior and posterior segments of the eye. In this group, 60 per cent lose all useful vision, and many require enucleation. Although many of these eyes are damaged beyond repair from expulsive haemorrhage at the time of injury, a proportion of these lose vision from the complications arising from intraocular fibrosis. Although much can be done at the time of primary repair, further surgery may be necessary. The recent development of vitrectomy machines, whereby damaged vitreous and lens can be cut and aspirated through a fine cannula, while replacing the intraocular volume with an infusion of a physiological solution, enables these damaged structures to be removed through a closed incision thus minimizing the risk of further bleeding. Reports are encouraging and we hope that these developments will lead to preservation of vision in some of these badly injured eyes (Benson and Machemer, 1976).

INTRAOCULAR FOREIGN BODIES

The intraocular foreign body causes one of the most commonly missed injuries. It is also one of the most serious, because a retained intraocular

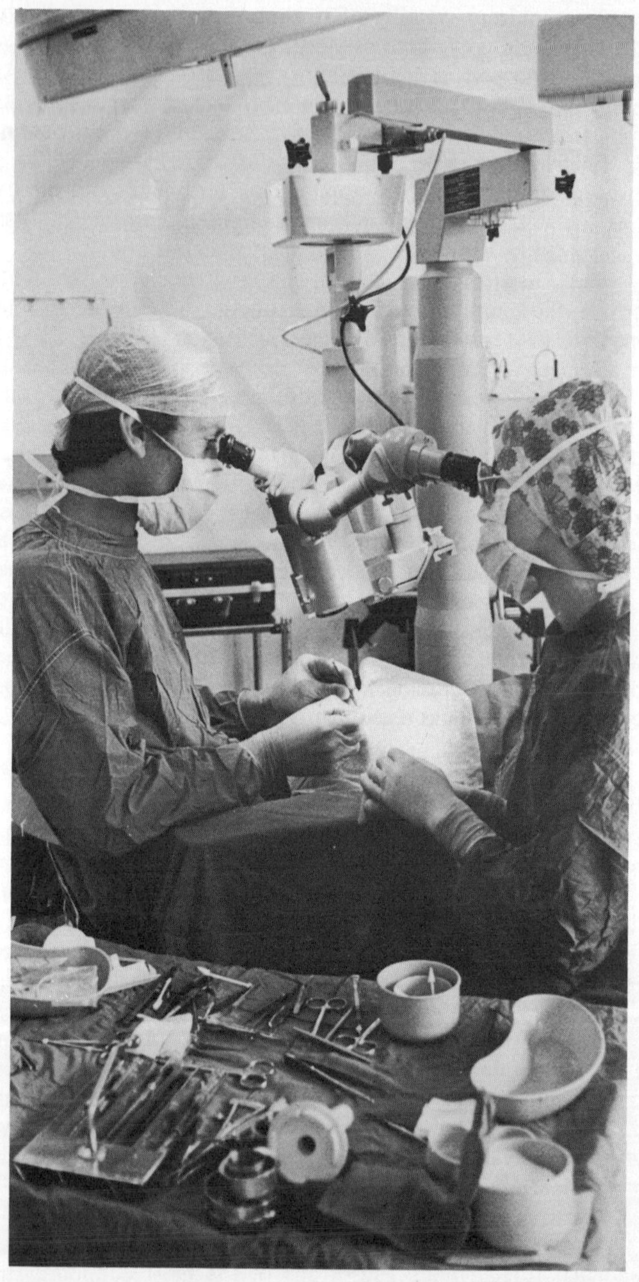

Fig. 9.2. The operating microscope.

foreign body causes insidious blindness. The most common cause of such an injury is hammering steel on steel; a chip flies off the hammer head or chisel and hits the eye at great speed. These particles are often small, usually 1–2 mm so the entry wound is difficult to see. Vision may be blurred if the foreign body has tracked through the lens of the eye, causing an incipient cataract, or the patient may describe black floaters from vitreous haemorrhage; there may, however, be no visual disturbance. Any explosive injury may result in an intraocular foreign body, and the steel particle may well become non-magnetic in this situation.

All hammer and chisel injuries, and any explosive injury, should be X-rayed in search of an intraocular foreign body; this is the only reliable way to be certain that such an injury has not occurred. Two A–P and two lateral views should be taken, so that artefacts are not mistaken for an intraocular foreign body.

Iron and copper are the two most noxious metals to the eye and both may cause severe intraocular inflammation, particularly the latter. The iron content of steel causes insidious blindness by intracellular deposition which affects the metabolism of the retina, lens and pigmented structures within the eye.

The successful removal of an intraocular foreign body depends on accurate identification of its position within the eye (*Fig. 9.3 and 9.4*). Radiographic localization is achieved by suturing a metallic ring around the cornea to act as a reference point for calculations of the foreign body's position. The image-intensifier may be used during surgery for further localization, particularly when non-magnetic foreign bodies are being removed by direct instrumentation within the eye.

Other methods can be very useful. In most patients, the foreign body can be seen using the powerful head-light on an indirect ophthalmoscope, which enables the retina to be examined even in the presence of an early cataract. An improved version of the electronic Roper-Hall foreign body locator has recently been developed (*Fig. 9.5*) which provides very accurate localization of the position and metallic nature of the foreign body, and is of great assistance during surgery (*Plate 7*).

Delayed recognition of an intraocular foreign body considerably reduces the chances of successful removal. Even with early removal, and an initial good visual outcome the later results may be disappointing, as one in five patients lose all useful vision from the development of retinal detachment. As with perforating injuries, the developments in vitreous surgery may improve on these figures (O'Neill and Eagling, 1978).

BURNS

Serious eye burns follow either thermal or chemical injury. The reflex lid closure offers considerable protection in thermal burns, so it is only the most severe facial burns that result in major ocular damage. The exception

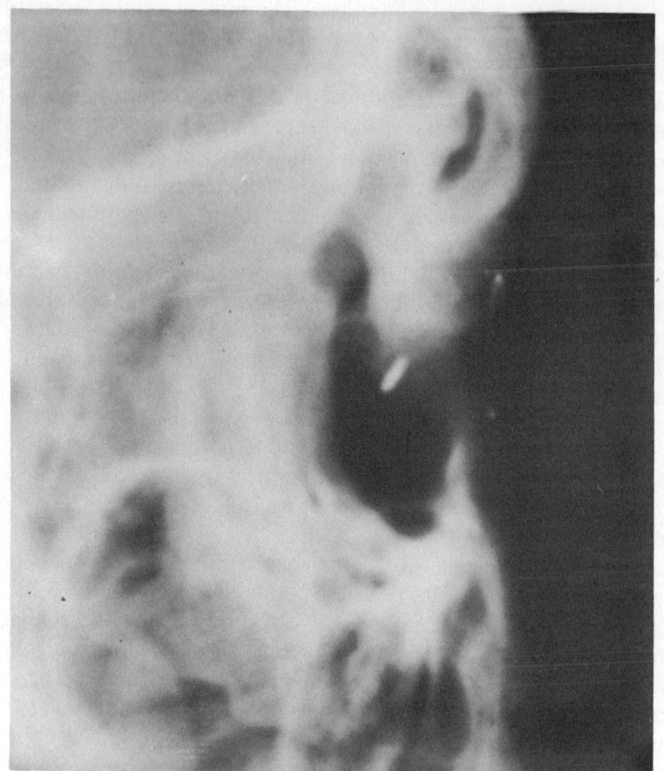

Fig. 9.3. X-ray of intraocular foreign body with surface ring marker.

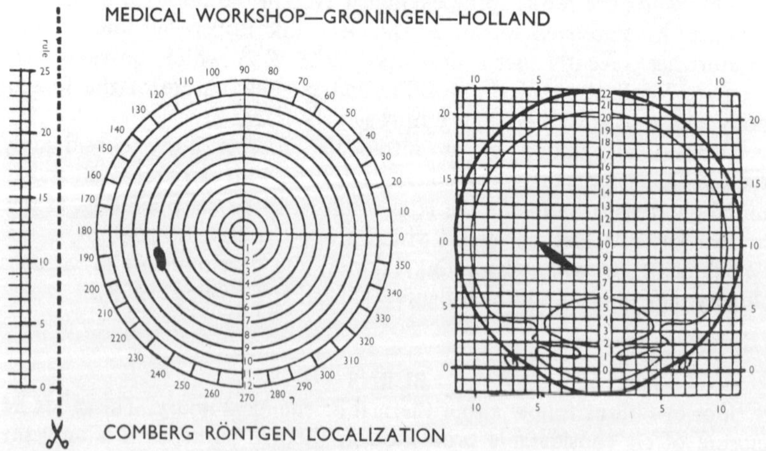

Fig. 9.4. Calculated position of foreign body, illustrated in X-ray above.

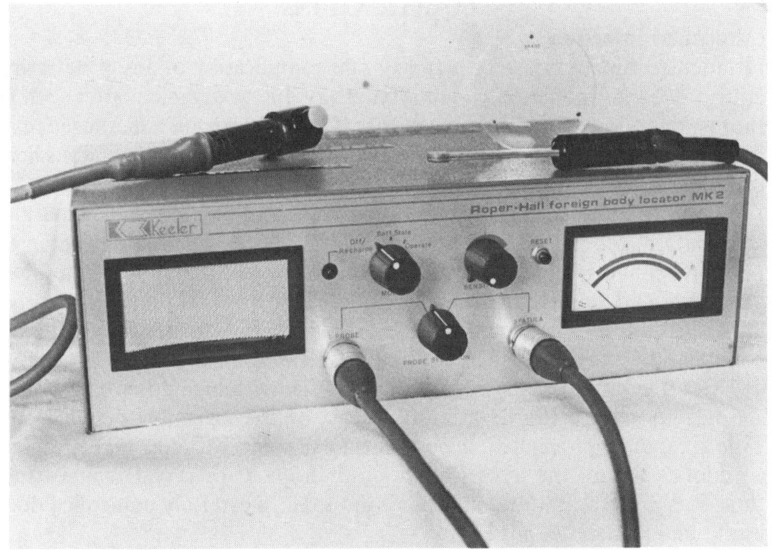

Fig. 9.5. The Roper-Hall foreign body locator.

to this is industrial accidents with molten metal burns, where the injury may be quite localized.

With chemical burns, alkalis are more serious than acids, as they are lipid-soluble and can penetrate deeply, whereas acids form a surface coagulum which resists penetration. Speed is essential in first-aid treatment; caustic alkalis penetrate the deeper tissues of the eye within seconds, and immediate irrigation is vital. This should be continued for at least twenty minutes before transferring the patient.

The changes in the cornea and surrounding conjunctiva will reflect the severity of the burn. If the cornea is clear with epithelial loss only and the conjunctiva is hyperaemic, complete recovery is likely. Varying degrees of haziness of the cornea and white ischaemia of the circumcorneal con-junctiva (*Plate 8*) indicate ischaemic changes in the burnt tissues, and scarring is inevitable; total opacification of the cornea means that perforation and loss of the eye is likely (*Plate 9*).

Treatment is directed towards preventing secondary infection and reducing the inflammatory effects of ischaemia. Healing is very slow, and fibrovascular scarring progresses for several months, followed by slow regression. Reconstructive surgery will have to be delayed for at least two years. As the healing process results in a heavily vascularized cornea, it is not suitable for corneal grafting; in selected cases, some success with an intracorneal perspex implant has been achieved.

COMPLICATIONS

Intraocular Infection

Intraocular infection is a surprisingly rare complication of any penetrating injury; it is most commonly seen after injury due to organic matter such as thorns, or following delayed diagnosis. It is rare with metallic intraocular foreign bodies, as the air friction during its passage causes tremendous heat resulting in sterilization.

Once established, however, intraocular infection is devastating; suppuration within the globe destroys vital tissues, eventually leading to perforation and loss of the eye. Vigorous treatment is required with both parenteral and subconjunctival antibiotic administration; unless a positive identification of the organism can be made after successful culture, a combination of bacteriocidal antibiotics active against both Gram-positive and Gram-negative organisms is given, together with high doses of systemic steroids to reduce the devastating effects of the inflammatory changes. Unless rapid improvement occurs, intraocular lavage with instillation of antibiotics within the eye offers the only hope of preserving some visual function. Since antibiotics may be retino-toxic, a carefully controlled dose is required (Forster et al., 1976).

Sympathetic Ophthalmitis

All penetrating injuries carry a potential risk of sympathetic ophthalmitis. This is thought to be an autoimmune condition in which a severe inflammation develops first in the injured or exciting eye, and subsequently in the uninjured or sympathizing eye, and may lead to blindness. The antigenic stimulus involved is uncertain, but both lens protein and retinal pigment epithelium are separated from immune-competent cells at an early stage in development, and damage to these structures with other adjuvants may be important in the development of the immune response leading to this most feared complication. A time factor is involved, and a policy of removing all eyes damaged beyond repair within two weeks of injury has helped reduce the incidence of this complication, which now affects less than 1 per cent of all injuries. High doses of systemic steroids are needed to control the established condition, but long-term treatment is required as relapse is common.

Traumatic Cataract

Traumatic cataract is common to both blunt and penetrating injuries (*Plate 10*) and presents some special problems with regard to restoring good visual function. Removal of a cataractous lens from one eye results in the loss of the major focusing power of the eye; spectacle correction requires a very powerful lens that gives such a magnification effect, that the image from this eye cannot be comfortably fused with that of the normal eye, resulting in double vision. This problem can be partly overcome by the use of a contact lens, which has a smaller magnification effect, and permits fusion of the two images in some patients. The recent development of high-water-content soft contact lenses allows continuous wear. Because this may allow development of normal vision this is of particular value in the treatment of children.

However, even with a contact lens, the difference in image size is still considerable, and a large proportion of patients abandon contact lenses either because of double vision, or because of discomfort. A better optical result is achieved by inserting a perspex intraocular lens at the time of cataract surgery; this is positioned either in the pupil plane supported by loops passing in front of and behind the iris, or behind the iris plane, where it is supported by a fine suture (*Plate 11*). It is designed to be of equivalent power to the normal lens of the eye, and good functional binocular vision can be achieved (Ridgway, 1977). However, not all patients with a traumatic cataract are suitable for this technique if other structures are damaged; in these patients, contact lens wear is the only alternative.

DIAGNOSIS

Special Equipment

The clinical assessment of a severely injured eye is often difficult in the early stages, as visibility is often obscured by haemorrhage. With the development of techniques for surgical reconstruction of badly injured eyes, other means of assessing visual potential are important. Special electrodiagnostic testing can now give valuable information about both the retinal function generally, and the function of the macula and higher visual pathways. Ultrasonic techniques have become more refined, and in conjunction with the electrodiagnostic tests, can help to distinguish vitreous membranes from a detached retina; this information is very valuable before embarking on vitreous surgery (Crews et al., 1975).

How to Examine an Eye Casualty

1. An accurate history is very important, as the type of damage can often be anticipated from the nature of the injury.

2. Test the distance vision of each eye, with glasses if normally worn. If formal testing with a Snellen visual acuity chart is not possible, estimate vision in terms of the ability to perceive light, to detect hand movements, to count fingers, to see features, or to see detail.

3. Examine the eye and extraocular structures in a logical sequence: lids and extraocular movements; cornea and conjunctiva; depth of anterior chamber; shape, and reaction of pupil to both direct and consensual stimulation; look for the clear red reflex through the pupil using an ophthalmoscope at arm's length; examine fundus.

4. Points relating to specific injuries.

Blunt Injuries

Look for ocular damage, particularly blood in the anterior chamber, and a sluggish pupil reaction. If there is a subconjunctival haemorrhage, examine the peripheral fundus carefully. Test eye movements in the four oblique positions of gaze, and question regarding double vision. Use X-rays to demonstrate orbital fractures.

Lacerations

Remember that facial lacerations may be complicated by an underlying ocular perforation. Blood and a jelly substance oozing from under eyelids indicate a major perforation – do not disturb further. Otherwise examine the eyes with a torch and gentle lid retraction using a gauze swab, instructing the patient to open both eyes: a corneal wound may be difficult to see, but if infected the margins become opaque. A dense subconjunctival haemorrhage may obscure a scleral perforation; such cases should be referred for exploration. Compare the anterior chamber depth in the two eyes, and note the pupils' shape and reaction; an iris or ciliary body prolapse is a dark knuckle herniating through the wound. If there is no obvious injury, test the red reflex and examine the fundus.

Foreign Bodies

If patients complain of a foreign body sensation instil a drop of fluorescein; this will stain an abrasion or ulcer bright green, while a superficial foreign body shows up as a black speck with a green halo. Instil antibiotic ointment and pad, and refer for treatment. If there is no stain, evert the upper lid by instructing the patient to look down, apply gentle traction to the lid margin and counter pressure with a glass rod to the skin above the tarsal plate; this is a common place for foreign bodies to be trapped and they can be removed with a cotton-wool bud. If the history suggests the possibility of intraocular foreign body (especially if using a hammer and chisel) *always X-ray*. There is no other safe way of excluding such an injury.

Burns

Irrigate chemical burns for 20 minutes with sterile saline before examining in detail. Fluorescein staining demonstrates the denuded surface; a major burn will show opacification of the cornea and conjunctiva. A common minor injury follows welding flash or exposure to ultraviolet light and gives rise to symptoms some hours after exposure. A severe foreign body sensation develops in both eyes, and fluorescein staining shows fine punctate erosions over both corneas. Healing occurs within 24 hours; instil local anaesthetic drops, antibiotic ointment, and double pad overnight.

Useful Eye Drops for a Casualty Department
Minims single-dose sterile application.
　　1. Fluorescein: for staining corneal abrasions, ulcers etc.

2. Benoxinate: local anaesthetic, effective within one minute.

3. Phenylephrine 10 per cent: to dilate pupil without affecting accommodation.

4. Cyclopertolate 10 per cent: powerful pupil dilator, but paralyses accommodation for three days.

5. Chloramphenicol: standard topical opthalmic antibiotic.

Summary

The modern approach to eye injuries can now achieve great success in restoring vision to a damaged eye. Early diagnosis and referral to a major centre with the necessary skills and equipment for dealing with such injuries provides the best chance of a favourable outcome.

REFERENCES

Benson W. E. and Machemer R. (1976) Severe perforating injuries treated with pars plana vitrectomy. *Am. J. Ophthalmol.* **81**, 728.

Coles W. H. and Haik G. M. (1972) Vitrectomy in intraocular trauma. *Arch. Ophthalmol.* 87, 621.

Crews S. J., Hillman J. S. and Thompson C. R. S. (1975) Electrodiagnosis and ultrasonography in the assessment of recent major trauma. *Trans. Ophthalmol. Soc. UK* 95, 315.

Eagling E. M. (1974) Ocular damage after blunt trauma to the eye. *Br. J. Ophthalmol.* 58, 126.

Eagling E. M. (1975) Perforating injuries involving the posterior segment. *Trans. Ophthalmol. Soc. UK* 95, 335.

Eagling E. M. (1976) Perforating injuries of the eye. *Br. J. Ophthalmol.* **60**, 732.

Emery J. M., von Noorden G. K. and Schlernitzauer D. A. (1972) Management of orbital floor fractures. *Am. J. Ophthalmol.* 74, 299.

Forster R. K., Zachary I. C. and Cottingham A. J. jun. (1976) Diagnosis and treatment of endophthalmitis. *Symposium on Ocular Therapy,* Vol. 9, p. 51. New York, Wiley.

MacKay G. M. (1975) Incidence of trauma to the eye of car occupants. *Trans. Opthalmol. Soc. UK* 95, 311.

O'Neill E. and Eagling E. M. (1978) Intraocular foreign bodies: indications for lensectomy and vitrectomy. *Trans. Ophthalmol. Soc. UK* 98, 47.

Putterman A. M., Stevens T. and Wist M. J. (1974) Non-surgical management of blow-out fractures of the orbital floor. *Am. J. Ophthalmol.* 77, 232.

Ridgway A. E. (1977) Binocular effects of intraocular lens insertion. *Trans. Ophthalmol. Soc. UK* 97, 96.

Roper-Hall M. J. (1959) The treatment of ocular injuries. *Trans. Ophthalmol. Soc. UK* 79, 57.

Soni K. G. (1973) Eye injuries in road traffic accidents. *Injury* 5, 41.

Töngum A. M. (1966) *Acta Opthalmol. (Kbh)* 44, 650.

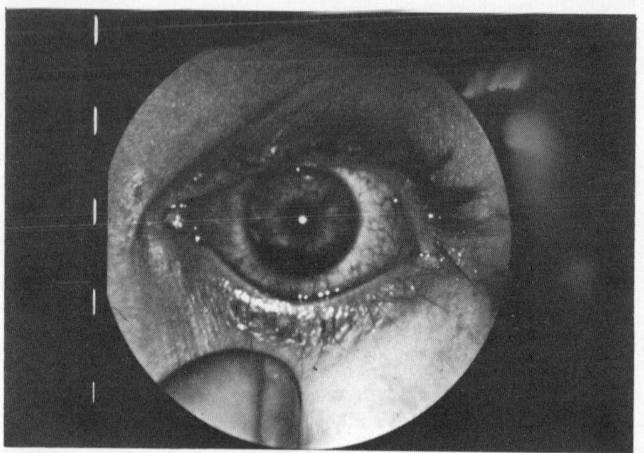

Plate 1. A hyphaema.

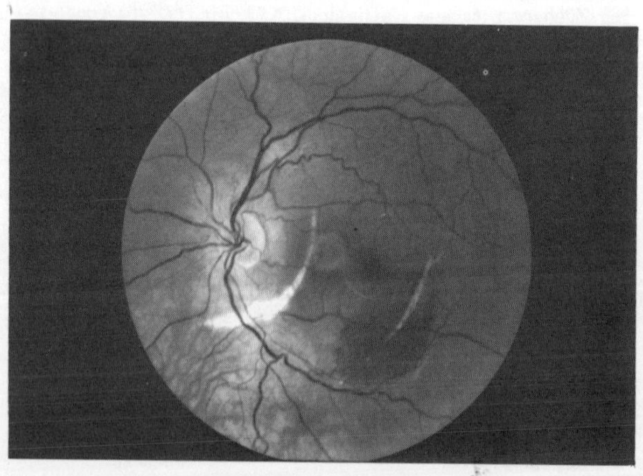

Plate 2. Choroidal ruptures.

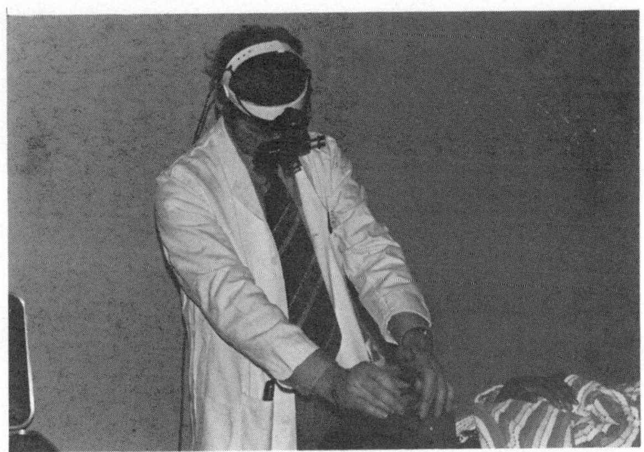

Plate 3. Indirect ophthalmoscopy.

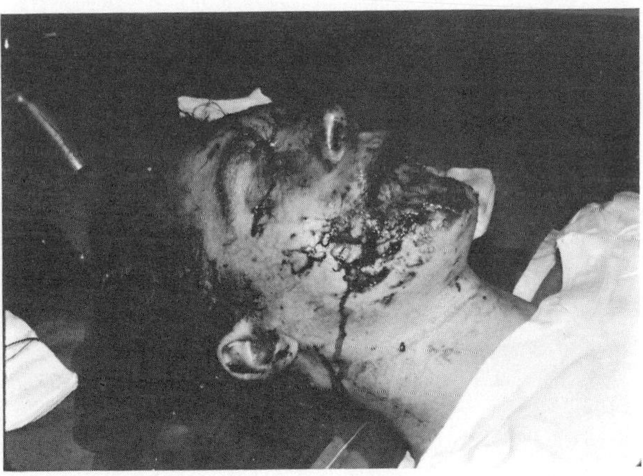

Plate 4. Facial lacerations and bilateral perforating eye injuries following a windscreen accident.

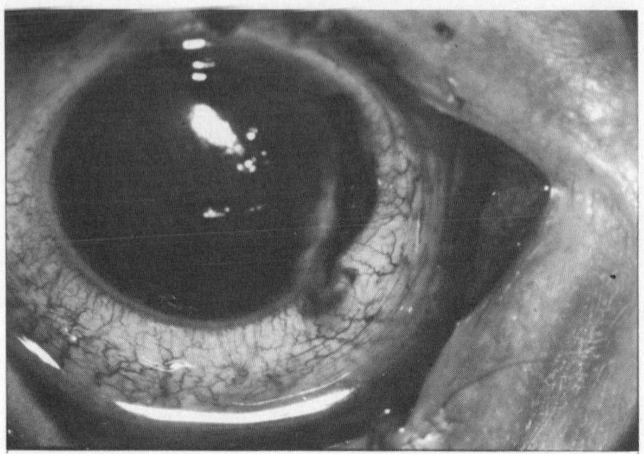

Plate. 5. Perforating injury from a wooden arrow, with prolapse of intraocular contents.

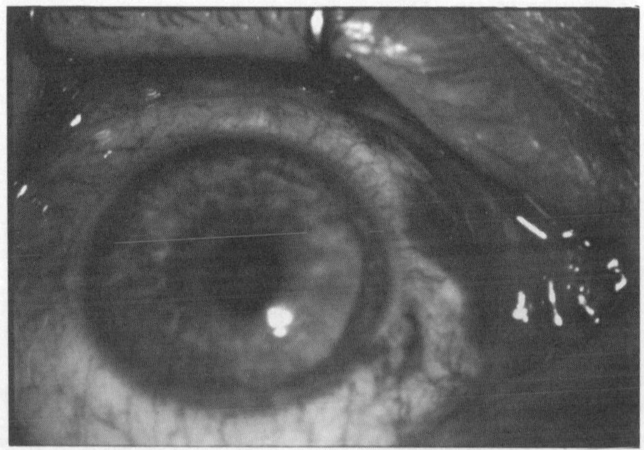

Plate 6. Corneal laceration with loss of anterior chamber.

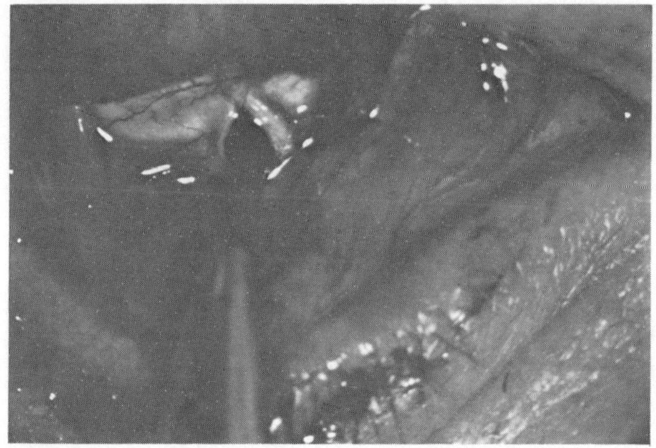

Plate 7. Magnetic removal of a large steel foreign body.

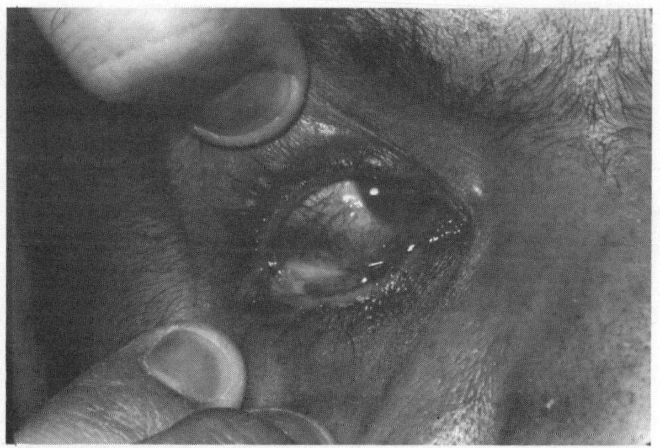

Plate 8. Hot metal burn of the lower conjunctival fornix.

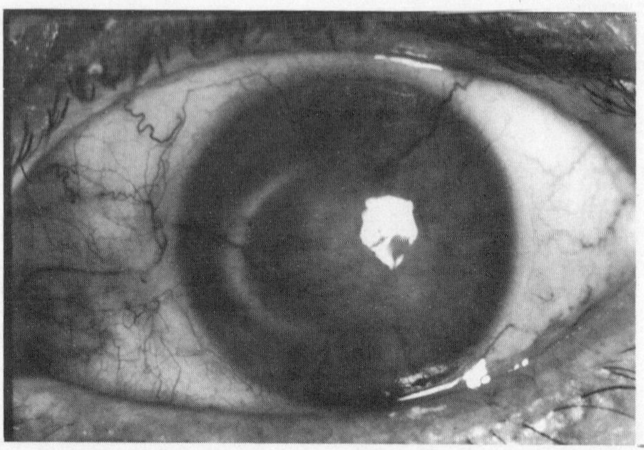

Plate 9. Corneal scarring following a severe chemical burn.

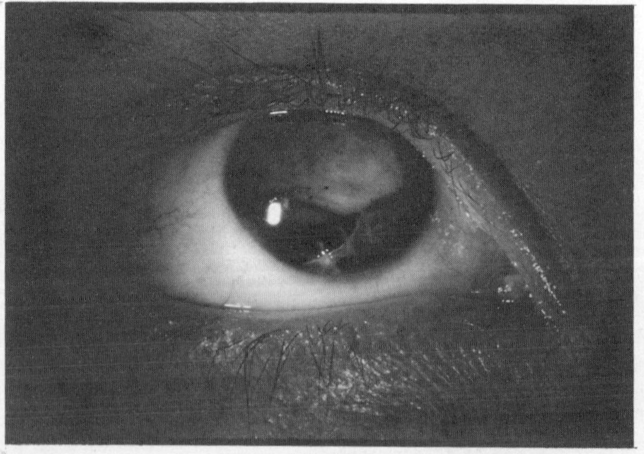

Plate 10. Traumatic cataract following a perforating injury.

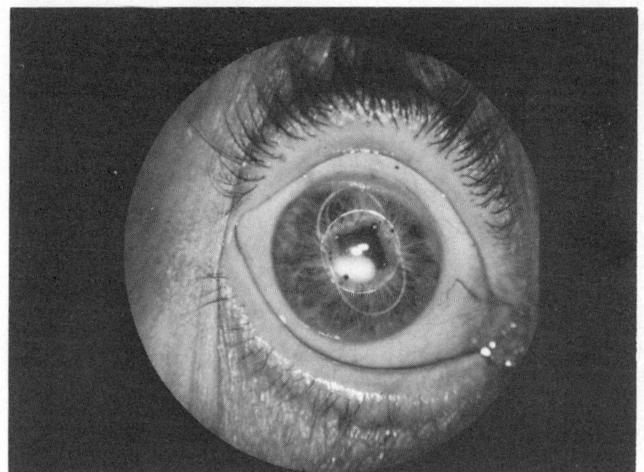

Plate 11. Binkhorst intraocular lens in place of a cataract.

Index